T0257762

Advanced Theory of Neural Stem Cells

Advanced Theory
of Neural Stem Cells

Edited by **Jose Clark**

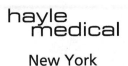

New York

Published by Hayle Medical,
30 West, 37th Street, Suite 612,
New York, NY 10018, USA
www.haylemedical.com

Advanced Theory of Neural Stem Cells
Edited by Jose Clark

International Standard Book Number: 978-1-63241-018-4 (Hardback)

Printed in the United States of America.

Contents

Preface

This book consists of a collection of research work by international veterans in the neural stem cell field and includes the characterization of adult and embryonic neural stem cells in both vertebrates as well as invertebrates. It focuses on the history and the latest discoveries in neural stem cells, and sums up the mechanisms of neural stem cell development. It is intended for basic readers, doctors, students and researchers who are interested in comprehending the principles and novel discoveries in neural stem cells.

After months of intensive research and writing, this book is the end result of all who devoted their time and efforts in the initiation and progress of this book. It will surely be a source of reference in enhancing the required knowledge of the new developments in the area. During the course of developing this book, certain measures such as accuracy, authenticity and research focused analytical studies were given preference in order to produce a comprehensive book in the area of study.

This book would not have been possible without the efforts of the authors and the publisher. I extend my sincere thanks to them. Secondly, I express my gratitude to my family and well-wishers. And most importantly, I thank my students for constantly expressing their willingness and curiosity in enhancing their knowledge in the field, which encourages me to take up further research projects for the advancement of the area.

Editor

Part 1

Characterization of Neural Stem Cells

Neural Stem Cells from Mammalian Brain: Isolation Protocols and Maintenance Conditions

Jorge Oliver-De la Cruz and Angel Ayuso-Sacido
Regenerative Medicine Program, Centro de Investigación Príncipe Felipe,
REIG and Ciberned
Spain

1. Introduction

Traditionally, the adult brain has been considered a quiescent organ, lacking the production of new cells, or more exactly, new mature and functional neurons. This dogma has been widely refused in the last decades with the discovery of proliferative cells with stem cell properties in the adult brain.

First evidences come from the demonstration of neurogenesis in non-mammal vertebrates such as birds or lizards (as reviewed in Garcia-Verdugo et al., 2002). Neurogenesis was also confirmed to occur in adult mammals, like mice and rats, and, finally, in primates and humans (for a complete revision see Gil-Perotín et al., 2009). Though the process of neurogenesis in the adult is primarily confined to the subventricular zone (SVZ) and the subgranular zone (SGZ) of the dentate gyrus, glial progenitors exist in other brain regions. These widespread glial progenitors remain quiescent and do not generate mature glial cells, but, in certain situations such as traumatic injury, they may act as true stem cells (Belachew et al., 2003; Rivers et al., 2008).

The terminology of stem cell, progenitor cell and precursor cell has been adapted from others tissues. Basically, a *bona fide* neural stem cell (NSC) must meet all these three features: capacity of self-renewal, capacity to differentiate into the three neural lineages (neuron, astrocyte and oligodendrocyte) and, finally, the ability to regenerate neural tissue. When cells show a limited self-renewal and are already committed toward a specific fate, they are classified as progenitor cells, while the term "precursor" represents intermediate stages.

Neural stem/progenitor cells (NSPc) primary cultures provide the best *in vitro* model to study proliferation and differentiation signaling pathways, a difficult issue to address *in vivo*. Additionally, these cells might be used in future replacement cell therapies, thus motivating the development of protocols aimed to isolate and expand these cells *in vitro*. These protocols display significant variations among them, and the introduction of new technologies has increased drastically their number. The differences in the protocols have rendered different results in terms of stem cell subpopulations, differentiation potential and the amount of cells. The last is especially relevant in the case of human samples because of their low availability.

Therefore, the aim of this chapter is to recapitulate some of these technical differences that could induce variances in the final results. We have analyzed the main isolation protocols from the two canonical neurogenic zones in the adult (subventricular zone and hippocampus), described for both animal models (mouse and rat) and human.

2. Neural stem/progenitor cell isolation

The NSPc isolation procedures follow common steps including tissue dissection, digestion and cell enrichment. However, comparing the different protocols found in the bibliography, it is notable the presence of significant differences between them even when they are consecutive works from the same group. The introduction of new technologies has also increased drastically the number and variety of protocols. Additionally, some tissues like normal human brain are particularly difficult to manage due to their low availability, which requires improvements in the protocol to include modifications that increase the rate of isolated cells. Interestingly, the diversity of isolation procedures results in the obtaining of different stem/progenitor cell subpopulations with distinct differentiation potential, and might be also responsible for the, sometimes contradictory, results observed in the literature.

Although the development of standard protocols would be the best option to assure that results can be easily compared, in the practice, this is almost impossible. Different groups have generated independently alternative procedures for the isolation, dissociation and enrichment of NSPc. Furthermore, the animal model, the specific location of the brain sample, or even the characteristics of the experiment have requirements that would make unmanageable the use of universal procedures. Usually, the same group employs very similar strategies to isolate cells from different samples, independently of their developmental stage or animal/human origin. Nevertheless, it will be interesting to establish flexible guidelines to indicate what can be modified from the standard procedures and how to do so.

The basic scheme followed by NSPc isolation protocols is reflected in figure 1, and we will discuss the specific methodology associated with every step in the following headings

2.1 Tissue dissection methods

The origin of the tissue influences the type of isolated cells as well as their proliferation and differentiation capacity. A number of profound differences have been reported between brain samples from different species (mouse, rat of human) or from different stages of development within a given specie (Gritti et al., 2009; Svendsen et al., 1997). However, the accurate dissection of specific regions of the brain has become more relevant as the knowledge on the NSPc biology and location increases. In fact, regardless of the animal model, one of the main factors that might determine the final results is the specific location of the brain tissue from where NSPc are isolated.

Different regions of the brain have been used as a primary source of NSPc and, consequently, discrepancies in the isolated cells have been reported. In this sense, analyzing the distinct approaches for the tissue dissection might be useful to contextualize such a controversy.

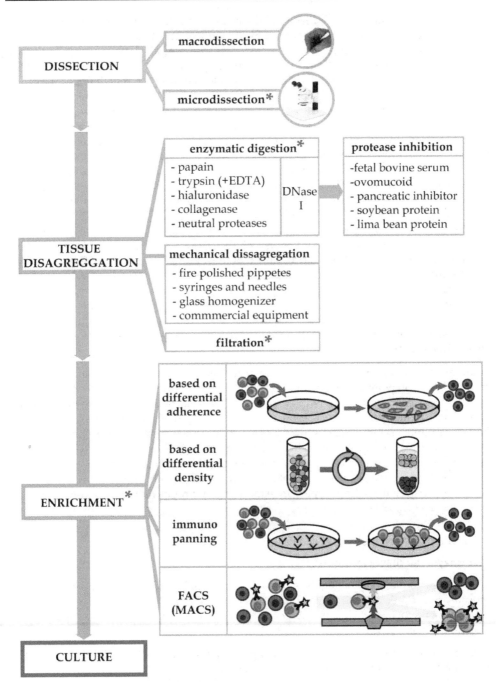

Fig. 1. Diagram depicting the main steps of standard neural stem/progenitor cell isolation protocol. Headings marked with an asterisk are not always included.

We might consider three different levels of dissection according to the amount and location of tissue, ranging from large unselected brain tissue to microdissection. In a first level, a number of works start from whole brain (e.g. Von Visger et al., 1994) or large areas that include heterogeneous regions (e.g. whole human temporal lobe, Kirschenbaum et al., 1994). In these cases, the results can be highly variable, because of the different types of progenitors coming from distinct locations and giving rise to an artefactual impression of cell heterogeneity. An intermediate step of complexity is found in those works that use tissue from specific areas, but without the exclusion of contiguous tissues, i.e. macrodissection. In this regard, some authors reported the presence of multipotent stem cells from different regions of the adult parenchyma that differ from canonical neurogenic zones (SVZ and SGZ), e.g. from striatum (Reynolds & Weiss, 1992). However, these cells might arise from the cross-contamination of adjacent neurogenic regions (Lois & Alvarez-Buylla, 1993). Likewise, as will be discussed later, the existence of real neural stem cells in adult dentate gyrus of hippocampus has become a controversial subject. Some authors claim that there are true stem cells from this zone. However, others state that these isolated cells should be considered progenitors because of their low proliferation *in vitro* and their doubtful multipotentiality. The main argument of these authors is the lack of fine dissection, and the inclusion of neural stem cells from other adjacent tissues, like SVZ. Therefore, considering the current knowledge on NPSc niches location, an exhaustive microdissection is essential to take out the region of interest in a reliable way before starting the isolation procedures. Then, it is highly recommendable the use of thin slices of tissue for the accurate microdissection of different compartments under a dissecting microscope (e.g. Seaberg & van der Kooy, 2002).

Tissue dissection is particularly challenging in the case of human surgical samples, where orientation and anatomical organization is usually altered after surgery, making difficult the recognition of particular zones and, consequently, a good dissection. Alternatively, some authors have demonstrated the isolation of viable cells from postmortem tissue, especially in the case of human samples (e.g. Schwartz et al., 2001). While these procedures might be the only way to access some type of tissues, there might be some logistical inconveniences, the main one being that collection of tissue and cell isolation protocols need to be performed within few hours, because the number of NSPc decreases with time (Leonard et al., 2009; Xu et al., 2003), especially when samples are exposed to environmental temperature instead of 4°C (Laywell et al., 1999).

2.2 Tissue digestion methods

2.2.1 Enzymatic dissociation

NSPc are surrounded by a highly structured extracellular matrix mainly composed by lecticans, hyaluronic acid, tenascin-C and tenascin-R (Rutka et al., 1988). These molecules interact among them and with membrane molecules on cell surfaces, and can regulate part of their behavior.

Therefore, one of the most successful strategies for removing NSPc from the rest of the tissue implies the use of proteases to degrade this matrix.

The first step, to prepare the tissue for enzymatic digestion, involves the mincing into small pieces (less than 1 mm^3) in order to provide more degradable surface for the action of proteases. In this sense, the use of two different enzymes stands over the rest in the literature: trypsin (examples of its applications in different samples and developmental stages can be read at Kirschenbaum et al., 1994; Kukekov et al., 1997, Reynolds et al., 1992; Reynolds&Weiss, 1992; Svendsen et al., 1998) and papain (Babu et al., 2007; Roy et al., 2000a; Wang et al., 2000; Windrem et al., 2004). Trypsin is the most employed one, and is often combined with ethylenediaminetetraacetic acid (EDTA), a Ca^{2+} chelating agent that weakens intercellular unions. Regarding the concentration and the incubation time, it is not always possible to compare between different protocols as the enzyme units are not always specified and the incubation time ranges from 10 to 90 minutes. Additionally, other enzymes can be found in the bibliography such as hialuronidase (e.g. Gritti et al., 1995; Weiss et al., 1996), collagenase (e.g. Uchida et al., 2000), and neutral protease (dispase) (e.g. Babu et al., 2007), alone or in combination with others.

Generally, the use of proteases is linked to the utilization of Desoxiribonuclease I (DNase I), usually from bovine origin, in order to eliminate the DNA mucus originated by cell lysis, which could hinder cell survival and further experiments.

In any case, the employment of enzyme specific buffers (with adjusted pH and containing activators) is necessary to allow the action of these enzymes. In some cases, antibiotic/ antimitotic is added to the digestion solution to prevent contamination. At this stage, some authors also include kynurenic acid in order to reduce glutamate excitotoxicity through NMDA receptor channels (e.g. Reynolds&Weiss, 1992). Afterward, the use of protease inhibitors is necessary to stop enzymatic reaction. Papain is usually neutralized with fetal bovine serum, whereas in the case of trypsin, the most employed method includes ovomucoid, although there are commercially available soy, lima bean, and basic pancreatic protein -based inhibitors.

The criterion for the choice of one or another enzyme is not clear, and frequently it has more to do with the previous experience and skills of the group. Nevertheless, as a general rule, embryo and early fetal samples require less amount of enzyme due to its laxity. For this reason, some protocols reduce protease concentrations and/or exposure time (e.g. Svendsen et al., 1998) or even recommend the use of mechanical disaggregation techniques alone (e.g. Ciccolini&Svendsen, 1998; Reynolds&Weiss, 1996).

The enzymatic digestion is a critical step because it affects directly to the NSPc survival rate. In this sense, some studies have been done to compare cell survival after dissociation with different protease. Maric et al., 1998, used murine embryonic tissue to evaluate the efficacy of papain, trypsin, and collagenase treatment, or mechanical disaggregation alone. The results indicate that papain dissociation is optimal, achieving the maximum reproducible cell recovery and viability. On the contrary, trypsin, collagenase, and mechanical dissociations resulted on suboptimal and highly variable yields. Another study, carried out by Panchision et al., 2007 also compared the results obtained for mouse embryonic stem cell isolation when using papain, Tryple™ (a commercial analog of trypsin), or collagenase/neutral protease commercial cocktails (Accutase™ and Liberase-1™). Data also confirmed that mechanic dissociation induced more variability, cell death and more number of aggregates. However, Tryple™ and papain produced more quantity of DNA mucus (but not an increased cell death) and a lower adherence to culture plate after planting. They conclude that the best results were obtained with papain, independently of the exposure time to the enzyme.

Moreover, this work also revealed another important factor to take into account when optimizing protease dissociation: cell surface markers can be altered by these enzymes, inducing false negatives when immunocytochemistry or Fluorescent Activated cell sorting is performed just after isolation. Table 1 includes a list of sensitive markers described in this paper and similar reports. In addition, another work detected that trypsin cleavage can lead to an increased positivity of some tumor –related surface markers, depending on the state of glycosylation (Corver et al., 1995).

	enzyme -sensitive	very weakly enzyme - sensitive
Trypsin	hCD133, CD31, O4, CD81, c14, Ca125, BMa180	A2B5, CD15
Papain	PSA-NCAM, CD24, BMP IA, BMP IB	CD15, O4, CD81
Liberase-1™	BMP IA, BMP IB	
Accutase™	none of the studied	
Tryple™	none of the studied	

Table 1. List of enzyme – sensitive markers that are reported in Corver et al., 1995; Panchision et al., 2007; and commercial report by Reiβ et al (Miltenyi). CD133 has been reported to be sensitive to trypsin treatment in human cells, but not in rodent cells.

2.2.2 Mechanical disaggregation

Usually, the enzymatic digestion is not enough to remove the NSPc from the remaining tissue. After or during enzymatic digestion, the tissue must be triturated to break up the digested pieces into a single cell suspension. It is a dramatic process that ends up with an important number of dead cells. However, different strategies have been described in the literature in order to reduce, to some extent, this number. The most common method consists in passing the suspension through fire polished glass pipettes, due to their high availability and lower price (e.g. Ciccolini & Svendsen, 1998; Gage et al., 1995; Reynolds&Weiss, 1992). Moreover, they can be narrowed into different diameters, adapting their thickness to samples of different size. Many protocols include the sequential trituration through pipettes with decreasing diameters in order to disaggregate the tissue in successive steps and reduce cell death (e.g. Wang et al., 2000). Nevertheless, this system also presents some technical problems. First, cells display a relative adherence to glass and might be lost. Furthermore, as glass pipettes are usually prepared specifically for each experiment, their diameter can vary, and therefore, different cell survival rates can be obtained. The cell adherence issues might be partially resolved by coating pipettes with silicone. Alternatively, some commercially available plastic pipettes (Kukekov et al., 1997) are treated to reduce the adherence, but they cannot be fire polished.

Another strategy is based on the utilization of sterile syringes and needles (e.g. Shi et al., 1998). In this sense, a large range of needle gauges is available commercially, ensuring the reproducibility of the technique; however, their edges are too sharp and that results in an increase in cell death. Although less frequent, it is worth mentioning the use of different devices like the glass homogenizer, used for embryonic neural stem cell isolation (Carpenter et al., 1999), and some commercial equipment that appeared in the last years, promising a higher efficiency via the automation of the isolation procedure (Reiβ et al (Miltenyi)).

2.2.3 Filters utility

Some groups, after enzymatic digestion and mechanical disaggregation, include a filtering step to remove the debris from the cell suspension. This additional step might eliminate undissociated tissue pieces as well as avoid the presence of necrotic particles in the final pellet that would potentially induce cell death. However, it also reduces the final number of viable cells trapped into the filter. In any case, the use of filters usually requires a DNase I treatment, to remove the mucus that can difficult the filtering, and it is strongly recommended the dilution of cell suspension in a considerable volume of medium. Regarding the type and size of the filters, some authors describe the use of cell strainers, whereas others prefer sterile gauze (e.g. Kukekov et al., 1997). The mesh size also differs among protocols (40 um (Wang et al., 2000), 70 um (Rietze et al., 2001), 100 um, etc), and should be chosen in accordance with the efficiency of preceding methodology.

2.3 Neural stem/progenitor cells enrichment procedures

The initial protocols for NSPc isolation were designed with the only purpose of isolating and culturing these cells to study their biology *in vitro*. However, as the knowledge on the biology and differentiation potential of NSPc increased, it was evident that cell cultures comprised a number of different subpopulations with different degree of stemness. Consistently with this reality, many authors have recently included separation steps into their NSPc isolation protocols. This separation is usually based on the NSPc phenotypic characteristics closely related to their stem cell features.

In this sense, the first works on NSPc isolation and culture described a selection based on their capacity to proliferate in the chosen medium and growth factors. Obviously, it was not enough to discriminate heterogeneity. Consequently, many technical approaches have been developed since then, for the enrichment of a specific subpopulation. This way, the biological significance behind the molecule chosen to enrich for a specific type of cell and the technology used for the procedure become an important step determining the differentiation potential of the final cell culture. The current techniques for the separation and enrichment of NSPc are described below.

2.3.1 Methods based on differential adherent properties of cells

One of the first methodologies for the enrichment of particular subpopulations was based on the differential attachment of cells to the culture plate due to their particular adhesion molecule patterns. By optimizing some parameters like substrates and time in culture it is possible to distinguish between different types of cells. Astroglial cells show the biggest adherence, even in untreated culture plate, whereas oligodendrocytes can be easily detached through the agitation on a rotary shaker at slow revolutions (200-300 rpm) for 12-20 h. This procedure has demonstrated to be useful, easy and affordable. As a consequence, it has been common in the purification of specific cell types like oligodendrocytes (McCarthy & de Vellis, 1980; Chen et al., 2007b).

Taking advantage of these properties, Lim&Alvarez-Buylla, 1999, reported the isolation of 4 cell fractions using serial streaming of medium or PBS over the surface of poly-D-lysine treated plates, and a final step with trypsin. The first fraction (or fraction 1), which contains the less adherent cells, was enriched in PSA-NCAM and Tuj1 (identified as migrating neuroblasts). On the contrary, cells from the most adherent fraction (fraction 4) were GFAP+ and show characteristics of neural stem cells (type B/C according to the model of SVZ organization (Fig.2). However, it is important to mention that this procedure does not allow the obtaining of high purity cultures.

2.3.2 Differential gradient centrifugation

Another group of technical approaches for NSPc enrichment is based on fractionating cell populations according to their buoyant density. Previously, the cells are dissolved in specific solvents that, after centrifugation, generate a density gradient. The cells distribute in this gradient and can be collected separately. The gradient might be formed by using different types of reagents, being Percoll the most widely used (e.g. Palmer et al., 1999; K. Chen et al., 2007a). It consists of colloidal silica particles coated with a layer of polyvinylpyrrolidone (PVP) that can be used to form solution densities between 1.00 and 1.20 g/ml. A combination of Percoll gradients can be generated in order to separate more subpopulations. Using a discontinuous density gradient, Maric et al., 1998 reported the isolation of 20 different bands and the delimitation of density bands can be facilitated by commercial color-coded density marker beads. While its application has become very common because of its low interaction with cells and low toxicity, it is restricted to research as it may contain variable quantities of endotoxin (PVP). Alternatively, density gradients can be also generated using sucrose solutions (Johansson et al., 1999) and Bovine Serum Albumin (Ericsson, 1977).

2.3.3 Immunopanning

Initial immunopanning applications were essentially directed to eliminate specific cell subpopulations by antibody union and complement-mediated lysis (e.g. Gard&Pfeiffer, 1993). Nevertheless, the present acceptation of the immunopanning technic comprises the purification of a cell population by exploiting their differential binding to the culture dishes previously coated with a cell-surface antibody. Cells expressing this surface antigen are retained on the dish and are thereby separated from the remaining cell population. It has been especially applied to the isolation of oligodendrocyte progenitor cells, using A2B5 or O4 (Barres et al., 1992; Wu et al., 2009; Mayer-Proschel, 2001) as molecular surface markers, but it can also be adapted to segregate immature neurons (PSA-NCAM) (Ben-Hur et al., 1998; Schmandt et al., 2005). Although the use of immunopanning has become less popular with the introduction of Fluorescence-activated cell sorting (FACS) technology, some authors had reported that immunopanning provides a higher survival (Mayer-Proschel, 2001).

2.3.4 Fluorescence activated cell sorting (FACS)

The main improvement in terms of separation and enrichment of specific NSPc comes with the introduction of the FACS technology. As a specialized form of flow citometry, it provides a method for sorting heterogeneous cells based upon the specific union of a fluorophore-labeled antibody to a cell surface maker. In addition to antibodies, other molecules like lectins can be used to recognize the glycosylation state of some membrane epitopes (as reviewed in Kitada et al., 2011).

The main advantage of this procedure is its high sensitivity, reaching values of purity above 95%. Moreover, the possibility of labeling cells with simultaneous antibodies allows the isolation of a particular subset of cells with a combination of membrane markers (e.g. Uchida *et al*, 2000). Moreover, the use of this technology makes possible the sorting of cells according to the expression of either cytoplasmic or nuclear markers. This advantage allowed the design of transgenic animal models that express a given fluorophore under the control of specific promoters. Additionally, the introduction of small DNA molecules can also induce the expression of a fluorescent molecule in both animal and human cells.

Alternatively, magnetic labeled antibodies might be used through a variation known as Magnetic-activated cell sorting (MACS). This technology uses a more reduced and affordable equipment, although it does not allow the labeling of more than one surface marker. Table 2 lists the stem cell markers used in the isolation of NSPc subpopulations by FACS or MACS.

NEURAL STEM CELLS	ANTIBODY	Integrin α1β5	Yoshida et al., 2003
		CD15	Capela et al., 2002; Corti et al., 2005; Panchision et al., 2007
		CD24LOW	Murayama et al., 2002; Rietze et al., 2001
		CD133	Cortie tal., 2005; Panchision et al., 2007; Uchida et al., 2000
		CXCR4	Corti et al., 2005
		EGFR1 (EGF)	Ciccolini et al., 2005; Pastrana et al., 2009
		NOTCH1	Johansson et al., 1999
	LECTINS	PHA-E4	Hamanoue et al., 2008
		WGA	Hamanoue et al., 2008
	FLUOROPHORE UNDER PROMOTOR CONTROL	p/GFAP	Doetsch et al., 1999; Pastrana et al., 2009
		p/MELK	Nakano et al., 2005
		p/MSI1	Keyoung et al., 2001
		p/Nestin	Kawaguchi et al., 2001; Keyoung et al., 2001; Roy et al., 2000a, 200b; Sawamoto et al., 2001; Yoshida et al., 2003
		p/SOX1	Barraud et al.,2005

				Brazelet al., 2005; Ellis et al., 2004; ; Keyoung et al., 2001; Suh et al., 2007; Wang et al., 2010
LINEAGE RESTRICTED PRECURSOR	glial	ANTIBODY	A2B5	Maric et al., 2003; Nunes et al., 2003; Windrem et al., 2002; Windremet al., 2004; Wright et al., 1997
			CD44	Liu et al., 2004
			GD3	Maric et al., 2003
			NG2	Aguirre et al., 2004
			O1	Duncan et al., 1992
		FLUOROPHORE UNDER PROMOTOR CONTROL	p/CNP	Aguirre et al., 2004; Nunes et al., 2004; Roy et al., 1999; Yuan et al., 2002
	neuronal	ANTIBODY	PSA-NCAM	Panchision et al., 2007:Windrem et al, 2004
		FLUOROPHORE UNDER PROMOTOR CONTROL	P/Tα1	Piper et al., 2001; Roy et al, 2000[a], 2000b; Sawamoto et al., 2001; Wang et al., 2000
			P/Neurogenin2	Thompson et al., 2006
		OTHERS	Cholera toxin	Maric et al., 2003
			Tetanus toxin	Maric et al., 2003

Table 2. Main markers used for NSPc isolation by FACS or MACS.

3. Primary neural stem/progenitor cell culture

3.1 Culture conditions

3.1.1 Culture media

The culture media commonly used to grow NSPc includes two components, the basal media and supplements and the use of growth factors. The basal culture media formulation does not change significantly between different groups. It is based on the use of Dulbecco's modified Eagle's Medium (DMEM), which is composed by a defined mixture of inorganic salts, amino acids and vitamins among other nutrients. DMEM is usually combined (1:1) with Ham's F-12 (F-12), which basically increases the level of some nutrients and provides different inorganic salts. Although less frequent, other alternatives with similar characteristics have been reported as basal media, such as Neurobasal™, or Ex Vivo™ 15 (e.g. Babu et al., 2007).

The basal media is frequently supplemented with N2 or B27 supplements which contain nutrients like insulin, transferrin or putrescine, among others. These supplements cannot be added to basal formulation until they are used because of their short life at 4°C. Although both of them might be used, even in combination, they have different properties that may influence cell culture behavior. B27 has a more complex composition than N2 supplement and only enhances cell survival during the period immediately following isolation (Svendsen et al., 1995), while N2 offers the same results, at a lower price. Babu et al. (2007) concluded that monolayer cells maintained with N2 supplement generated more neurons after differentiation, whereas B27 supplement promoted proliferation.

3.1.2 Serum and growth factors

Although basal media and supplements are quite similar in most cases, the most important issue in terms of culture media is the use of either specific growth factors or serum. The first works on NSPc isolation and maintenance described the use of serum in their culture media. However, as the knowledge on NSPc biology increased, researchers found that the use of serum, generally fetal bovine serum (FBS), had several disadvantages. As a complex solution of undefined composition that can vary drastically among batches, the use of serum does not contribute to improve our knowledge about trophic signals requirements. Additionally, it is not a physiological condition, since neural stem cells are not exposed directly to serum *in vivo*. Finally, serum includes a combination of different growth factors that are able to maintain stem cell phenotype and also induce differentiation. All these reasons made the authors substitute serum for a specific combination of purified growth factors. The utilization of two main growth factors stands out from the rest: fibroblast growth factor 2 (FGF-2, also called basic FGF or bFGF) and epidermal growth factor (EGF), alone or in combination. Moreover, FGF-2 must be used in combination with heparin, which mediates the binding of the growth factor to its receptor (Yayon et al., 1991).

Initial works (Reynolds, 1992; Reynolds & Weiss, 1992) described the isolation of an EGF-responsive neural stem cell population from striata/lateral ventricle, although some authors reported that similar cell cultures could be also maintained with FGF (Gritti et al., 1995; Vescovi et al., 1993). Similarly, some works also found a synergic effect of both EGF and FGF in proliferation, but only at low cell densities (Svendsen, 1997; Tropepe, 1999). Finally, a series of studies (Martens et al., 2000; Tropepe et al., 1999; Ciccolini, 2001; Maric et al., 2003) demonstrated that FGF- responsive cells arise earlier at development, and then give rise to both EGF/FGF- responsive cells. Moreover, it was revealed that the acquisition of EGF responsiveness is promoted by FGF *in vitro* (Ciccolini & Svendsen, 1998). First isolations could be explained with the discovery of a small autocrine/paracrine FGF production by neural stem cells, allowing the survival of FGF-2 dependent cells without FGF until the acquisition of EGF responsiveness (Maric et al., 2003).

Other growth factors that have been reported to support cell culture are Transforming growth factor alpha (TGF-α) (Reynolds et al., 1992), Leukemia inhibitory factor (LIF) and its equivalent Ciliary neurotrophic factor (CNTF) (Carpenter et al., 1999), or Brain-derived neurotrophic factor (BDNF), although its capacity to enhance later neuronal production and survival has been questioned (Kirschenbaum & Goldman, 1995; Ahmed et al., 1995; Reynolds & Weiss, 1996).

Platelet-derived growth factor alpha (PDGFα) is frequently used in the maintenance media for oligodendrocyte progenitor cells. The signaling pathway through the PDGFα/PDGFRα has different effects depending on the stage of differentiation of these progenitors: it provides signals favoring proliferation and migration in murine and human oligodendrocyte progenitors (Wilson et al., 2003; Calver et al., 1998), whereas later in development is related with cell survival (Gogate et al, 1994). Similarly, FGF promotes proliferation and blocks differentiation of oligodendrocyte progenitors, in part through the modulation of PDGFRα receptors expression (McKinnon et al., 1990).

Finally, some works have attempted to co-culture NSPc in the presence of other supportive cells like astrocytes (Richards et al., 1992; Lim et al., 1999), that seem to favor the NSPc growth by physical contact, or endothelial cells, that also enhance cell proliferation via VEGF production (Sun et al., 2010).

3.1.3 pH and oxygen levels

The metabolic processes undergone by the cells in culture give rise to acidic components that eventually are released to the media, thus decreasing the pH. This alteration, easily followed by the inclusion of a pH indicator like phenol red, has a direct influence in the behavior of the cells. Therefore, buffering agents are commonly added to medium formulation in order to control variations in the pH. In this sense, two main systems are routinely used in the elaboration of the media: sodium bicarbonate buffer, which is dependent on the CO_2 concentration present in the incubator, and HEPES (4-(2-hydroxyethyl)-1-piperazineethanesulfonic acid), independent of atmospheric CO_2. Although HEPES is better at maintaining physiological pH controls, the exposure of HEPES-containing media to light must be reduced as HEPES-containing media generates hydrogen peroxide when exposed to ambient light ({Zigler et al., 1985).

In contrast, the level of O_2 tension remains to be optimized for NSPc cultures. The standard conditions to culture NSPc had included atmospheric levels of O_2 (21%), although physiological levels are much lower (around 3%). Several studies have confirmed that NSPc expansion under low level of O_2 correlates with the expression of stemness markers and higher survival rate both *in vitro* and *in vivo* after engraftment (reviewed in De Filippis & Delia, 2011).

3.2 Monolayer versus neurosphere cultures

To maintain and propagate stem cell cultures different authors have published two alternative methods of NSPc culture and expansion: as free-floating cell clusters (neurospheres) or as adherent cultures forming a monolayer on the plate surface.

The neurosphere assay has been the most extended method to demonstrate the presence of NSPc in culture (Reynolds et al., 1992) and it is still used with different modifications (Rietze& Reynolds, 2006). Some authors claim that each neurosphere represents a microenvironment that recapitulates neurogenic niche and allows survival of stem cells *in vitro* (Bez et al., 2003) through direct cell-to-cell interaction. Nevertheless, a single neurosphere contains only a small percentage of true stem cells, whereas the remaining cells are in different stages of differentiation. Necrotic and apoptotic cells are also present (Lobo et al., 2003). Interestingly, it has been reported that committed progenitors, like oligodendrocyte precursors, can generate cell clusters similar to neurospheres (Chen Y. et al., 2007).

This culture method has also several technical disadvantages. First, when neurospheres become larger, the diffusion of nutrients and growth factors through the neurosphere is compromised (Svendsen et al., 1997b), which makes difficult the interpretation of some experimental results. Second, packed neurospheres do not allow the tracking of individual cells, which also hinders studies relating to differentiation processes. Finally, recent publications demonstrate that neurospheres are not static particles originated from a single cell and isolated from the rest of the neurospheres and cells (Rietze, 2006). On the contrary, they are dynamic structures within the culture, were cells are exchangeable from one to another sphere. This effect, may be circumvented by either using a limiting dilution analysis to obtain a single cell in each well or using semisolid cultures by adding methylcellulose (Gritti et al., 1999; Kukekov et al., 1997) or collagen (Neural Colony-Forming Cell Assay (Louis et al., 2008).

By contrast, monolayer cultures obviate some of these restrictions. They can be used to study the properties of stem cells at individual cell level, although it does not allow cell interaction during differentiation. Moreover, cells are exposed homogeneously to growth factors and serum, with the consequent reduction in cell heterogeneity.

In all, there is not a prevalent method over the other. It has not been demonstrated a total equivalence between both type of cultures and the two methods have advantages and limitations that researchers should take into consideration in the experimental design. The formation of neurospheres may be promoted by following several strategies, being the most common one the use of nonadherent surfaces like poly-2-hydroxyethyl methacrylate (Kukekov et al, 1999). Furthermore, it has been also reported the addition of mercaptoethanol to avoid cell attachment (Kukekov et al., 1997). However, not all attempts to transform an adherent culture into neurospheres have been successful (Walton et al., 2006). Alternatively, cell attachment may be induced by coating the plate surface with charged molecules such as poly-l-ornithine, poly-d-lysine or laminin.

3.3 Cell passaging

Before cells become totally confluent, it is necessary to subculture them after disaggregation of cell clusters into single cell suspensions. Regardless of the type of culture, monolayer or suspension, passaging should be performed before cells achieve their maximum confluence (monolayer) or cell cluster become necrotic (neurospheres) in order to avoid senescence associated with prolonged high cell density. The methodology employed for the disaggregation step depends on the cell type.

Adherent cells are usually detached from the surface of the culture vessel by enzymatic means. Trypsin, alone or in combination with EDTA, has been the most used protease (e.g. Palmer et al., 1997); but in the last years it has been substituted in current protocols by Tryple™, since this commercial product is free of animal- and human- derived components, less damaging to cells, and does not require the use of inhibitors.

In the case of neurospheres, cell disaggregation is performed by using mechanical procedures which involve triturating spheres with fire polished pipettes. However, this is an aggressive method that renders high levels of cell death. Enzymatic digestion can be also used before triturating, however, this may alter the experimental results if FACS assays are conducted right after disaggregation.

An alternative method was reported by Svendsen & ter Borg, 1998 for passaging neurospheres isolated from human fetal tissue. Briefly, neurospheres were cut into 4 pieces instead of standard trituration into single cell suspension. According to their data, this sectioning method reduces cellular trauma and preserves cell interaction, allowing NSPc to proliferate more replication rounds *in vitro*.

3.4 Cryopreservation

Cryopreservation allows the maintenance of NSPc in a suspension mode awaiting for future experiments and saving expensive culture reagents. Considering the low number of cells obtained from each sample, especially in human tissue, increasing the survival ratio after long-term preservation of NSPc becomes a major concern. The main cryopreservation protocols employ dimethylsulfoxyde (DMSO) diluted at 10-20% in culture media to avoid ice crystallization, accompanied by a slow cooling step in isopropanol recipients. Although less popular, glycerol can be used instead of DMSO. Cellular viability can be improved adding animal serum to freezing medium, but it can potentially introduce contaminants, and induce differentiation. In any case, cryopreservation must follow some general rules to ensure the successful preservation of cells. It must be performed during the logarithmic growth phase and high cell density in each ampoule seems to facilitate cell recuperation. Smaller neurospheres survive better than larger, so triturating cells until getting a suspension of small neurospheres improves cell survival.

Recently, a new alternative preservation method, named vitrification, has been adapted for NSPc (Tan et al., 2007). In brief, cells are sequentially submerged in a series of freezing solutions with increasing concentrations of cryoprotectant (ethylene glycol and sucrose), and finally transferred into borosilicate glass capillaries, snap-frozen and stored in liquid nitrogen. The results showed that vitrification offered the best combination of cell viability, multipotency, and preservation of structural integrity of neurospheres.

3.5 Differentiation

After isolation of proliferating cells, it is necessary to confirm the stemness characteristics of the cells, that is, the multipotent and self-renewal capacities. In this sense, cells with lower self-renewal or with potential to generate just one type of cell should be considered as progenitor cells. To evaluate the differentiation capacity, cells are exposed to differentiation signals coming from animal serum or chemically defined compounds.

The use of serum has the same problems highlighted above. Nevertheless, this is still the standard methodology, because the specific signals inducing NSPc differentiation into a specific lineage remains largely unknown. Cells maintained in defined medium tend to differentiate when exposed to serum in a variable concentration (from 1% up to 10%)(e.g. Ciccolini & Svendsen, 1998; Palmer et al., 1999; Roy et al., 2000; Wanget al., 2000), although a preference towards astroglial differentiation has been reported (Palmer et al., 1995). The use of serum is usually accompanied by the addition of molecules such as Poly-L-ornithine, laminin or matrigel to promote adhesion to substrate, which seem to enhance differentiation of neurospheres cultures (Ciccolini & Svendsen, 1998; Reynolds & Weiss, 1996; Tropepe et al., 1999). In some cases, the removal of growth factors in conjunction with an adherent substrate has been also used to differentiate NSPc (Gritti et al., 1996).

Alternatively, media previously exposed to other cell cultures (conditioned medium) may be used to induce differentiation. Probably the most employed one is B104 conditioned medium, which is exposed to a neuroblastoma cell line and induces oligodendroglial differentiation (Young & Levinson, 1997).

Few authors have conducted NSPc differentiation assays by using growth factor cocktails in the absence of serum. Uchida et al., 2000 reported that a combination of BDNF and glial-derived growth factor (GDNF) was enough to differentiate CD133+ cells from human fetal tissue. Ling et al., 1998 reported a more specific differentiation protocol, proving that the combination of Interlekine-1b, Intelkeulin-11 and GDNF promoted the appearance of dopaminergic neurons (tyrosine hydroxylase -positive cells).

Furthermore, a number of chemical signals have been also reported to stimulate the differentiation toward a particular neural lineage.

In the case of neuronal maturation, BDNF, retinoic acid, Neurotrophin (NT3), and Sonic Hedgehog (SHH) have been associated to an enhanced neural obtaining (Babu et al., 2007; Bull & Bartlett, 2005; Dutton et al., 1999; Roy et al., 2000a, 2000b).

Oligodendroglial differentiation can be also enhanced using PDGFa, which promotes their survival (Gogate et al., 1994) in collaboration with NT3 and Triiodothyronine (T3), factors necessary for the correct development of oligodendrocytes and the expression of myelin proteins (Billon et al., 2002; Park et al., 2001).

4. Isolation from neurogenic zones

Neural stem cells seem to reside within specific niches of the adult brain. These regions are located in the subventricular zone of the lateral ventricles and the subgranular zone in the hippocampus. The origin of NSPc in these two areas has been the focus of intense debates in the literature and the isolation procedures of such cells from these specific locations need special attention.

Since the discovery of adult neural stem cells, the isolation procedures have been modified along with the increased knowledge of NSPc biology. Initially, these cells were supposed to be scattered within the brain parenchyma. However, soon after it was restricted to the SVZ, although the individual cell identity is still a source of division among researchers due to the lack of a specific marker to label neural stem cells. The nature and origin of the neural stem cell in the SGZ of the hippocampus has been also a subject of an intense debate, questioning whether they could be considered true neural stem cells or committed progenitors. Additionally, other types of neural progenitors like oligodendrocyte progenitor cells (OPCs) seem to be dispersed through the white matter, and their isolation procedures and characterization have become recently relevant in the context of demyelinating diseases.

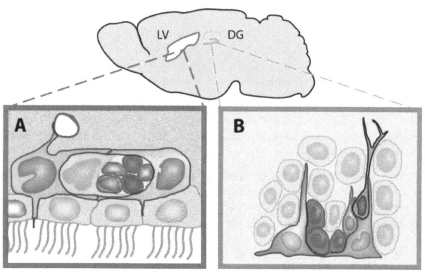

Fig. 2. Schematic representation of both adult neurogenic niches and their location in a sagittal section of rodent brain. A) The subventricular zone (SVZ) of the lateral ventricles (LV) contains an astrocyte-like stem cell population termed as type B1 cells (blue) that, unlike ependymal cells (grey), contact with lumen occasionally, showing a single cilium. Through asymmetrical divisions, Type B1 cells generate rapidly dividing, transit-amplifying cells, termed as Type C (green) which, in turn, give rise to immature neuroblasts or Type A cells (red). Those neuroblasts migrate through an astroglial scaffold toward the olfactory bulb, where they fully differentiate into granular neurons. B) The subgranular zone (SGZ) of the dentate gyrus of hippocampus also harbors an astroglial stem cell subpopulation (green). These cells generate directly immature neuroblasts , which can divide once (Type D1, red), migrate while undergoing differentiation (Type D2, type D3,pink) and integrate as granular neurons (brown).

4.1 Subventricular zone

The first population of adult neural stem cells in mammals is located in a specific niche along the SVZ of the lateral ventricles. Several types of cells can be distinguished within these niches including type B cells (slowly dividing astroglial cells and the *bona fide* adult neural stem cells), type C cells (transit-amplifying cells derived from asymmetric division of Type B cells), type A cells (immature neuroblasts derived from Type C cells) and ependymal cells lining the lumen of the ventricle. Although this is a general model found in rodents, some differences have been described in primates and humans (for a complete revision see Quiñones-Hinojosa et al., 2006). However, the accumulating knowledge on the neural stem cells biology, and their interaction with other elements of the niches, has transformed the description of the neurogenic regions into a dynamic process were the acquisition of new findings changes the model over the time. The evolution of this model has also derived in the inclusion of changes in the NSC isolation and maintenance protocols.

Once the presence of neural stem cells was demonstrated within the adult brain of mammals, the first question to address was the location of such cells and the neurogenic region. Early studies reported the isolation of NSC from the striatal tissue of both rat (Gritti et al., 1995; Reynolds & Weiss, 1992;) and mouse (Richards et al., 1992). Nevertheless, the striatum is a relatively large region that is not consistent with data about NSC biology. Afterwards the investigations in this field confirmed that only SVZ tissue was able to generate cell cultures with stem cell properties, whether via explants (Kirschenbaum et al., 1994; Kirschenbaum & Goldman, 1995; Lois & Alvarez-Buylla, 1993) or neurospheres cultures (Morshead et al., 1994) were used. Subsequent articles which described the isolation of neural stem cells from striatum specified the inclusion of the SVZ region within the dissected tissue (Weiss et al., 1996) and confirmed that the results of neural stem cell isolation exclusively from SVZ were identical to those obtained from extensive anatomical regions containing the SVZ (Kukekov et al., 1997). These initial works emphasized the relevance of a fine orientated dissection for a successful NSC isolation protocol.

Nonetheless, the SVZ comprises a heterogeneous population, and those early reports did not reveal the cellular identity of the NSC. Probably, the first work addressing the NSC identity *in vitro,* was performed by Johansson et al., 1999. Marking ventricular cells with DiI (a lipophilic membrane stain that diffuses laterally to stain the entire cell), they concluded that NSC were actually ciliated ependymal cells. By contrast, Doetsch et al. (1999) reported that only GFAP expressing cells (marked via adenovirus which allowed the expression of the green fluorescent protein (GFP) under the control of glial fibrillary acidic protein (GFAP) promoter) give rise to neurospheres culture. Moreover, it was previously described that those astrocyte-like cells occasionally contacted the ventricle and displayed a single cilium, suggesting that DiI isolated cultures could be originated from them instead of ependymal cells (a more complete model can be consulted at Mirzadeh et al. (2008)). Following previous findings, two new studies described that both types of cells were able to proliferate *in vitro,* but only SVZ astrocytes generated neurospheres with self-renewal and mutipotential capacity (Chiasson et al., 1999; Laywell et al., 2000). These findings also marked the need for an identification and selection step in the NSPc isolation protocol. With the introduction of FACS technology, two phenotypical features of NSC supported the astrocyte-like theory, the isolation of a CD15+ population with stem cell characteristics (Capela & Temple, 2002), a carbohydrate only expressed in astrocytes, and the identification of NSC as CD24^{low} (Rietze et al, 2001), whereas ependymal cells are CD24+. Using an opposite strategy to deplete adult GFAP+ cells, two independent studies demonstrated that the ablation of adult astrocytes resulted in the loss of multipotent neurosphere formation (Morshead et al, 2003; Imura et al., 2003). However, with the controversy surrounding the identity of NSCs, two later studies reported the isolation of CD133+ cells from adult brain, as previously reported by Uchida et al. (2000) for fetal tissue. Nevertheless, opposite results were obtained from each one. The first one (Corti et al., 2007) concluded that CD133 stained a small number of cells underlying the ependymal layer, and the sorting of those CD133+ cells leads to the isolation of a NSC population. Interestingly, Mirzadeh et al. (2008) found that 29% of the apical processes of B1 cells were positive for CD133. By contrast, Coskun et al. (2008) found that both CD133+ ependymal cells and NSC originate from ependymal cells. In any case, it will be necessary to find new markers in order to improve the identification and selection of either the real adult neural stem cells and the different range of progenitor cells. This will allow the study of their specific biological features and maybe modulate their behavior *in vivo.*

4.2 Subgranular zone

In the adult hippocampus, NSCs are located in the SGZ, a cellular layer found between the granule cell layer and the hilus, in the dentate gyrus. Similarly to SVZ, NSCs have been identified as astrocyte-like cells, with cell bodies located in the SGZ and vertical processes extended through the molecular layer. However, unlike what happens in the SVZ, these astrocytic cells generate an earlier immature neuroblast that divides only once and expresses neuronal markers (PSA-NCAM and doublecourtin) (Type D1 cells). Those cells migrate short distances within the granule cell layer while undergoing morphological changes (type D2 and Type D3 cells) until they reach a final position and differentiate into mature granular neurons.

The first data from adult hippocampal cell cultures were published by Palmer et al., 1995. They isolated a monolayer culture from adult female rat hippocampus. These cells were capable of proliferating in serum free media supplemented with FGF. In Gage et al., 1995, they were also able to derivate a FGF-2 -dependent adherent culture that differentiates into mature neurons when engrafted into adult rat brain. Short after, *in vitro* differentiation was attempted by Palmer et al., 1997. Using several combinations of growth factors, they demonstrated the multipotency of those progenitor cells, and the enhancement of neuronal maturation when BDNF was added (similarly to NT3 and retinoic acid results), whereas serum addition promoted astroglial differentiation.

As described previously for initial reports on SVZ, those studies also isolated cells with similar features from non-neurogenic zones, including the septum of striatum. However a few years later was published the first work that isolated specific hippocampal neural stem cells from adult human samples (Kukekov et al., 1999). They observed the presence of neurospheres when cultured in non-adherent conditions by using mercaptoethanol, similarly to previous studies carried out with SVZ samples (Kukekov et al., 1997). Following the enrichment step based on the expression of GFP under the control of an specific promoter (P/Tα1:hGFP and E/nestin:EGFP), described previously to identify NSC from the SVZ, Roy et al., 2000b, isolated, for the first time, neural stem cells from human hippocampal samples. However, these results did not reproduce in mice and later works criticized the gross microdissection done in these publications. Afterwards, Seaberg & van der Kooy, 2002 tried to generate neurospheres from microdissected mouse dentate gyrus. They were unable to generate neurospheres capable of self-renewal, and multipotency was also compromised. Nevertheless, hippocampus obtained with gross dissection was able to generate neurospheres, suggesting that previous results could be explained if the dissection procedure included contaminating cells from the ventricular layer next to the hippocampus, or even white matter progenitors. They also assayed different culture conditions and dissection techniques, including dentate gyrus microdissection, and were unable to obtain proliferating neurospheres. After a number of publications showing controversial results in this regard Babu et al., 2007, using dentate gyrus microdissection from p/Nestin:EGFP transgenic mouse, were able to obtain monolayer cultures with self-renewal (up to 66 passages) and multipotency characteristics. Moreover, they observed spheres-like colonies when performing a modified neurosphere assay using semisolid medium. Additionally, after trying different media and supplements they concluded that although B27 and EGF promoted a slightly higher proliferation, N2 supplement and bFGF maintained cells differentiate better into mature neurons. Moreover, they reconfirmed that BDNF, NT3, SHH promoted neuronal differentiation, while LIF and Bone morphogenetic protein 2 (BMP-2) promoted glial differentiation

More recent works found that isolated neural progenitor/stem cells display paracrinal production of BMP, and the addition of noggin to culture media favors the formation of multipotential and self-renewal neurospheres (Bonaguidi et al., 2005; Bonaguidi et al., 2008).

The differences, in terms of culture media requirements, between NSC isolated from the SVZ and those from the SGZ might be due to their behavior *in vivo*. NSPc from lateral ventricle are prepared to migrate a larger distance to the olfactory lobes, while new neurons produced from dentate gyrus integrate nearby the stem cell niche and, therefore, are not prepared to maintain their stemness capacity in the absence of the niche signals.

5. Conclusions

Cell isolation and culture provides a powerful tool for the study of neural stem and progenitor cells. Although *in vitro* analysis has several limitations, and results cannot be directly extrapolated to the *in vivo* behavior of the isolated cells, it allows the analysis of their features and potential capacities in a controlled environment that can be modified and monitored more accurately.

Every step of the isolation procedure is likely to be optimized. Any protocol amendment should be tested and not considered trivial, as it can have a high impact on the cell population obtained. Consequently, isolation methods should be planned according to further experimental applications and not based on the routine practices of each research group, especially in the case of adaptation of protocols used previously for tissues collected from different species.

Moreover, it should be considered that the final purpose of most experiments is to improve our knowledge about stem cells and their clinical applications. For this reason, steps in the protocol which include reagents with undefined composition or with the possibility of introducing contaminants, such as serum, must be redesigned, because it is the only way to understand the chemical signals underlying the biological behavior of neural stem or progenitor cells.

6. Acknowledgements

We are especially grateful to Mario Soriano Navarro and Josefa Carrión Navarro for their assistance. Jorge Oliver De La Cruz is a recipient of a Predoctoral Fellowship from The FPU program (AP2008/02823), Ministerio de Educacion y Ciencia, Spain. This work was supported in part by grants from Alicia Koplowitz Foundation (JMGC, AAS, JOC) The Gent x Gent Foundation (AAS) and Fondo de Investigaciones Sanitarias (FIS) del Instituto de Salud Carlos III (PI10/01069)(AAS).

7. References

Aguirre, A. A., Chittajallu, R., Belachew, S., et al. (2004). NG2-expressing cells in the subventricular zone are type C-like cells and contribute to interneuron generation in the postnatal hippocampus. *J Cell Biol*, Vol. 165, No. 4 (May 2004), pp. (575-589), ISSN 0021-9525

Ahmed, S., Reynolds, B. A.&Weiss, S. (1995). BDNF enhances the differentiation but not the survival of CNS stem cell-derived neuronal precursors. *J Neurosci,* Vol. 15, No. 8 (August 1995), pp. (5765-5778), ISSN 0270-6474

Babu, H., Cheung, G., Kettenmann, H., et al. (2007). Enriched monolayer precursor cell cultures from micro-dissected adult mouse dentate gyrus yield functional granule cell-like neurons. *PLoS One,* Vol. 2, No. 4, (2007), pp. (e388), ISSN 1932-6203

Barres, B. A., Hart, I. K., Coles, H. S., et al. (1992). Cell death and control of cell survival in the oligodendrocyte lineage. *Cell,* Vol. 70, No. 1, (July 1992), pp. (31-46), ISSN 0092-8674

Belachew, S., Chittajallu, R., Aguirre, A. A., et al. (2003). Postnatal NG2 proteoglycan-expressing progenitor cells are intrinsically multipotent and generate functional neurons. *J Cell Biol,* Vol. 161, No. 1, (April 2003), pp. (169-186), ISSN 0021-9525

Ben-Hur, T., Rogister, B., Murray, K., et al. (1998). Growth and fate of PSA-NCAM+ precursors of the postnatal brain. *J Neurosci,* Vol. 18, No. 15 (August 1998), pp. (5777-5788), ISSN 0270-6474

Bez, A., Corsini, E., Curti, D., et al. (2003). Neurosphere and neurosphere-forming cells: morphological and ultrastructural characterization. *Brain Res,* Vol. 993, No. 1-2, (December 2003), pp. (18-29), ISSN 0006-8993

Billon, N., Jolicoeur, C., Tokumoto, Y., et al. (2002). Normal timing of oligodendrocyte development depends on thyroid hormone receptor alpha 1 (TRalpha1). *EMBO J,* Vol. 21, No. 23, (December 2002), pp. (6452-6460), ISSN 0261-4189

Bonaguidi, M. A., McGuire, T., Hu, M., et al. (2005). LIF and BMP signaling generate separate and discrete types of GFAP-expressing cells. *Development,* Vol. 132, No. 24, (December 2005), pp. (5503-5514), ISSN 0950-1991

Bonaguidi, M. A., Peng, C. Y., McGuire, T., et al. (2008). Noggin expands neural stem cells in the adult hippocampus. *J Neurosci,* Vol. 28, No. 37, (September 2008), pp. (9194-9204), ISSN 1529-2401

Brazel, C. Y., Limke, T. L., Osborne, J. K., et al. (2005). Sox2 expression defines a heterogeneous population of neurosphere-forming cells in the adult murine brain. *Aging Cell,* Vol. 4, No. 4, (August 2005), pp. (197-207), ISSN 1474-9718

Bull, N. D.&Bartlett, P. F. (2005). The adult mouse hippocampal progenitor is neurogenic but not a stem cell. *J Neurosci,* Vol. 25, No. 47 (November 2005), pp. (10815-10821), ISSN 1529-2401

Calver, A. R., Hall, A. C., Yu, W. P., et al. (1998). Oligodendrocyte population dynamics and the role of PDGF in vivo. *Neuron,* Vol. 20, No. 5, (May 1998), pp. (869-882), ISSN 0896-6273

Capela, A.&Temple, S. (2002). LeX/ssea-1 is expressed by adult mouse CNS stem cells, identifying them as nonependymal. *Neuron,* Vol. 35, No. 5, (August 2002), pp. (865-875), ISSN 0896-6273

Carpenter, M. K., Cui, X., Hu, Z. Y., et al. (1999). In vitro expansion of a multipotent population of human neural progenitor cells. *Exp Neurol,* Vol. 158, No. 2, (August 1999), pp. (265-278), ISSN 0014-4886

Ciccolini, F.&Svendsen, C. N. (1998). Fibroblast growth factor 2 (FGF-2) promotes acquisition of epidermal growth factor (EGF) responsiveness in mouse striatal precursor cells: identification of neural precursors responding to both EGF and FGF-2. *J Neurosci,* Vol. 18, No. 19, (October 1998), pp. (7869-7880), ISSN 0270-6474

Ciccolini, F. (2001). Identification of two distinct types of multipotent neural precursors that appear sequentially during CNS development. *Mol Cell Neurosci*, Vol. 17, No. 5, (May 2001), pp. (895-907), ISSN 1044-7431

Ciccolini, F., Mandl, C., Holzl-Wenig, G., et al. (2005). Prospective isolation of late development multipotent precursors whose migration is promoted by EGFR. *Dev Biol*, Vol. 284, No. 1, (August 2005), pp. (112-125), ISSN 0012-1606

Corti, S., Locatelli, F., Papadimitriou, D., et al. (2005). Multipotentiality, homing properties, and pyramidal neurogenesis of CNS-derived LeX(ssea-1)+/CXCR4+ stem cells. *FASEB J*, Vol. 19, No. 13, (November 2005), pp. (1860-1862), ISSN 1530-6860

Corti, S., Nizzardo, M., Nardini, M., et al. (2007). Isolation and characterization of murine neural stem/progenitor cells based on Prominin-1 expression. *Exp Neurol*, Vol. 205, No. 2, (June 2007), pp. (547-562), ISSN 0014-4886

Corver, W. E., Cornelisse, C. J., Hermans, J., et al. (1995). Limited loss of nine tumor-associated surface antigenic determinants after tryptic cell dissociation. *Cytometry*, Vol. 19, No. 3, (March 1995), pp. (267-272), ISSN 0196-4763

Coskun, V., Wu, H., Blanchi, B., et al. (2008). CD133+ neural stem cells in the ependyma of mammalian postnatal forebrain. *Proc Natl Acad Sci U S A*, Vol. 105, No. 3, (January 22 2008), pp. (1026-1031), ISSN 1091-6490

Chen, K., Hughes, S. M.&Connor, B. (2007). Neural progenitor cells derived from the adult rat subventricular zone: characterization and transplantation. *Cell Transplant*, Vol. 16, No. 8, (2007), pp. (799-810), ISSN 0963-6897

Chen, Y., Balasubramaniyan, V., Peng, J., et al. (2007). Isolation and culture of rat and mouse oligodendrocyte precursor cells. *Nat Protoc*, Vol. 2, No. 5 (2007), pp. (1044-1051), ISSN 1750-2799

Chiasson, B. J., Tropepe, V., Morshead, C. M., et al. (1999). Adult mammalian forebrain ependymal and subependymal cells demonstrate proliferative potential, but only subependymal cells have neural stem cell characteristics. *J Neurosci*, Vol. 19, No. 11, (June 1999), pp. (4462-4471), ISSN 1529-2401

De Filippis, L.&Delia, D. (2011). Hypoxia in the regulation of neural stem cells. *Cell Mol Life Sci*, Vol. 68, No. 17, (September 2011), pp. (2831-2844), ISSN 1420-9071

Doetsch, F., Caille, I., Lim, D. A., et al. (1999). Subventricular zone astrocytes are neural stem cells in the adult mammalian brain. *Cell*, Vol. 97, No. 6, (June 1999), pp. (703-716), ISSN 0092-8674

Duncan, I. D., Paino, C., Archer, D. R., et al. (1992). Functional capacities of transplanted cell-sorted adult oligodendrocytes. *Dev Neurosci*, Vol. 14, No. 2 (1992), pp. (114-122), ISSN 0378-5866

Dutton, R., Yamada, T., Turnley, A., et al. (1999). Sonic hedgehog promotes neuronal differentiation of murine spinal cord precursors and collaborates with neurotrophin 3 to induce Islet-1. *J Neurosci*, Vol. 19, No. 7, (April 1 1999), pp. (2601-2608), ISSN 0270-6474

Ellis, P., Fagan, B. M., Magness, S. T., et al. (2004). SOX2, a persistent marker for multipotential neural stem cells derived from embryonic stem cells, the embryo or the adult. *Dev Neurosci*, Vol. 26, No. 2-4, (March-August 2004), pp. (148-165),ISSN 0378-5866

Ericsson, R. J. (1977). Isolation and storage of progressively motile human sperm. *Andrologia*, Vol. 9, No. 1, (January-March 1977), pp. (111-114),ISSN 0303-4569

Gage, F. H., Coates, P. W., Palmer, T. D., et al. (1995). Survival and differentiation of adult neuronal progenitor cells transplanted to the adult brain. *Proc Natl Acad Sci U S A,* Vol. 92, No. 25, (December 1995), pp. (11879-11883), ISSN 0027-8424

Garcia-Verdugo, J. M., Ferron, S., Flames, N., et al. (2002). The proliferative ventricular zone in adult vertebrates: a comparative study using reptiles, birds, and mammals. *Brain Res Bull,* Vol. 57, No. 6, (April 2002), pp. (765-775) ,ISSN 0361-9230

Gard, A. L.&Pfeiffer, S. E. (1993). Glial cell mitogens bFGF and PDGF differentially regulate development of O4+GalC- oligodendrocyte progenitors. *Dev Biol,* Vol. 159, No. 2, (October 1993), pp. (618-630), ISSN 0012-1606

Gil-Perotin, S., Alvarez-Buylla, A.&Garcia-Verdugo, J. M. (2009). *Identification and characterization of neural progenitor cells in the adult mammalian brain.* Springer, ISBN 3540887180, Berlin, Germany

Gogate, N., Verma, L., Zhou, J. M., et al. (1994). Plasticity in the adult human oligodendrocyte lineage. *J Neurosci,* Vol. 14, No. 8, (August 1994), pp. (4571-4587), ISSN 0270-6474

Gritti, A., Cova, L., Parati, E. A., et al. (1995). Basic fibroblast growth factor supports the proliferation of epidermal growth factor-generated neuronal precursor cells of the adult mouse CNS. *Neurosci Lett,* Vol. 185, No. 3, (February 1995), pp. (151-154), ISSN 0304-3940

Gritti, A., Parati, E. A., Cova, L., et al. (1996). Multipotential stem cells from the adult mouse brain proliferate and self-renew in response to basic fibroblast growth factor. *J Neurosci,* Vol. 16, No. 3, (February 1996), pp. (1091-1100), ISSN 0270-6474

Gritti, A., Frolichsthal-Schoeller, P., Galli, R., et al. (1999). Epidermal and fibroblast growth factors behave as mitogenic regulators for a single multipotent stem cell-like population from the subventricular region of the adult mouse forebrain. *J Neurosci,* Vol. 19, No. 9, (May 1999), pp. (3287-3297), ISSN 0270-6474

Gritti, A., Dal Molin, M., Foroni, C., et al. (2009). Effects of developmental age, brain region, and time in culture on long-term proliferation and multipotency of neural stem cell populations. *J Comp Neurol,* Vol. 517, No. 3 (November 2009), pp. (333-349), ISSN 1096-9861

Hamanoue, M., Sato, K.&Takamatsu, K. (2008). Lectin panning method: the prospective isolation of mouse neural progenitor cells by the attachment of cell surface N-glycans to Phaseolus vulgaris erythroagglutinating lectin-coated dishes. *Neuroscience,* Vol. 157, No. 4, (December 2008), pp. (762-771), ISSN 0306-4522

Imura, T., Kornblum, H. I.&Sofroniew, M. V. (2003). The predominant neural stem cell isolated from postnatal and adult forebrain but not early embryonic forebrain expresses GFAP. *J Neurosci,* Vol. 23, No. 7, (April 2003), pp. (2824-2832), ISSN 1529-2401

Johansson, C. B., Momma, S., Clarke, D. L., et al. (1999). Identification of a neural stem cell in the adult mammalian central nervous system. *Cell,* Vol. 96, No. 1, (January 1999), pp. (25-34), ISSN 0092-8674

Kawaguchi, A., Miyata, T., Sawamoto, K., et al. (2001). Nestin-EGFP transgenic mice: visualization of the self-renewal and multipotency of CNS stem cells. *Mol Cell Neurosci,* Vol. 17, No. 2, (February 2001), pp. (259-273), ISSN 1044-7431

Keyoung, H. M., Roy, N. S., Benraiss, A., et al. (2001). High-yield selection and extraction of two promoter-defined phenotypes of neural stem cells from the fetal human brain. *Nat Biotechnol*, Vol. 19, No. 9, (September 2001), pp. (843-850), ISSN 1087-0156

Kirschenbaum, B., Nedergaard, M., Preuss, A., et al. (1994). In vitro neuronal production and differentiation by precursor cells derived from the adult human forebrain. *Cereb Cortex*, Vol. 4, No. 6, (November-December 1994), pp. (576-589),ISSN 1047-3211

Kirschenbaum, B.&Goldman, S. A. (1995). Brain-derived neurotrophic factor promotes the survival of neurons arising from the adult rat forebrain subependymal zone. *Proc Natl Acad Sci U S A*, Vol. 92, No. 1 (January 1995), pp. (210-214), ISSN 0027-8424

Kitada, M., Kuroda, Y.&Dezawa, M. (2011). Lectins as a tool for detecting neural stem/progenitor cells in the adult mouse brain. *Anat Rec (Hoboken)*, Vol. 294, No. 2, (February 2011), pp. (305-321), ISSN 1932-8494

Kukekov, V. G., Laywell, E. D., Thomas, L. B., et al. (1997). A nestin-negative precursor cell from the adult mouse brain gives rise to neurons and glia. *Glia*, Vol. 21, No. 4, (December 1997), pp. (399-407), ISSN 0894-1491

Kukekov, V. G., Laywell, E. D., Suslov, O., et al. (1999). Multipotent stem/progenitor cells with similar properties arise from two neurogenic regions of adult human brain. *Exp Neurol*, Vol. 156, No. 2, (April 1999), pp. (333-344), ISSN 0014-4886

Laywell, E. D., Kukekov, V. G.&Steindler, D. A. (1999). Multipotent neurospheres can be derived from forebrain subependymal zone and spinal cord of adult mice after protracted postmortem intervals. *Exp Neurol*, Vol. 156, No. 2, (April 1999), pp. (430-433), ISSN 0014-4886

Laywell, E. D., Rakic, P., Kukekov, V. G., et al. (2000). Identification of a multipotent astrocytic stem cell in the immature and adult mouse brain. *Proc Natl Acad Sci U S A*, Vol. 97, No. 25, (December 2000), pp. (13883-13888), ISSN 0027-8424

Leonard, B. W., Mastroeni, D., Grover, A., et al. (2009). Subventricular zone neural progenitors from rapid brain autopsies of elderly subjects with and without neurodegenerative disease. *J Comp Neurol*, Vol. 515, No. 3, (July2009), pp. (269-294), ISSN 1096-9861

Lim, D. A.&Alvarez-Buylla, A. (1999). Interaction between astrocytes and adult subventricular zone precursors stimulates neurogenesis. *Proc Natl Acad Sci U S A*, Vol. 96, No. 13, (June 1999), pp. (7526-7531), ISSN 0027-8424

Ling, Z. D., Potter, E. D., Lipton, J. W., et al. (1998). Differentiation of mesencephalic progenitor cells into dopaminergic neurons by cytokines. *Exp Neurol*, Vol. 149, No. 2 (February 1998), pp. (411-423), ISSN 0014-4886

Liu, Y., Han, S. S., Wu, Y., et al. (2004). CD44 expression identifies astrocyte-restricted precursor cells. *Dev Biol*, Vol. 276, No. 1, (December 2004), pp. (31-46), ISSN 0012-1606

Lobo, M. V., Alonso, F. J., Redondo, C., et al. (2003). Cellular characterization of epidermal growth factor-expanded free-floating neurospheres. *J Histochem Cytochem*, Vol. 51, No. 1, (January 2003), pp. (89-103), ISSN 0022-1554

Lois, C.&Alvarez-Buylla, A. (1993). Proliferating subventricular zone cells in the adult mammalian forebrain can differentiate into neurons and glia. *Proc Natl Acad Sci U S A*, Vol. 90, No. 5 (March1993), pp. (2074-2077), ISSN 0027-8424

Louis, S. A.&Reynolds, B. A. (2005). Generation and differentiation of neurospheres from murine embryonic day 14 central nervous system tissue. *Methods Mol Biol,* Vol. 290, (2005) , pp. (265-280), ISSN 1064-3745

Louis, S. A., Rietze, R. L., Deleyrolle, L., et al. (2008). Enumeration of neural stem and progenitor cells in the neural colony-forming cell assay. *Stem Cells,* Vol. 26, No. 4, (April 2008), pp. (988-996), ISSN 1549-4918

Maric, D., Maric, I.&Barker, J. L. (1998). Buoyant density gradient fractionation and flow cytometric analysis of embryonic rat cortical neurons and progenitor cells. *Methods,* Vol. 16, No. 3, (November 1998), pp. (247-259), ISSN 1046-2023

Maric, D., Maric, I., Chang, Y. H., et al. (2003). Prospective cell sorting of embryonic rat neural stem cells and neuronal and glial progenitors reveals selective effects of basic fibroblast growth factor and epidermal growth factor on self-renewal and differentiation. *J Neurosci,* Vol. 23, No. 1, (January 2003), pp. (240-251), ISSN 1529-2401

Martens, D. J., Tropepe, V.&van Der Kooy, D. (2000). Separate proliferation kinetics of fibroblast growth factor-responsive and epidermal growth factor-responsive neural stem cells within the embryonic forebrain germinal zone. *J Neurosci,* Vol. 20, No. 3, (February 2000), pp. (1085-1095),ISSN 1529-2401

Mayer-Proschel, M. (2001). Isolation and generation of oligodendrocytes by immunopanning. *Curr Protoc Neurosci,* Vol. Chapter 3, No. (May 2001), pp. (Unit 3 13),ISSN 1934-8576

McCarthy, K. D.&de Vellis, J. (1980). Preparation of separate astroglial and oligodendroglial cell cultures from rat cerebral tissue. *J Cell Biol,* Vol. 85, No. 3, (June 1980), pp. (890-902), ISSN 0021-9525

McKinnon, R. D., Matsui, T., Dubois-Dalcq, M., et al. (1990). FGF modulates the PDGF-driven pathway of oligodendrocyte development. *Neuron,* Vol. 5, No. 5, (November 1990), pp. (603-614), ISSN 0896-6273

Mirzadeh, Z., Merkle, F. T., Soriano-Navarro, M., et al. (2008). Neural stem cells confer unique pinwheel architecture to the ventricular surface in neurogenic regions of the adult brain. *Cell Stem Cell,* Vol. 3, No. 3, (September 2008), pp. (265-278),ISSN 1875-9777

Morshead, C. M., Reynolds, B. A., Craig, C. G., et al. (1994). Neural stem cells in the adult mammalian forebrain: a relatively quiescent subpopulation of subependymal cells. *Neuron,* Vol. 13, No. 5, (November 1994), pp. (1071-1082), ISSN 0896-6273

Morshead, C. M., Garcia, A. D., Sofroniew, M. V., et al. (2003). The ablation of glial fibrillary acidic protein-positive cells from the adult central nervous system results in the loss of forebrain neural stem cells but not retinal stem cells. *Eur J Neurosci,* Vol. 18, No. 1, (July 2003), pp. (76-84), ISSN 0953-816X

Murayama, A., Matsuzaki, Y., Kawaguchi, A., et al. (2002). Flow cytometric analysis of neural stem cells in the developing and adult mouse brain. *J Neurosci Res,* Vol. 69, No. 6, (September 2002), pp. (837-847), ISSN 0360-4012

Nakano, I., Paucar, A. A., Bajpai, R., et al. (2005). Maternal embryonic leucine zipper kinase (MELK) regulates multipotent neural progenitor proliferation. *J Cell Biol,* Vol. 170, No. 3, (August 2005), pp. (413-427), ISSN 0021-9525

Nunes, M. C., Roy, N. S., Keyoung, H. M., et al. (2003). Identification and isolation of multipotential neural progenitor cells from the subcortical white matter of the adult human brain. *Nat Med*, Vol. 9, No. 4, (April 2003), pp. (439-447), ISSN 1078-8956

Palmer, T. D., Ray, J.&Gage, F. H. (1995). FGF-2-responsive neuronal progenitors reside in proliferative and quiescent regions of the adult rodent brain. *Mol Cell Neurosci*, Vol. 6, No. 5, (October 1995), pp. (474-486), ISSN 1044-7431

Palmer, T. D., Takahashi, J.&Gage, F. H. (1997). The adult rat hippocampus contains primordial neural stem cells. *Mol Cell Neurosci*, Vol. 8, No. 6, (1997), pp. (389-404), ISSN 1044-7431

Palmer, T. D., Markakis, E. A., Willhoite, A. R., et al. (1999). Fibroblast growth factor-2 activates a latent neurogenic program in neural stem cells from diverse regions of the adult CNS. *J Neurosci*, Vol. 19, No. 19, (October 1999), pp. (8487-8497), ISSN 1529-2401

Panchision, D. M., Chen, H. L., Pistollato, F., et al. (2007). Optimized flow cytometric analysis of central nervous system tissue reveals novel functional relationships among cells expressing CD133, CD15, and CD24. *Stem Cells*, Vol. 25, No. 6 (June 2007), pp. (1560-1570), ISSN 1066-5099

Park, S. K., Solomon, D.&Vartanian, T. (2001). Growth factor control of CNS myelination. *Dev Neurosci*, Vol. 23, No. 4-5, (2001), pp. (327-337), ISSN 0378-5866

Pastrana, E., Cheng, L. C.&Doetsch, F. (2009). Simultaneous prospective purification of adult subventricular zone neural stem cells and their progeny. *Proc Natl Acad Sci U S A*, Vol. 106, No. 15, (April 2009), pp. (6387-6392), ISSN 1091-6490

Piper, D. R., Mujtaba, T., Keyoung, H., et al. (2001). Identification and characterization of neuronal precursors and their progeny from human fetal tissue. *J Neurosci Res*, Vol. 66, No. 3, (November 2001), pp. (356-368), ISSN 0360-4012

Quinones-Hinojosa, A., Sanai, N., Soriano-Navarro, M., et al. (2006). Cellular composition and cytoarchitecture of the adult human subventricular zone: a niche of neural stem cells. *J Comp Neurol*, Vol. 494, No. 3, (January 2006), pp. (415-434), ISSN 0021-9967

Reynolds, B. A., Tetzlaff, W.&Weiss, S. (1992). A multipotent EGF-responsive striatal embryonic progenitor cell produces neurons and astrocytes. *J Neurosci*, Vol. 12, No. 11, (November 1992), pp. (4565-4574), ISSN 0270-6474

Reynolds, B. A.&Weiss, S. (1992). Generation of neurons and astrocytes from isolated cells of the adult mammalian central nervous system. *Science*, Vol. 255, No. 5052, (March 1992), pp. (1707-1710), ISSN 0036-8075

Reynolds, B. A.&Weiss, S. (1996). Clonal and population analyses demonstrate that an EGF-responsive mammalian embryonic CNS precursor is a stem cell. *Dev Biol*, Vol. 175, No. 1, (April 1996), pp. (1-13),ISSN 0012-1606

Richards, L. J., Kilpatrick, T. J.&Bartlett, P. F. (1992). De novo generation of neuronal cells from the adult mouse brain. *Proc Natl Acad Sci U S A*, Vol. 89, No. 18, (September 1992), pp. (8591-8595), ISSN 0027-8424

Rietze, R. L., Valcanis, H., Brooker, G. F., et al. (2001). Purification of a pluripotent neural stem cell from the adult mouse brain. *Nature*, Vol. 412, No. 6848, (August 2001), pp. (736-739),ISSN 0028-0836

Rietze, R. L.&Reynolds, B. A. (2006). Neural stem cell isolation and characterization. *Methods Enzymol*, Vol. 419, (2006), pp. (3-23), ISSN 0076-6879

Rivers, L. E., Young, K. M., Rizzi, M., et al. (2008). PDGFRA/NG2 glia generate myelinating oligodendrocytes and piriform projection neurons in adult mice. *Nat Neurosci,* Vol. 11, No. 12, (December 2008), pp. (1392-1401), ISSN 1546-1726

Roy, N. S., Wang, S., Harrison-Restelli, C., et al. (1999). Identification, isolation, and promoter-defined separation of mitotic oligodendrocyte progenitor cells from the adult human subcortical white matter. *J Neurosci,* Vol. 19, No. 22, (November1999), pp. (9986-9995), ISSN 1529-2401

Roy, N. S., Benraiss, A., Wang, S., et al. (2000a). Promoter-targeted selection and isolation of neural progenitor cells from the adult human ventricular zone. *J Neurosci Res,* Vol. 59, No. 3, (February 2000), pp. (321-331), ISSN 0360-4012

Roy, N. S., Wang, S., Jiang, L., et al. (2000b). In vitro neurogenesis by progenitor cells isolated from the adult human hippocampus. *Nat Med,* Vol. 6, No. 3, (March 2000), pp. (271-277), ISSN 1078-8956

Rutka, J. T., Apodaca, G., Stern, R., et al. (1988). The extracellular matrix of the central and peripheral nervous systems: structure and function. *J Neurosurg,* Vol. 69, No. 2 (August 1988), pp. (155-170), ISSN 0022-3085

Sawamoto, K., Yamamoto, A., Kawaguchi, A., et al. (2001). Direct isolation of committed neuronal progenitor cells from transgenic mice coexpressing spectrally distinct fluorescent proteins regulated by stage-specific neural promoters. *J Neurosci Res,* Vol. 65, No. 3, (August 2001), pp. (220-227), ISSN 0360-4012

Schmandt, T., Meents, E., Gossrau, G., et al. (2005). High-purity lineage selection of embryonic stem cell-derived neurons. *Stem Cells Dev,* Vol. 14, No. 1 (February 2005), pp. (55-64), ISSN 1547-3287

Schwartz, P. H., Bryant, P. J., Fuja, T. J., et al. (2003). Isolation and characterization of neural progenitor cells from post-mortem human cortex. *J Neurosci Res,* Vol. 74, No. 6, (December 2003), pp. (838-851), ISSN 0360-4012

Seaberg, R. M.&van der Kooy, D. (2002). Adult rodent neurogenic regions: the ventricular subependyma contains neural stem cells, but the dentate gyrus contains restricted progenitors. *J Neurosci,* Vol. 22, No. 5, (March 2002), pp. (1784-1793), ISSN 1529-2401

Shi, J., Marinovich, A.&Barres, B. A. (1998). Purification and characterization of adult oligodendrocyte precursor cells from the rat optic nerve. *J Neurosci,* Vol. 18, No. 12, (June 15 1998), pp. (4627-4636), ISSN 0270-6474

Suh, H., Consiglio, A., Ray, J., et al. (2007). In vivo fate analysis reveals the multipotent and self-renewal capacities of Sox2+ neural stem cells in the adult hippocampus. *Cell Stem Cell,* Vol. 1, No. 5, (November 2007), pp. (515-528), ISSN 1934-5909

Sun, J., Zhou, W., Ma, D., et al. (2010). Endothelial cells promote neural stem cell proliferation and differentiation associated with VEGF activated Notch and Pten signaling. *Dev Dyn,* Vol. 239, No. 9, (September 2010), pp. (2345-2353), ISSN 1097-0177

Svendsen, C. N., Fawcett, J. W., Bentlage, C., et al. (1995). Increased survival of rat EGF-generated CNS precursor cells using B27 supplemented medium. *Exp Brain Res,* Vol. 102, No. 3, (1995), pp. (407-414), ISSN 0014-4819

Svendsen, C. N., Caldwell, M. A., Shen, J., et al. (1997a). Long-term survival of human central nervous system progenitor cells transplanted into a rat model of Parkinson's disease. *Exp Neurol,* Vol. 148, No. 1, (November 1997), pp. (135-146),I SSN 0014-4886

Svendsen, C. N., Skepper, J., Rosser, A. E., et al. (1997b). Restricted growth potential of rat neural precursors as compared to mouse. *Brain Res Dev Brain Res*, Vol. 99, No. 2, (April 1997), pp. (253-258), ISSN 0165-3806

Svendsen, C. N., ter Borg, M. G., Armstrong, R. J., et al. (1998). A new method for the rapid and long term growth of human neural precursor cells. *J Neurosci Methods*, Vol. 85, No. 2, (December 1998), pp. (141-152), ISSN 0165-0270

Tan, F. C., Lee, K. H., Gouk, S. S., et al. (2007). Optimization of cryopreservation of stem cells cultured as neurospheres: comparison between vitrification, slow-cooling and rapid cooling freezing protocols. *Cryo Letters*, Vol. 28, No. 6, (November-December 2007), pp. (445-460), ISSN 0143-2044

Thompson, L. H., Andersson, E., Jensen, J. B., et al. (2006). Neurogenin2 identifies a transplantable dopamine neuron precursor in the developing ventral mesencephalon. *Exp Neurol*, Vol. 198, No. 1, (March 2006), pp. (183-198), ISSN 0014-4886

Tropepe, V., Sibilia, M., Ciruna, B. G., et al. (1999). Distinct neural stem cells proliferate in response to EGF and FGF in the developing mouse telencephalon. *Dev Biol*, Vol. 208, No. 1, (April 1999), pp. (166-188), ISSN 0012-1606

Uchida, N., Buck, D. W., He, D., et al. (2000). Direct isolation of human central nervous system stem cells. *Proc Natl Acad Sci U S A*, Vol. 97, No. 26, (December2000), pp. (14720-14725), ISSN 0027-8424

Vescovi, A. L., Reynolds, B. A., Fraser, D. D., et al. (1993). bFGF regulates the proliferative fate of unipotent (neuronal) and bipotent (neuronal/astroglial) EGF-generated CNS progenitor cells. *Neuron*, Vol. 11, No. 5, (November 1993), pp. (951-966), ISSN 0896-6273

Von Visger, J. R., Yeon, D. S., Oh, T. H., et al. (1994). Differentiation and maturation of astrocytes derived from neuroepithelial progenitor cells in culture. *Exp Neurol*, Vol. 128, No. 1, (July 1994), pp. (34-40), ISSN 0014-4886

Walton, N. M., Sutter, B. M., Chen, H. X., et al. (2006). Derivation and large-scale expansion of multipotent astroglial neural progenitors from adult human brain. *Development*, Vol. 133, No. 18, (September 2006), pp. (3671-3681), ISSN 0950-1991

Wang, S., Roy, N. S., Benraiss, A., et al. (2000). Promoter-based isolation and fluorescence-activated sorting of mitotic neuronal progenitor cells from the adult mammalian ependymal/subependymal zone. *Dev Neurosci*, Vol. 22, No. 1-2, (2000), pp. (167-176), ISSN 0378-5866

Wang, S., Chandler-Militello, D., Lu, G., et al. (2010). Prospective identification, isolation, and profiling of a telomerase-expressing subpopulation of human neural stem cells, using sox2 enhancer-directed fluorescence-activated cell sorting. *J Neurosci*, Vol. 30, No. 44, (November 2010), pp. (14635-14648), ISSN 1529-2401

Weiss, S., Dunne, C., Hewson, J., et al. (1996). Multipotent CNS stem cells are present in the adult mammalian spinal cord and ventricular neuroaxis. *J Neurosci*, Vol. 16, No. 23, (December 1 1996), pp. (7599-7609), ISSN 0270-6474

Wilson, H. C., Onischke, C.&Raine, C. S. (2003). Human oligodendrocyte precursor cells in vitro: phenotypic analysis and differential response to growth factors. *Glia*, Vol. 44, No. 2, (November 2003), pp. (153-165), ISSN 0894-1491

Windrem, M. S., Roy, N. S., Wang, J., et al. (2002). Progenitor cells derived from the adult human subcortical white matter disperse and differentiate as oligodendrocytes within demyelinated lesions of the rat brain. *J Neurosci Res*, Vol. 69, No. 6, (September 2002), pp. (966-975), ISSN 0360-4012

Windrem, M. S., Nunes, M. C., Rashbaum, W. K., et al. (2004). Fetal and adult human oligodendrocyte progenitor cell isolates myelinate the congenitally dysmyelinated brain. *Nat Med*, Vol. 10, No. 1, (January 2004), pp. (93-97), ISSN 1078-8956

Wright, A. P., Fitzgerald, J. J.&Colello, R. J. (1997). Rapid purification of glial cells using immunomagnetic separation. *J Neurosci Methods*, Vol. 74, No. 1, (June 6 1997), pp. (37-44), ISSN 0165-0270

Wu, C., Chang, A., Smith, M. C., et al. (2009). Beta4 tubulin identifies a primitive cell source for oligodendrocytes in the mammalian brain. *J Neurosci*, Vol. 29, No. 24, (June 2009), pp. (7649-7657),ISSN 1529-2401

Xu, Y., Kimura, K., Matsumoto, N., et al. (2003). Isolation of neural stem cells from the forebrain of deceased early postnatal and adult rats with protracted post-mortem intervals. *J Neurosci Res*, Vol. 74, No. 4, (2003), pp. (533-540), ISSN 1097-4547

Yayon, A., Klagsbrun, M., Esko, J. D., et al. (1991). Cell surface, heparin-like molecules are required for binding of basic fibroblast growth factor to its high affinity receptor. *Cell*, Vol. 64, No. 4, (February 1991), pp. (841-848), ISSN 0092-8674

Yoshida, N., Hishiyama, S., Yamaguchi, M., et al. (2003). Decrease in expression of alpha 5 beta 1 integrin during neuronal differentiation of cortical progenitor cells. *Exp Cell Res*, Vol. 287, No. 2, (July 2003), pp. (262-271), ISSN 0014-4827

Young, G. M.&Levison, S. W. (1997). An improved method for propagating oligodendrocyte progenitors in vitro. *J Neurosci Methods*, Vol. 77, No. 2, (December 1997), pp. (163-168),ISSN 0165-0270

Yuan, X., Chittajallu, R., Belachew, S., et al. (2002). Expression of the green fluorescent protein in the oligodendrocyte lineage: a transgenic mouse for developmental and physiological studies. *J Neurosci Res*, Vol. 70, No. 4, (November 2002), pp. (529-545), ISSN 0360-4012

Zigler, J. S., Jr., Lepe-Zuniga, J. L., Vistica, B., et al. (1985). Analysis of the cytotoxic effects of light-exposed HEPES-containing culture medium. *In Vitro Cell Dev Biol*, Vol. 21, No. 5, (May 1985), pp. (282-287), ISSN 0883-8364

2

Neurogenesis in Adult Hippocampus

Xinhua Zhang and Guohua Jin
Nantong University
China

1. Introduction

Hippocampus as a whole has the shape of a curved tube including CA1-CA4 regions with a single layer of densely packed pyramidal neurons which curl into a tight "U" shape. One edge of the "U", field CA4, is embedded into a backward facing strongly flexed V-shaped cortex, the dentate gyrus (DG) which comprises molecular, granular, subgranular cell layers and poly-morph layer called hilus (Figure 1). The ability to learn or form a memory requires a neuron to translate a transient signal into gene expression changes that have a long-lasting effect on synapse activity and connectivity. There are many neural circuits formed by multi-class neurons in hippocampus. One of them is the trisynaptic circuit (Figure 1) that is made up of three major cell groups: granule cells, CA3 pyramidal neurons, and CA1 pyramidal cells. The axons of layer II neurons in the entorhinal cortex (EC) project to the dentate gyrus through the perforant pathway. The dentate gyrus sends projections to the pyramidal cells in CA3 through mossy fibres. CA3 pyramidal neurons relay the information to CA1 pyramidal neurons through Schaffer collaterals. CA1 pyramidal neurons send back projections into deep-layer neurons of the EC. This kind of circuit is involved in long term potentiation (LTP) mediating learning and memory. CA3 also directly receives the projections from EC layer II neurons through the perforant pathway. CA1 receives direct input from EC layer III neurons through the temporoammonic pathway. The dentate granule cells also project to the mossy cells in the hilus and hilar interneurons, which send excitatory and inhibitory projections, respectively, back to the granule cells. The complicated neural circuits in hippocampus form the foundation of hippocampal functions.

The external relation between hippocampus and other brain regions also plays an important role in cognition and attentional behaviors. Hippocampal afferents are from the septal area, the locus coeruleus, and the raphe nuclei via 3 anatomically distinct pathways, cingular bundle (CB), Fimbria Fornix (FiFx) and a ventral pathway whose exact anatomical location is not well defined but is thought to reach the hippocampus after passing in the vicinity of the amygdalar complex (Cassel et al., 1997; Eckenstein et al., 1988; Gage et al., 1994; Hong & Jang, 2010; Saper, 1984). Afferent fibers via the FiFx and CB provide the hippocampus with cholinergic, extrinsic GABAergic, noradrenergic and serotonergic inputs. A very important projection comes from the medial septal area, which sends cholinergic and GABAergic fibers to all parts of the hippocampus. The inputs from the septal area play a key role in controlling the physiological state of the hippocampus: destruction of the septal area abolishes the hippocampal theta rhythm, and severely impairs certain types of memory. Hippocampal efferents carry fibers from hippocampal pyramidal CA2-CA4 cells projecting to the anterior thalamic nucleus, medial mamillary nucleus, cingular gyrus, and the nucleus basalis of Meynert (Cassel et al., 1997). Cholinergic projections comprise a complex neural network that supports higher brain functions, and the FiFx and CB are the principal cholinergic pathways that communicate between the basal forebrain and hippocampus and cortex.

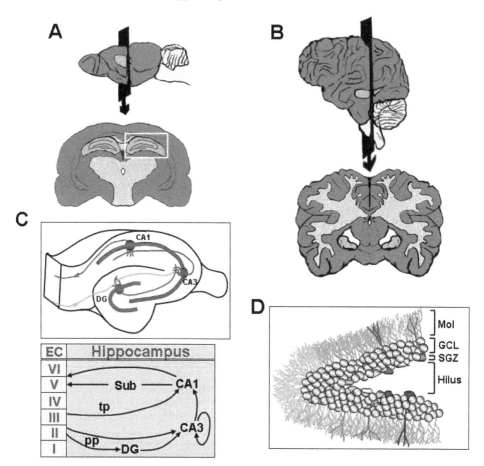

A) Hippocampus (orange region) sits below the surface of the neocortex in rodent brain. The lower is a coronal section through hippocampus. B) Hippocampus (orange region) in human brain is also located under the surface of the neocortex. The lower is a coronal typical section through hippocampus. C) Basic circuit of the hippocampus. Neurons in EC II project to the DG through the perforant pathway (pp). DG sends projections to pyramidal cells in CA3 through mossy fibres. CA3 also receives the projections from EC II neurons through the perforant pathway. CA3 pyramidal neurons send axons to CA1 pyramidal neurons. CA1 also directly receives input from EC III neurons through the temporoammonic pathway (tp). CA1 pyramidal neurons send back projections into deep layers of EC. D) The details of cell layers in rodent DG indicate the neurogenic cells migrate along SGZ and into GCL, and finally form mature granule cells projecting processes into Mol. Abbreviation: DG, dentate gyrus; EC, entorhinal cortex; GCL, granule cell layer; Mol, molecular layer; SGZ, subgranular zone; Sub, subiculum.

Fig. 1. Location and inner structure of the hippocampus.

2. Distribution and fate of neural progenitor cells in hippocampus

Findings of new neurons in the adult brain challenge the dogma that cells of the central nervous system (CNS) are incapable of regeneration. It is well established that the DG in the hippocampus is one of two adult well-accepted regions with continuous addition of new neurons throughout life (Gage, 2000; Kempermann & Gage, 2000). The adult hippocampal neurogenesis is a complex process that originates from proliferation of neural progenitor cells (NPCs) located in the subgranular zone (SGZ), a germinal layer between the granular layer and hilus. The majorities of NPC progenies are specified to become dentate granule cells (DGCs) and go through the initial differentiation and migrate into the inner granule cell layer within a week of their birth. The adult immature DGCs generated from NPCs in SGZ undergo maturation and make important contributions to learning and memory (Deng et al., 2009).

Subventricular zone (SVZ) is another adult region continuously generating new neurons. SVZ NPCs give rise to neuroblasts that migrate in chains to the olfactory bulb through the rostral migratory stream (RMS) where they differentiate into granule and periglomerular neurons (Bovetti et al., 2007; Corotto et al., 1993; Lois & Alvarez-Buylla, 1994; Lois et al., 1996). In the adult DG, new neurons from NPCs are born in the SGZ and migrate a short distance to differentiate into granule cells that project their dendrites into the molecular layer (ML) and axons to the CA3 pyramidal cell layer via the mossy fiber pathway (Markakis & Gage, 1999; Stanfield & Trice, 1988) and establish synaptic connection with local neurons (McDonald & Wojtowicz, 2005).

There are four main cell types in the SVZ: neuroblasts (Type A cells), SVZ astrocytes (Type B cells), immature precursors (Type C cells) and ependymal cells (Doetsch et al., 1997). The neuroblasts (Type A cells) which are from the focal clusters of rapidly dividing precursors (Type C cells) along the SVZ network of chains divide as they migrate as chains through glial tunnels formed by the processes of slowly dividing SVZ astrocytes (Type B cells).

As in the SVZ, there are four types of cells in dentate gyrus: SGZ astrocytes (Type B cells), immature dividing cells (type D cells), granule neurons (type G cells) and endothelial cells. SGZ astrocytes are in close proximity to blood vessels and extend basal processes under the blades of the dentate gyrus and an apical process into the granule cell layer. It is the same as SVZ that SGZ astrocytes are the primary precursors of neurons. The SGZ astrocytes divide to give rise to immature dividing D cells and generate granule neurons. So the type D cells are adjacent to SGZ astrocytes. Neurogenesis in the SGZ occurs in foci formed by these cells suggesting mutual co-regulation between them (Palmer et al., 2000). Endothelial cells are likely an important source of signals for neurogenesis.

Accumulating evidences lead to a detailed classification of the SGZ cells characterized by their properties and specific markers (Figure 2). Adult hippocampal neurons originate from a radial glia-like precursor cell (type-1) which is glial fibrous acid protein (GFAP) positive but negative to S100 beta, doublecortin (DCX) and polysialic acid-neural cell adhesion molecule (PSA-NCAM) in the SGZ of DG through a number of intermediate cell types (type-2, GFAP-, S100-, DCX+, PSA-NCAM+ and type 3 with DCX expression). Type-1 cells correspond to type B cells because they have a proliferative capacity and are marked by GFAP (Seri et al., 2004; Suh et al., 2007; Zhao et al., 2006). Nestin, Sox2, and brain lipid-binding protein (BLBP) are also expressed in type-1 cells suggesting their radial glial features and the expression persists into the type-2 cell stages (Steiner et al., 2006). Although type 1 cells have a proliferative capacity, their cycles are much slower than the followed type-2 progenitor cells supposed to be the type D cells (Filippov et al., 2003; Fukuda et al., 2003; Kronenberg et al., 2003; Steiner et al., 2004). Type-2 cell stage marks the transition between cells with astrocytic phenotype (type-2a cells, the early stage of type-2 cells) and cells with early features of the neuronal lineage (type-2b cells, the later stage of type-2 cells). A panel of different markers (Sox2, BLBP, DCX, and NeuroD) discriminates between the type 2a and type 2b cells. Type-2a cells feature, to some degree, properties of radial glia-like cells marked with BLBP and Sox2. NeuroD and DCX, the markers of immature neurons, appear in type-2b cells and persist into postmitotic but immature granule cell precursors with transient Calretinin-expression. That is to say, type-2b cells are committed to the neuronal lineage. The type-3 cells are the terminal postmitotic differentiation of granule cells that exits from the cell cycle (Kempermann et al., 2004; Steiner et al., 2006). Finally, these cells mature into granule cell neurons in the DG that express specifically NeuN, calbindin and Prox1 (Figure 2). These newborn granule cells elongate their dendrites and axons integrating into the DG circuitry (Jessberger & Kempermann, 2003; Song et al., 2005; van Praag et al., 2002).

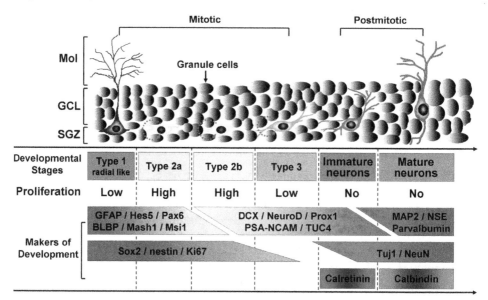

Adult hippocampal neurons originate from type-1 cell with radial glia properties through a number of intermediate type-2 and type 3 cells. Type 2 cells with transit rapid proliferation have two types 2a and 2b. The neuronal determination is at stage type 2b. Type 3 cells gradually exit from the cell cycle and then subsequently form the immature and mature neurons. These newborn granule cells elongate their dendrites and axons integrating into the molecular layer. Cells in different stages of neurogenesis express neural specific markers highlighted in this figure.

Fig. 2. Proposed course of adult hippocampal neurogenesis.

Recent studies in increasing detail showed that a sequence of markers express in the SGZ cells of various stages during the adult hippocampal neurogenesis in mice and rats (Kempermann et al., 2004; Kim et al., 2008; Steiner et al., 2006; Steiner et al., 2008). The stage-specific expressions of neural markers are summarized in Figure 2. In an addition to the putative markers described above, other genes are expressed in different stages of hippocampal neurogenesis. The neuronal marker Hu appears in the GFAP positive intermediate progenitors committed to the neuronal lineage, while Hu is undetectable in primary progenitors and astrocytes, indicating that Hu is a useful marker for discriminating GFAP+ astrocytes and GFAP+ neural progenitors that generate neurons (Liu et al., 2010). The transcription factor Pax6 is expressed not only in precursor cells during embryonic development of the central nervous system but also in the adult SGZ (Sakurai & Osumi, 2008). It plays an important role in the regulation of cell proliferation and neuronal fate determination (Englund et al., 2005; Gotz et al., 1998; Heins et al., 2002). About half of the Pax6-positive cells in the SGZ display a radial glial phenotype which is marked for GFAP, whereas about 30% of the Pax6-positive cells are immunoreactive to PSA-NCAM or DCX (Maekawa et al., 2005; Nacher et al., 2005). In addition, more than 50% of Pax6-positive cells are immunoreactive to NeuroD (Nacher et al., 2005). Thus, Pax6 may represent a suitable marker for type 1 and type 2a cells. The transcription factor NeuroD is expressed in later stages of neuronal commitment (Lee et al., 1995) and during neurogenesis in the adult DG (Kawai et al., 2004). It is important for the proper development of the DG, the proliferation and postnatal differentiation of neuronal progenitors (Liu et al., 2000; Miyata et al., 1999). Thus it could serve as a specific marker. TUC-4 is not only expressed in postmitotic neurons during brain development as they begin their migration but also re-expressed in adult neurogenesis again. Its expression pattern during neurogenesis resembles that of PSA-NCAM and DCX. Thus, TUC-4 can be used as a marker for different stages of adult neurogenesis in the DG. Calretinin is expressed in specific non-pyramidal γ-aminobutyric acid (GABA)-ergic neurons within the adult hippocampus. At late phases of neurogenesis, new neurons express calretinin and doublecortin or NeuN but do not express GABA (Brandt et al., 2003). At later time-points, the newly generated neurons stop expressing calretinin and start to express calbindin, a marker of mature dentate granule cells (Brandt et al., 2003). So that calretinin expression within the DG is restricted to a short postmitotic time window in which axonal and dendritic target their destination regions (Kempermann et al., 2004; Ming & Song, 2005). FABP7 (BLBP) is expressed in the type 1, 2a, and 2b cells, since FABP7 (BLBP) were found in bromodeoxyuridine (BrdU)-positive newly generated cells whereas Tuj1 or PSA-NCAM positive newborn neurons in the vicinity of the astrocytes express none of the FABPs. (Boneva et al., 2011). Musashi1 (Msi1) is a neural RNA binding protein (Sakakibara et al., 1996) that expressed in early-stage NPCs (Kaneko et al., 2000; Sakakibara et al., 1996). The clarity of the development stage-specific markers is not only helpful for gaining further insights into the genesis of new neurons in the hippocampus, but also might be applicable to the development of strategies for therapeutic interventions.

3. Survival and differentiation of grafted NSCs in hippocampus

In CNS the mature neurons lose the ability to undergo cell division once they fully differentiate. Therefore, cell replacement is recognized as a potential strategy to treat neurodegenerative diseases.

The past studies showed that hippocampus is vulnerable to many pathogenic factors or chemical substances. Since that, the hippocampus is preferred as pathological model to investigate the mechanisms and therapies of nervous disorders, such as ischemia, epilepsy, aging and excitotoxicity, all of which disturb the physiological balances in the circuits of hippocampus. For example, cholinergic input plays an important role in cognition and attentional behaviors, and cholinergic dysfunction is a prominent feature of dementias including Alzheimer's disease (AD).

Although the pharmacotherapy, such as acetylcholinesterase inhibitors (Gauthier, 2002), secretase inhibitors (Lanz et al., 2003), transition metal chelators (Gnjec et al., 2002) and Aβ immunization (Ferrer et al., 2004; Heppner et al., 2004), has exerted curative effects to some extent on the amelioration of hippocampal neurodegeneration syndromes, but can not completely rescue or replace the dying neurons. Neuro-transplantation has been proposed recent years as a potential treatment for neurodegenerative disorders (Bachoud-Levi et al., 2000; Gaura et al., 2004). Grafts of neural stem/progenitor cells (NSCs/NPCs) present a potential and innovative strategy for the treatment of many disorders of central nervous system, with the possibility of providing a more permanent remedy than present drug treatments.

Cholinergic projections comprise a complex neural network that supports higher brain functions. FiFx and CB are the principal cholinergic pathways that communicate signals between the basal forebrain and hippocampus and cortex. Lesions of the FiFx plus CB lead to substantially reduced cholinergic innervation (Gage et al., 1994) and produce lasting impairments of spatial learning and memory (Liu et al., 2002), all of which are among the earliest events in the pathogenesis of AD (Geula & Mesulam, 1989; Schliebs & Arendt, 2006; Szenborn, 1993). Selective depletion of cholinergic neurons in the basal forebrain elevated APP immunoreactivity in the cerebral cortex and hippocampus, and increased APP levels correlated with decreased cholinergic activity (Leanza, 1998; Lin et al., 1998). The increased expression of APP after cholinergic lesion can potentially lead to increased Aβ production, thereby possibly causing Aβ accumulation and deposition, which is one of the main pathological features.

In our study [(Zhang et al., 2007) and Figure 3] we transplanted SVZ progenitors directly into the denervated and contralateral hippocampi of the AD rat models and determined the effect of different hippocampal environment on the fate of NPCs. The donor neural progenitors in this study were derived from the neonatal SVZ for their features prior to and following transplantation that make them candidates for cell replacement therapy. The grafted cells survived well even through the longest span, 2 months after implantation, and migrate along the subgranular layer after. The same model was treated through neural stem cell transplantation by Xuan and his colleagues (Xuan et al., 2009). The results indicate that the deafferented hippocampus provided proper microenvironment for the survival and neuronal differentiation of neural progenitors and transplanted NSCs can differentiate into cholinergic neurons and enhance the learning and memory abilities. Another kind of AD model produced by injections of amyloid-β peptide (1-40) ($A\beta_{1-40}$) received neural stem cell transplantation into the hippocampus dentate gyrus. The grafted cells can survive, and differentiate with high yield into immunohistochemically mature glial cells and neurons of diverse neurotransmitter-subtypes. More importantly, transplanted cells demonstrate characteristics of proper synapse formation between host and grafted neural cells (Li et al., 2010).

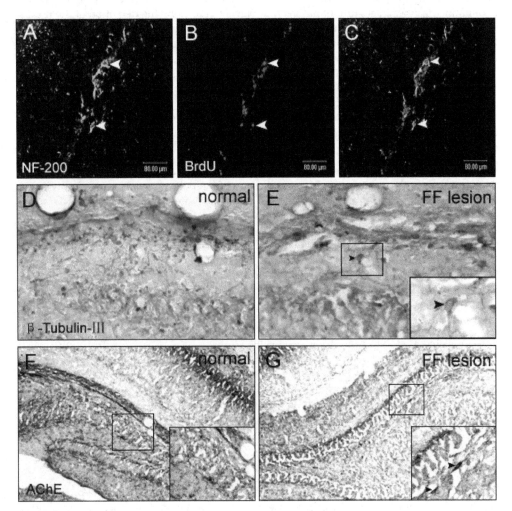

(A–C) Cofocal images of NF-200 positive (green) and BrdU positive (red) neurons in denervated hippocampus at day 30 after transplantation. Arrow showed the neurons double positive to BrdU and NF200. (D and E) β-Tubulin-III (Tuj1, brown) and BrdU (blue) immunohistochemistry on the normal (D) and denervated (E) hippocampus. Arrow showed the β-Tubulin-III and BrdU positive neurons in denervated hippocampus. (F and G) AChE histochemistry on the normal (F) and denervated (G) hippocampus. Arrow showed the AChE positive neurons in denervated hippocampus which may be from differentiation of the grafted cells or endogenous NPCs because there originally are no cholinergic neurons in normal hippocampus.

Fig. 3. Immunodetection to the neuronal differentiation of SVZ NPCs grafted into adult hippocampus.

Prophylactic cranial radiotherapy involves giving radiotherapy to a person's head to prevent or delay the possible spread of cancer cells to the brain, but induces progressive and debilitating declines in cognition that may, in part, be caused by the depletion of the normal neural cells or NSC in hippocampus. Acharya and his colleagues (Acharya et al., 2011) used NSC replacement as a strategy to combat radiation-induced cognitive decline by intrahippocampal transplantation with human neural stem cells (hNSC). Unbiased stereology revealed that 23% and 12% of the engrafted cells survived 1 and 4 months after transplantation, respectively. Engrafted cells migrated extensively, differentiated along glial and neuronal lineages, and expressed the activity-regulated cytoskeleton-associated protein (Arc), suggesting their capability to functionally integrate into the hippocampus. Behaviorally the irradiated animals engrafted with hNSCs showed significantly less decline in cognitive function.

After transplantation if these cells survive the injured and/or degenerative insult(s), they may migrate within damaged areas and promote repair or neuroprotection via cell replacement, integration or neuroprotection. The neuroprotection from grafted NPCs may be the results of in situ release of immunomodulatory molecules (e.g., anti-inflammatory cytokines) and neurotrophic factors [e.g., nerve growth factor (NGF), fibroblast growth factor (FGF)-2, ciliary neurotrophic factor (CNTF) and brain-derived neurotrophic factor (BDNF)] (Martino & Pluchino, 2006; Pluchino et al., 2005). On the other hand, transplanted NPCs may also differentiate into local specific cells to replace the dying cells and integrate within the host neural cells. Thus, we can propose the concept of 'therapeutic plasticity', which can be viewed as the capacity of somatic stem cells to adapt their fate and function(s) to specific environmental needs occurring as a result of different pathological conditions.

It is indicated that NPCs afford a promising strategy for functionally restoring defects induced by hippocampal degenerations or injuries. However, neural transplantation to correct congenital or acquired disorders using multipotent progenitor cells has several major limitations: migration of the transplanted cells is limited; the cells seldom develop into neurons; the limited sources of donor cells and many ethical concerns and political restrictions. Motivating endogenous neural progenitors may be another good strategy for the neurodegenerative disorders.

4. Adult neurogenesis of endogenous NSCs in hippocampus

During the past decade, the progress in the field of stem cells has fueled the hope to cure currently intractable diseases by cell replacement. In regard of ethical concerns and political restrictions that have been raised regarding the use and manipulation of fetal tissue and embryonic stem cells and the limitation of heterogeneous graft, adult endogenous NPCs have been prefered as a cellular source for the treatment of CNS diseases. The use of endogenous sources for cell replacement offer a potential advantage over other cell sources: Immunological reactions are avoided.

After injury or during neurodegenerative processes in restricted brain regions the NPCs frequently reside in niches that regulate their self-renewal, activation and differentiation. Within the niche, both environmental cues and intrinsic genetic programs are two factors required to direct/regulate stem and precursor cell proliferation, differentiation and integration. The adult born functional neurons in the neural networks is believed to experience sequential steps in a highly regulated fashion: proliferation of the NSC, generation of a rapidly amplifying progenitor cell, differentiation into an immature neuron, migration to the final location, growth of axons and dendrites and formation of synapses with other neurons in the circuits, and ultimately maturation into a fully functional neuron. Although these steps are equivalent to the ones that newborn neurons undergo during development, the fundamental difference between the developmental and adult neurogenesis is that new adult neurons undergo these processes in an already mature environment and integrate into preexisting circuits in adult hippocampal neurogenesis. During this period, the newborn neurons undergo dying, surviving, migrating into the granular layer, sending axons to the CA3 region to form mossy fibers and projecting dendrites to the outer molecular layer (Hastings & Gould, 1999; Kempermann et al., 2003; Markakis & Gage, 1999; Seri et al., 2001; van Praag et al., 2002). Simultaneously, the newly generated neurons receive synaptic inputs from the other region within four to six weeks after birth (van Praag et al., 2002). The complexity and density of their dendritic spines have to continuously grow for several months. Thus, the course of neuronal development for granule neurons born in the adult hippocampus appears much more protracted than those generated during embryonic stages.

The endogenous NPCs in the SVZ and SGZ are the source of adult neurogenesis and remodeling which are implicated in responses to multiple insults including ischemia (Arvidsson et al., 2002; Jin et al., 2001; Miles & Kernie, 2008; Nakatomi et al., 2002), trauma (Johansson et al., 1999; Yoshimura et al., 2001), seizure (Parent et al., 1997; Parent & Murphy, 2008) and neurodegeneration (Fallon et al., 2000; Magavi & Macklis, 2002). Adult neurogenesis in hippocampus can be regulated by numerous factors associated with an animal's behavioural and cognitive states. Indeed, an animal's experiences on cognition and mood, including hippocampus-dependent learning, environmental enrichment, voluntary running and chronic treatment with antidepressants, can affect the rate of neurogenesis. The factors enhancing hippocampal neurogenesis are summarized in the following and Figure 5 which also enumerates the factors decreasing adult hippocampal neurogenesis.

4.1 Enriched environment

Gage and his colleagues have demonstrated that mice placed in an enriched environment where there are more social interactions, inanimate objects for play and a wheel for voluntary exercise have an increased rate of neurogenesis relative to mice that are kept in standard cages (Kempermann et al., 1997). Subsequently, the similar experiments have been repeated and proven by other laboratories (Beauquis et al., 2010; Brown et al., 2003; Ehninger & Kempermann, 2003; Kempermann et al., 2002; Kohl et al., 2002; Llorens-Martin et al., 2010; Olson et al., 2006; Steiner et al., 2008). The dual-birthdating analysis used to study two subpopulations of newborn neurons born at the beginning and end of enrichment suggested that enriched environment induces differential effects on distinct subpopulations of newborn neurons depending on the age of the immature cells and on the duration of the enriched environment itself (Llorens-Martin et al., 2010). This work points to a hypothesis that the effects of physical-cognitive activity on neurogenesis depend on the interaction of two critical parameters: the age/differentiation status of the immature neuron plus the time the individual is under the effects of an enriched environment.

4.2 Exercise

Studies of voluntary exercise demonstrate that running on wheel without other components of enriched environment is sufficient to increase proliferation and recruitment of granule cells into the adult DG (van Praag et al., 1999a; van Praag et al., 1999b). Although the exact mechanism underlying the exercise-induced up-regulation of neurogenesis remains unclear, exercise is reported to increase the expression of certain trophic factors, such as BDNF and FGF-2 (Ding et al., 2011; Gomez-Pinilla et al., 1997; Griffin et al., 2011; Russo-Neustadt et al., 1999), which have also been shown to increase neurogenesis during development or in adult brain (Ding et al., 2011; Zigova et al., 1998).

4.3 Psychotropic drugs

Serotonergic antidepressant drugs have been commonly used to treat mood and anxiety disorders. In experimental animals, chronic antidepressant treatments can facilitate neurogenesis in the DG of the adult hippocampus (Dagyte et al., 2010; Kitamura et al., 2011; Malberg et al., 2000; Nasrallah et al., 2011). The adult hippocampal neurogenesis has been implicated in some of the behavioral effects of antidepressants (Airan et al., 2007; Santarelli et al., 2003; Wang et al., 2008). Two molecular mechanisms are possibly involved in the antidepressant drug-induced hippocampal neurogenesis. One is the increased BDNF in hippocampus. Previous studies have demonstrated that repeated antidepressant administration increases the expression of BDNF in hippocampus (Duman et al., 1997; Duman et al., 2000; Lee & Kim, 2010; Pilar-Cuellar et al., 2011; Reus et al., 2011; Rogoz et al., 2008). In contrast, stress decreases BDNF expression in this brain region (de Lima et al., 2011; Murakami et al., 2005) and causes atrophy of hippocampal neurons and decreased neurogenesis (Gould et al., 1998; Yap et al., 2006). All these results have contributed to a neurotrophic hypothesis of depression and antidepressant action. Antidepressant treatment may block or even reverse these effects of stress via increased expression of BDNF. The other is the Notch1 signaling. New evidences indicated that fluoxetine (antidepressant) administration increased mRNA and protein expression of Notch1 signaling components (including Jag1, NICD, Hes1 and Hes5) and simultaneously up-regulated hippocampal cell proliferation and survival, suggesting that activation of Notch1 signaling might partly contribute to increased neurogenesis in hippocampus (Sui et al., 2009). In addition to promotion of neurogenesis, the psychotropic drugs significantly increased the survival of newborn neurons in dorsal hippocampus by approximately 50% (Su et al., 2009). Results from Kobayashi and his colleagues (Kobayashi et al., 2010) showed that serotonergic antidepressants can reverse the established state of neuronal maturation in the adult hippocampus, termed "dematuration" of mature granule cells, and up-regulate 5-HT4 receptor-mediated signaling which may play a critical role in this distinct action of antidepressants. Such reversal of neuronal maturation could affect proper functioning of the mature hippocampal circuit. Together with these results support the hypothesis that antidepressants exert therapeutic effects on neuropsychiatric disease via not only activating the hippocampal neurogenesis but also reinstating neuronal functions of the matured granular cells.

Evidences have not show the confirmed effects on the repeated antipsychotic drug administration because of the contradictory results that Dawirs et al. work (Dawirs et al., 1998) demonstrated granular cell proliferation by chronic administration of haloperidol while Backhouse et al., (Backhouse et al., 1982) reported a decrease in hippocampal cell proliferation. Abuse of drugs including opiates and psychostimulants can influence cognition, learning and memory, which is accompanied by decrease of the proliferation of granule cells in adult rat hippocampus (Eisch et al., 2000).

4.4 Ischemia

Studies have noted that ischemia also produces enhanced neurogenesis in neuroproliferative regions of the adult rodent brain, including the SVZ of the lateral ventricles and SGZ of DG (Burns et al., 2009; Jin et al., 2001; Parent et al., 2002; Yagita et al., 2001). Proliferation induced by transient focal or global ischemia peaks 7 to 10 days after ischemia and returns to baseline levels within several weeks. Some of the new cells die but others survive to adopt a neuronal fate in the ischemic and uninjured dentate gyrus. Newborn cells labeled EGFP retroviral reporter are found to move from the subgranular proliferative zone to the DGC layer, shift from coexpression of immature to mature neuronal markers, and increase in dendritic length (Tanaka et al, 2004), suggesting that newly generated DGCs in the ischemic brain follow a time course of neuronal maturation. A new report from Liu and his colleagues (Wang et al., 2011) indicated that transient brain ischemia initiates a sustained increase in neurogenesis for at least 6 months and promotes the normal development of the newly generated neurons in the adult DG.

4.5 Traumatic Brain Injury (TBI)

The hippocampus, a region responsible for memory and learning, is particularly vulnerable to brain trauma. Learning and memory deficits are the most enduring and devastating consequences following TBI on hippocampus. A slow but significant improvement in cognitive function after TBI indicates that innate mechanisms for repair exist in the brain (Schmidt et al., 1999). Although the mechanisms underlying this innate recovery remain largely unknown, the findings that NSCs persist in the hippocampal DG throughout life (Gage, 2000; Kempermann & Gage, 2000) and exhibit high activation of proliferation and neurogenesis in response to brain trauma (Chirumamilla et al., 2002; Dash et al., 2001; Urrea et al., 2007; Yu et al., 2008) suggest that neurogenesis may contribute to the cognitive recovery observed following TBI.

In our laboratory transection of FiFx plus CB is deemed as a kind of TBI to produce deafferented hippocampus. The denervated hippocampus provided a proper microenvironment for the survival and neuronal differentiation of exogenous neural progenitors (Zhang et al., 2007). Subsequently, we determined the endogenous NPCs in DG of adult hippocampus after denervation trauma. The results showed that traumatic injury by transecting FiFx and CB which carry cholinergic inputs promoted proliferation of the local NPCs and increased the number of newborn neurons in SGZ of hippocampus (Figure 4). Indicating that the changes in the deafferented hippocampus provided a suitable microenvironment for neurogenesis of endogenous progenitors of adult hippocampus. However, Christiana et al. (Cooper-Kuhn et al., 2004) produced a cholinergic depletion model by infusion of the immunotoxin 192IgG-saporin into lateral ventricle to selectively lesion cholinergic neurons of the cholinergic basal forebrain. Oppositely, their results showed a significant declination of neurogenesis in the granule cell layer of the dentate gyrus and olfactory bulb. Furthermore, immunotoxic lesions led to increased numbers of apoptotic cells specifically in the SGZ and the periglomerular layer of the olfactory bulb. The model of TBI created by distinct ways may contribute to the conflict results because the immunotoxin might exert negative effects on the neural progenitors and newborn neurons.

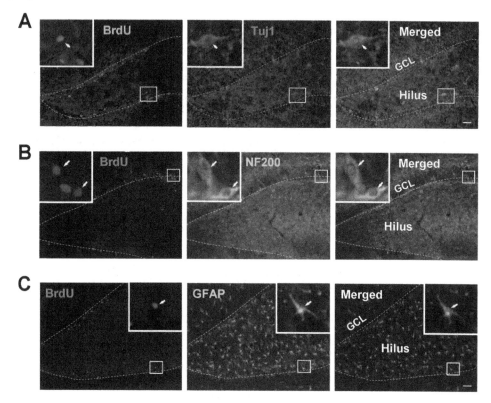

A) Immunofluorescence micrographs of anti–BrdU (Blue), β-tubulin III (Tuj1, red) in coronal sections of the hippocampus at day 35 after denervation operation. Arrows show the cells immunoreactive to BrdU and Tuj1. B) Microscope images of sections through deafferented hippocampus stained by BrdU and NF-200 antibodies on day 42 after transection. Arrows show the BrdU and NF-200 double positive neurons. (C) Microscope image of BrdU positive (red) and GFAP positive (green) astrocytes in denervated hippocampus 28 days after transection. Arrow showed the BrdU and GFAP positive astrocytes.

Fig. 4. Endogenous NPCs labeled with BrdU differentiate into neurons and astrocytes in deafferented hippocampus.

4.6 Seizures

Seizures characterize the periodic and unpredictable occurrences of epilepsy. Accumulating evidences indicate that seizures alter not only the amount, but also the pattern of neurogenesis, though the overall effect depends on the type of seizures. Acute seizures abnormally increase the amount of hippocampal neurogenesis and induce aberrant migration of newly born neurons into the dentate hilus and the dentate molecular layer

(Bengzon et al., 1997; Jessberger et al., 2005; Kralic et al., 2005; Parent et al., 1997). Examination of the hippocampus from young temporal lobe epilepsy patients (<4 years of age) suggested increased cell proliferation of neural precursor cells (Blumcke et al., 2001). However, recurrent spontaneous seizures typically observed in chronic temporal lobe epilepsy lead to a radically waned neurogenesis (Hattiangady et al., 2004; Kralic et al., 2005), which, interestingly, coexists with learning and memory impairments and depression. Heinrich et al. (Heinrich et al. 2006) reported a gradual fall in neurogenesis at 1 week and virtual loss of all neurogenesis by 4-6 weeks after the initial seizure episode. However, a modest increase in neurogenesis was observed even at 2 months post status epilepticus in a lithium-pilocarpine model of epilepsy using postnatal day 20 rats (Cha et al., 2004). It emerges that decreased levels of hippocampal neurogenesis in chronic epilepsy depend on the model and the age of the animal at the time of the initial seizure episode.

4.7 Others

Lithium was noticed to have mood stabilizing properties in the late 1800s when doctors were using it to treat gout. Australian psychiatrist John Cade published the first paper on the use of lithium in the treatment of acute mania. Lithium, as a mood stabilizer, is used as an add-on treatment for clinical depression. Recent reports have described that lithium increases cell proliferation and/or promotion of neuronal differentiation of NPCs (Boku et al., 2011; Chen et al., 2000; Fiorentini et al., 2010; Hanson et al., 2011; Kim et al., 2004; Kitamura et al., 2011; Son et al., 2003; Wexler et al., 2008) and blocks the effects of stress on depression-like behaviors through increasing hippocampal neurogenesis in adult rodent models (Silva et al., 2008). Results of these studies suggest that adult hippocampal neurogenesis plays an important role in the therapeutic action of mood stabilizers as well. Inhibition of GSK-3β and subsequent activation of Wnt/β-catenin signalling may underlie lithium-induced hippocampal neurogenesis and therapeutic effect (Boku et al., 2010; Fiorentini et al., 2010; Wexler et al., 2008).

Acupuncture or electroacupuncture, the ancient Chinese treatments through stimulating the acu-points, can ameliorate syndromes of many illnesses pain, metabolic and pathological brain disease, and even mental disorders, such as major depression. Although the mechanisms underlying treatment of acupuncture on these diseases remain unclear till now, neurogenesis must be considered as a potential one of mechanisms in the process of therapy. It has been reported that acupuncture and electroacupuncture in the acu-points ST36 (*Zusanli*) and GV20 (*Baihui*) increase significantly neurogenesis in the normal DG, while electroacupuncture has greater effects on neuroblast plasticity in the DG than acupuncture (Hwang et al., 2010). In addition to normal status, relieves of illnesses were paralleled with the hippocampal neurogenesis in DG. For example, decreased cell proliferation in the DG of dementia model was improved by *Yiqitiaoxue* and *Fubenpeiyuan* acupuncture (Cheng et al., 2008). In addition, electroacupuncture at GV20 and EX17 increased hippocampal progenitor cell proliferation in adult rats exposed to chronic unpredictable stress (Liu et al., 2007). In ischemic models (Kim et al., 2001) and streptozotocin-induced diabetic models (Kim et al., 2002), acupuncture (ST36)-induced alleviation is paralleled with increased cell proliferation in the DG. Acupuncture at *Tanzhong* (CV17), *Zhongwan* (CV12), *Qihai* (CV6), ST36, and *Xuehai* (SP10) improve spatial memory impairment (Yu et al., 2005), maintain oxidant-antioxidant balance, and regulate cell proliferation in a rodent dementia model (Cheng et al., 2008; Liu et al., 2006).

After comparing the cell proliferation in DG of adult mice fed on hard and soft diet, Yamamoto et al. (Yamamoto et al., 2009) found that sufficient mastication activity enhanced hippocampal neurogenesis since that the total number of BrdU-labeled cells was fewer in the soft-diet group than in the hard-diet group at 3 and 6 months of age.

Additionally, Leuner et al. (Leuner et al., 2010) found that sexual experience that the adult male rats were exposed to a sexually-receptive female increased circulating corticosterone levels and the number of new neurons in the hippocampus and stimulated the growth of dendritic spines and dendritic architecture, suggesting that a rewarding experience actually promotes adult-born neuronal growth.

The persistence of neurogenesis in the adult mammalian forebrain suggests that endogenous precursors provide a potential source of neurons for the replacement of the dying or lost neurons due to brain damage or neurodegeneration. Based on the multiple stimuli inducing hippocampal neurogenesis, strategies that are designed to increase adult hippocampal neurogenesis specifically, by targeting the cell death of adult-born neurons or by other mechanisms, may have therapeutic potential for reversing impairments in pattern separation and DG dysfunction such as those seen during normal ageing.

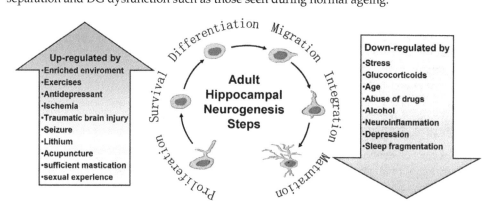

Fig. 5. Adult hippocampal neurogenesis can be up- or down-regulated by various stimuli. This summarizes the sequent steps of adult hippocampal neurogenesis and a variety of stimuli positively or negatively influencing adult hippocampal neurogenesis.

5. Signal pathways involved in hippocampal neurogenesis

Understanding the mechanisms underlying adult neurogenesis and differentiation of NPCs is crucial to delineate the function of NPCs and their progeny and ultimately their therapeutic potential. The initial investigations on environmental niches and intrinsic genetic programs that regulate early and adult neurogenesis have revealed many extrinsic and intrinsic elements playing critical roles in differential phrases of neurogenesis, such as proliferation, migration, differentiation, integration and maturation. The following lists the signal molecules involved in adult hippocampus neurogenesis.

5.1 Wnt (wingless)

Traditionally, Wnt proteins are assumed to act as stem cell growth factors, promoting the maintenance and proliferation of stem cells (Willert et al., 2003) and inducing of neural specification (Muroyama et al., 2002). Interaction of Wnts with their receptors can trigger several signaling pathways, including the β-catenin dependent pathway. Studies of Lie et al. (Lie et al., 2005) show that Wnt signalling components and their receptors were expressed in the adult hippocampal progenitor cells. Overexpression of Wnt3 is sufficient to increase neurogenesis of adult hippocampal progenitors in vitro and in vivo. By contrast, blockade of Wnt signalling reduces neurogenesis of adult hippocampal progenitor cells in vitro and abolishes neurogenesis almost completely in vivo. Evidence also suggests that β-catenin, which is present in neural progenitors and newborn granule neurons, plays an important role in the dendritic development of adult born hippocampal neurons (Gao et al., 2007). These data show that Wnt signalling is a principal regulator of adult hippocampal neurogenesis.

5.2 Notch

Notch (1 – 4 in mammals) signaling pathway is crucial for maintenance of stem cell self renewal, proliferation, and specification of cell fate (Mason et al., 2006). Notch signaling is highly activated in type-B cells of the SVZ of the lateral ventricle and type-1 cells of the SGZ of the DG (Ehm et al., 2010; Imayoshi et al., 2010; Lugert et al., 2010). In postnatal and adult mice, Overexpression of Notch1 in postnatal and adult mice increased hippocampal cell proliferation and maintained GFAP-expressing NSCs, while depletion of Notch signaling led to a decrease in cell proliferation and a shift in the differentiation of newly born cells towards a neuronal lineage suggesting that Notch1 signaling is required to maintain a reservoir of undifferentiated cells and ensure continuity of adult hippocampal neurogenesis (Ables et al., 2010; Breunig et al., 2007). In addition, Notch1 signaling modulates the dendritic morphology of newborn granule cells by increasing dendritic arborization (Breunig et al., 2007). These evidences suggest that Notch1 signaling is involved in the cell proliferation, fate determination, and maturation of adult hippocampal neurogenesis. Pathologically, antidepressant therapy chronic fluoxetine administration increased expression of Notch1 signaling components including Jag1, NICD, Hes1 and Hes5 in the hippocampus, accompanied by cell proliferation and survival (Sui et al., 2009). This indicated that activation of the Notch1 pathway might partly contribute to chronic antidepressant therapy-increased neurogenesis in hippocampus.

5.3 Bone Morphogenetic Protein (BMP)

BMP proteins, the extracellular signaling molecules, regulate cell proliferation and fate commitment throughout development and within the adult SVZ and SGZ neurogenic niches (Bonaguidi et al., 2005; Bonaguidi et al., 2008; Mehler et al., 2000). The cysteine knot proteins noggin, chordin and follistatin regulate BMP actions via competitively binding BMPs in the extracellular space to prevent receptor activation and the downstream signaling activity (Dal-Pra et al., 2006; Ebara & Nakayama, 2002). The inhibition of noggin in vivo by RNA interference decreased hippocampal cell proliferation (Fan et al., 2004). Study of Gobeske et al. indicated that BMP signaling mediates effects of exercise on hippocampal neurogenesis and cognition in mice (Gobeske et al., 2009).

5.4 Sonic hedgehog (Shh)

Shh is reported to be crucial in the expansion and establishment of postnatal hippocampal progenitors (Palma et al., 2005). The Shh receptors patched (Ptc) and smoothened (Smo) are expressed in the dentate gyrus subfield including the neurogenic niche of SGZ and in neural progenitor cells derived from hippocampus (Lai et al., 2003; Traiffort et al., 1998). Recently, it is addressed that Shh signaling regulates adult hippocampal neurogenesis (Han et al., 2008; Lai et al., 2003; Palma et al., 2005). In rats, overexpression of Shh in the DG increased cell proliferation and survival (Lai et al., 2003). On the other hand, inhibition of Shh signaling by injections of inhibitor cyclopamine reduced cell proliferation (Banerjee et al., 2005; Lai et al., 2003). Removal of Shh signaling in these animals resulted in dramatic reduction in number of neural progenitors in both the postnatal SVZ and hippocampus. Consistently, conditional null alleles of hedgehog signaling also resulted in abnormalities in the DG and olfactory bulb (Machold et al., 2003). These studies emphasize the importance of the Shh signaling pathway in adult neurogenesis. Findings from Banerjee et al. (Banerjee et al., 2005) demonstrated that Shh pathway may be involved in electroconvulsive seizure-enhanced adult hippocampal neurogenesis. The primary cilia are important sites of signal transduction which unite the receptors and the signal-transduction components, such as Wnt and Hedgehog (Hh) signaling cascades (Huangfu et al., 2003; Huangfu & Anderson, 2005). It is demonstrated that, in the absence of cilia, there is a dramatic diminution in Shh signaling, decreased early proliferation and a consequent loss of quiescent precursor cell (Breunig et al., 2008).

5.5 PI3K-Akt

PI3K-Akt signalling pathway is the downstream of neurotrophic and growth factor receptors, as well as monoamine receptors (Datta et al., 1999). It is potentially implicated in a number of different functions and especially associated with cell survival by inhibiting the activation of proapoptotic proteins and transcription factors (Aberg et al., 2003). Akt has three different isoforms, Akt1, -2, -3, each encoded by independent genes (Coffer et al., 1998). It was shown that Akt1 and Akt2 knockout mice had lower levels of hippocampal cell proliferation compared to wild type animals (Balu et al., 2008). However, only Akt2KO mice had impairment in the survival of adult born hippocampal progenitors (Balu et al., 2008). Subsequent report also showed the nonredundant roles of Akt in the regulation of hippocampal neurogenesis since that physical exercise activated Akt and three downstream targets, BAD, GSK3b and FOXO1 and inhibition of PI3K-Akt signaling blocks exercise-mediated enhancement of adult neurogenesis and synaptic plasticity in the DG (Bruel-Jungerman et al., 2009).

6. Conclusion

These findings have fuelled the hope of using neurogenesis, exogenous or endogenous, in regenerative medicine for neurological diseases, arguably the most difficult diseases to treat. The proposed regenerative approaches to neurological diseases include (1) cell therapy approaches in which donated cells are delivered by intracerebral injection or infusion through an intravenous or intra-arterial route; (2) stem cell mobilization approaches in which endogenous stem or progenitor cells are activated by cytokines or chemokines; (3) trophic and growth factor support in which the factors, such as BDNF and GDNF, were delivered through grafted stem cells modulated genetically into the brain to support the injured neurons. These approaches may be used together to maximize therapeutic effects. Although the mechanisms underlying these therapeutic processes are still unclear, the neurogenic cells must survival various complicated and difficult barriers from proliferation to maturation. Understanding the factors in NPC niches and intracellular molecules regulating/directing adult neurogenesis will largely speed the steps to make use of exogenous or endogenous NPCs in treatment of neural disorders. The past evidences indicate that cell therapy to the injured tissue and brain may be contributed by several processes including angiogenesis, neurogenesis and trophic or 'chaperone' support.

7. References

Aberg MA, Aberg ND, Palmer TD, Alborn AM, Carlsson-Skwirut C, Bang P, Rosengren LE, Olsson T, Gage FH & Eriksson PS. (2003). IGF-I has a direct proliferative effect in adult hippocampal progenitor cells. Mol Cell Neurosci 24(1):23-40.

Ables JL, Decarolis NA, Johnson MA, Rivera PD, Gao Z, Cooper DC, Radtke F, Hsieh J & Eisch AJ. (2010). Notch1 is required for maintenance of the reservoir of adult hippocampal stem cells. J Neurosci 30(31):10484-92.

Acharya MM, Christie LA, Lan ML, Giedzinski E, Fike JR, Rosi S & Limoli CL. (2011). Human neural stem cell transplantation ameliorates radiation-induced cognitive dysfunction. Cancer Res 71(14):4834-45.

Airan RD, Meltzer LA, Roy M, Gong Y, Chen H & Deisseroth K. (2007). High-speed imaging reveals neurophysiological links to behavior in an animal model of depression. Science 317(5839):819-23.

Arvidsson A, Collin T, Kirik D, Kokaia Z & Lindvall O. (2002). Neuronal replacement from endogenous precursors in the adult brain after stroke. Nat Med 8(9):963-70.

Bachoud-Levi AC, Remy P, Nguyen JP, Brugieres P, Lefaucheur JP, Bourdet C, Baudic S, Gaura V, Maison P, Haddad B and others. (2000). Motor and cognitive improvements in patients with Huntington's disease after neural transplantation. Lancet 356(9246):1975-9.

Backhouse B, Barochovsky O, Malik C, Patel AJ & Lewis PD. (1982). Effects of haloperidol on cell proliferation in the early postnatal rat brain. Neuropathol Appl Neurobiol 8(2):109-16.

Balu DT, Easton RM, Birnbaum MJ & Lucki I. 2008. Deletion of Akt Isoforms Reduce Hippocampal Neurogenesis, Fear Conditioning and Antidepressant Behavioral Responses. Society for Neuroscience. Washington, DC.

Banerjee SB, Rajendran R, Dias BG, Ladiwala U, Tole S & Vaidya VA. (2005). Recruitment of the Sonic hedgehog signalling cascade in electroconvulsive seizure-mediated regulation of adult rat hippocampal neurogenesis. Eur J Neurosci 22(7):1570-80.

Beauquis J, Roig P, De Nicola AF & Saravia F. (2010). Short-term environmental enrichment enhances adult neurogenesis, vascular network and dendritic complexity in the hippocampus of type 1 diabetic mice. PLoS One 5(11):e13993.

Bengzon J, Kokaia Z, Elmer E, Nanobashvili A, Kokaia M & Lindvall O. (1997). Apoptosis and proliferation of dentate gyrus neurons after single and intermittent limbic seizures. Proc Natl Acad Sci U S A 94(19):10432-7.

Blumcke I, Schewe JC, Normann S, Brustle O, Schramm J, Elger CE & Wiestler OD. (2001). Increase of nestin-immunoreactive neural precursor cells in the dentate gyrus of pediatric patients with early-onset temporal lobe epilepsy. Hippocampus 11(3):311-21.

Boku S, Nakagawa S & Koyama T. (2010). Glucocorticoids and lithium in adult hippocampal neurogenesis. Vitam Horm 82:421-31.

Boku S, Nakagawa S, Masuda T, Nishikawa H, Kato A, Toda H, Song N, Kitaichi Y, Inoue T & Koyama T. (2011). Effects of mood stabilizers on adult dentate gyrus-derived neural precursor cells. Prog Neuropsychopharmacol Biol Psychiatry 35(1):111-7.

Bonaguidi MA, McGuire T, Hu M, Kan L, Samanta J & Kessler JA. (2005). LIF and BMP signaling generate separate and discrete types of GFAP-expressing cells. Development 132(24):5503-14.

Bonaguidi MA, Peng CY, McGuire T, Falciglia G, Gobeske KT, Czeisler C & Kessler JA. (2008). Noggin expands neural stem cells in the adult hippocampus. J Neurosci 28(37):9194-204.

Boneva NB, Kaplamadzhiev DB, Sahara S, Kikuchi H, Pyko IV, Kikuchi M, Tonchev AB & Yamashima T. (2011). Expression of fatty acid-binding proteins in adult hippocampal neurogenic niche of postischemic monkeys. Hippocampus 21(2):162-71.

Bovetti S, Bovolin P, Perroteau I & Puche AC. (2007). Subventricular zone-derived neuroblast migration to the olfactory bulb is modulated by matrix remodelling. Eur J Neurosci 25(7):2021-33.

Brandt MD, Jessberger S, Steiner B, Kronenberg G, Reuter K, Bick-Sander A, von der Behrens W & Kempermann G. (2003). Transient calretinin expression defines early postmitotic step of neuronal differentiation in adult hippocampal neurogenesis of mice. Mol Cell Neurosci 24(3):603-13.

Breunig JJ, Silbereis J, Vaccarino FM, Sestan N & Rakic P. (2007). Notch regulates cell fate and dendrite morphology of newborn neurons in the postnatal dentate gyrus. Proc Natl Acad Sci U S A 104(51):20558-63.

Breunig JJ, Sarkisian MR, Arellano JI, Morozov YM, Ayoub AE, Sojitra S, Wang B, Flavell RA, Rakic P & Town T. (2008). Primary cilia regulate hippocampal neurogenesis by mediating sonic hedgehog signaling. Proc Natl Acad Sci U S A 105(35):13127-32.

Brown J, Cooper-Kuhn CM, Kempermann G, Van Praag H, Winkler J, Gage FH & Kuhn HG. (2003). Enriched environment and physical activity stimulate hippocampal but not olfactory bulb neurogenesis. Eur J Neurosci 17(10):2042-6.

Bruel-Jungerman E, Veyrac A, Dufour F, Horwood J, Laroche S & Davis S. (2009). Inhibition of PI3K-Akt signaling blocks exercise-mediated enhancement of adult neurogenesis and synaptic plasticity in the dentate gyrus. PLoS One 4(11):e7901.

Burns TC, Verfaillie CM & Low WC. (2009). Stem cells for ischemic brain injury: a critical review. J Comp Neurol 515(1):125-44.

Cassel JC, Duconseille E, Jeltsch H & Will B. (1997). The fimbria-fornix/cingular bundle pathways: a review of neurochemical and behavioural approaches using lesions and transplantation techniques. Prog Neurobiol 51(6):663-716.

Cha BH, Akman C, Silveira DC, Liu X & Holmes GL. (2004). Spontaneous recurrent seizure following status epilepticus enhances dentate gyrus neurogenesis. Brain Dev 26(6):394-7.

Chen G, Rajkowska G, Du F, Seraji-Bozorgzad N & Manji HK. (2000). Enhancement of hippocampal neurogenesis by lithium. J Neurochem 75(4):1729-34.

Cheng H, Yu J, Jiang Z, Zhang X, Liu C, Peng Y, Chen F, Qu Y, Jia Y, Tian Q and others. (2008). Acupuncture improves cognitive deficits and regulates the brain cell proliferation of SAMP8 mice. Neurosci Lett 432(2):111-6.

Chirumamilla S, Sun D, Bullock MR & Colello RJ. (2002). Traumatic brain injury induced cell proliferation in the adult mammalian central nervous system. J Neurotrauma 19(6):693-703.

Coffer PJ, Jin J & Woodgett JR. (1998). Protein kinase B (c-Akt): a multifunctional mediator of phosphatidylinositol 3-kinase activation. Biochem J 335 (Pt 1):1-13.

Cooper-Kuhn CM, Winkler J & Kuhn HG. (2004). Decreased neurogenesis after cholinergic forebrain lesion in the adult rat. J Neurosci Res 77(2):155-65.

Corotto FS, Henegar JA & Maruniak JA. (1993). Neurogenesis persists in the subependymal layer of the adult mouse brain. Neurosci Lett 149(2):111-4.

Dagyte G, Trentani A, Postema F, Luiten PG, Den Boer JA, Gabriel C, Mocaer E, Meerlo P & Van der Zee EA. (2010). The novel antidepressant agomelatine normalizes hippocampal neuronal activity and promotes neurogenesis in chronically stressed rats. CNS Neurosci Ther 16(4):195-207.

Dal-Pra S, Furthauer M, Van-Celst J, Thisse B & Thisse C. (2006). Noggin1 and Follistatin-like2 function redundantly to Chordin to antagonize BMP activity. Dev Biol 298(2):514-26.

Dash PK, Mach SA & Moore AN. (2001). Enhanced neurogenesis in the rodent hippocampus following traumatic brain injury. J Neurosci Res 63(4):313-9.

Datta SR, Brunet A & Greenberg ME. (1999). Cellular survival: a play in three Akts. Genes Dev 13(22):2905-27.

Dawirs RR, Hildebrandt K & Teuchert-Noodt G. (1998). Adult treatment with haloperidol increases dentate granule cell proliferation in the gerbil hippocampus. J Neural Transm 105(2-3):317-27.

de Lima MN, Presti-Torres J, Vedana G, Alcalde LA, Stertz L, Fries GR, Roesler R, Andersen ML, Quevedo J, Kapczinski F and others. (2011). Early life stress decreases hippocampal BDNF content and exacerbates recognition memory deficits induced by repeated d-amphetamine exposure. Behav Brain Res 224(1):100-6.

Deng W, Saxe MD, Gallina IS & Gage FH. (2009). Adult-born hippocampal dentate granule cells undergoing maturation modulate learning and memory in the brain. J Neurosci 29(43):13532-42.

Ding Q, Ying Z & Gomez-Pinilla F. (2011). Exercise influences hippocampal plasticity by modulating brain-derived neurotrophic factor processing. Neuroscience.

Doetsch F, Garcia-Verdugo JM & Alvarez-Buylla A. (1997). Cellular composition and three-dimensional organization of the subventricular germinal zone in the adult mammalian brain. J Neurosci 17(13):5046-61.

Duman RS, Heninger GR & Nestler EJ. (1997). A molecular and cellular theory of depression. Arch Gen Psychiatry 54(7):597-606.

Duman RS, Malberg J, Nakagawa S & D'Sa C. (2000). Neuronal plasticity and survival in mood disorders. Biol Psychiatry 48(8):732-9.

Ebara S & Nakayama K. (2002). Mechanism for the action of bone morphogenetic proteins and regulation of their activity. Spine (Phila Pa 1976) 27(16 Suppl 1):S10-5.

Eckenstein FP, Baughman RW & Quinn J. (1988). An anatomical study of cholinergic innervation in rat cerebral cortex. Neuroscience 25(2):457-74.

Ehm O, Goritz C, Covic M, Schaffner I, Schwarz TJ, Karaca E, Kempkes B, Kremmer E, Pfrieger FW, Espinosa L and others. (2010). RBPJkappa-dependent signaling is essential for long-term maintenance of neural stem cells in the adult hippocampus. J Neurosci 30(41):13794-807.

Ehninger D & Kempermann G. (2003). Regional effects of wheel running and environmental enrichment on cell genesis and microglia proliferation in the adult murine neocortex. Cereb Cortex 13(8):845-51.

Eisch AJ, Barrot M, Schad CA, Self DW & Nestler EJ. (2000). Opiates inhibit neurogenesis in the adult rat hippocampus. Proc Natl Acad Sci U S A 97(13):7579-84.

Englund C, Fink A, Lau C, Pham D, Daza RA, Bulfone A, Kowalczyk T & Hevner RF. (2005). Pax6, Tbr2, and Tbr1 are expressed sequentially by radial glia, intermediate progenitor cells, and postmitotic neurons in developing neocortex. J Neurosci 25(1):247-51.

Fallon J, Reid S, Kinyamu R, Opole I, Opole R, Baratta J, Korc M, Endo TL, Duong A, Nguyen G and others. (2000). In vivo induction of massive proliferation, directed migration, and differentiation of neural cells in the adult mammalian brain. Proc Natl Acad Sci U S A 97(26):14686-91.

Fan XT, Xu HW, Cai WQ, Yang H & Liu S. (2004). Antisense Noggin oligodeoxynucleotide administration decreases cell proliferation in the dentate gyrus of adult rats. Neurosci Lett 366(1):107-11.

Ferrer I, Boada Rovira M, Sanchez Guerra ML, Rey MJ & Costa-Jussa F. (2004). Neuropathology and pathogenesis of encephalitis following amyloid-beta immunization in Alzheimer's disease. Brain Pathol 14(1):11-20.

Filippov V, Kronenberg G, Pivneva T, Reuter K, Steiner B, Wang LP, Yamaguchi M, Kettenmann H & Kempermann G. (2003). Subpopulation of nestin-expressing progenitor cells in the adult murine hippocampus shows electrophysiological and morphological characteristics of astrocytes. Mol Cell Neurosci 23(3):373-82.

Fiorentini A, Rosi MC, Grossi C, Luccarini I & Casamenti F. (2010). Lithium improves hippocampal neurogenesis, neuropathology and cognitive functions in APP mutant mice. PLoS One 5(12):e14382.

Fukuda S, Kato F, Tozuka Y, Yamaguchi M, Miyamoto Y & Hisatsune T. (2003). Two distinct subpopulations of nestin-positive cells in adult mouse dentate gyrus. J Neurosci 23(28):9357-66.

Gage FH. (2000). Mammalian neural stem cells. Science 287(5457):1433-8.

Gage SL, Keim SR, Simon JR & Low WC. (1994). Cholinergic innervation of the retrosplenial cortex via the fornix pathway as determined by high affinity choline uptake, choline acetyltransferase activity, and muscarinic receptor binding in the rat. Neurochem Res 19(11):1379-86.

Gao X, Arlotta P, Macklis JD & Chen J. (2007). Conditional knock-out of beta-catenin in postnatal-born dentate gyrus granule neurons results in dendritic malformation. J Neurosci 27(52):14317-25.

Gaura V, Bachoud-Levi AC, Ribeiro MJ, Nguyen JP, Frouin V, Baudic S, Brugieres P, Mangin JF, Boisse MF, Palfi S and others. (2004). Striatal neural grafting improves cortical metabolism in Huntington's disease patients. Brain 127(Pt 1):65-72.

Gauthier S. (2002). Advances in the pharmacotherapy of Alzheimer's disease. Cmaj 166(5):616-23.

Geula C & Mesulam MM. (1989). Cortical cholinergic fibers in aging and Alzheimer's disease: a morphometric study. Neuroscience 33(3):469-81.

Gnjec A, Fonte JA, Atwood C & Martins RN. (2002). Transition metal chelator therapy--a potential treatment for Alzheimer's disease? Front Biosci 7:d1016-23.

Gobeske KT, Das S, Bonaguidi MA, Weiss C, Radulovic J, Disterhoft JF & Kessler JA. (2009). BMP signaling mediates effects of exercise on hippocampal neurogenesis and cognition in mice. PLoS One 4(10):e7506.

Gomez-Pinilla F, Dao L & So V. (1997). Physical exercise induces FGF-2 and its mRNA in the hippocampus. Brain Res 764(1-2):1-8.

Gotz M, Stoykova A & Gruss P. (1998). Pax6 controls radial glia differentiation in the cerebral cortex. Neuron 21(5):1031-44.

Gould E, Tanapat P, McEwen BS, Flugge G & Fuchs E. (1998). Proliferation of granule cell precursors in the dentate gyrus of adult monkeys is diminished by stress. Proc Natl Acad Sci U S A 95(6):3168-71.

Griffin EW, Mulally S, Foley C, Warmington SA, O'Mara SM & Kelly AM. (2011). Aerobic exercise improves hippocampal function and increases BDNF in the serum of young adult males. Physiol Behav.

Han YG, Spassky N, Romaguera-Ros M, Garcia-Verdugo JM, Aguilar A, Schneider-Maunoury S & Alvarez-Buylla A. (2008). Hedgehog signaling and primary cilia are required for the formation of adult neural stem cells. Nat Neurosci 11(3):277-84.

Hanson ND, Nemeroff CB & Owens MJ. (2011). Lithium, but not fluoxetine or the corticotropin-releasing factor receptor 1 receptor antagonist R121919, increases cell proliferation in the adult dentate gyrus. J Pharmacol Exp Ther 337(1):180-6.

Hastings NB & Gould E. (1999). Rapid extension of axons into the CA3 region by adult-generated granule cells. J Comp Neurol 413(1):146-54.

Hattiangady B, Rao MS & Shetty AK. (2004). Chronic temporal lobe epilepsy is associated with severely declined dentate neurogenesis in the adult hippocampus. Neurobiol Dis 17(3):473-90.

Heinrich C, Nitta N, Flubacher A, Müller M, Fahrner A, Kirsch M, Freiman T, Suzuki F, Depaulis A, Frotscher M, Haas CA. (2006). Reelin deficiency and displacement of mature neurons, but not neurogenesis, underlie the formation of granule cell dispersion in the epileptic hippocampus. J Neurosci 26(17):4701-13.

Heins N, Malatesta P, Cecconi F, Nakafuku M, Tucker KL, Hack MA, Chapouton P, Barde YA & Gotz M. (2002). Glial cells generate neurons: the role of the transcription factor Pax6. Nat Neurosci 5(4):308-15.

Heppner FL, Gandy S & McLaurin J. (2004). Current concepts and future prospects for Alzheimer disease vaccines. Alzheimer Dis Assoc Disord 18(1):38-43.

Hong JH & Jang SH. (2010). Neural pathway from nucleus basalis of Meynert passing through the cingulum in the human brain. Brain Res:(Epub ahead of print).

Huangfu D, Liu A, Rakeman AS, Murcia NS, Niswander L & Anderson KV. (2003). Hedgehog signalling in the mouse requires intraflagellar transport proteins. Nature 426(6962):83-7.

Huangfu D & Anderson KV. (2005). Cilia and Hedgehog responsiveness in the mouse. Proc Natl Acad Sci U S A 102(32):11325-30.

Hwang IK, Chung JY, Yoo DY, Yi SS, Youn HY, Seong JK & Yoon YS. (2010). Comparing the effects of acupuncture and electroacupuncture at Zusanli and Baihui on cell proliferation and neuroblast differentiation in the rat hippocampus. J Vet Med Sci 72(3):279-84.

Imayoshi I, Sakamoto M, Yamaguchi M, Mori K & Kageyama R. (2010). Essential roles of Notch signaling in maintenance of neural stem cells in developing and adult brains. J Neurosci 30(9):3489-98.

Jessberger S & Kempermann G. (2003). Adult-born hippocampal neurons mature into activity-dependent responsiveness. Eur J Neurosci 18(10):2707-12.

Jessberger S, Romer B, Babu H & Kempermann G. (2005). Seizures induce proliferation and dispersion of doublecortin-positive hippocampal progenitor cells. Exp Neurol 196(2):342-51.

Jin K, Minami M, Lan JQ, Mao XO, Batteur S, Simon RP & Greenberg DA. (2001). Neurogenesis in dentate subgranular zone and rostral subventricular zone after focal cerebral ischemia in the rat. Proc Natl Acad Sci U S A 98(8):4710-5.

Johansson CB, Momma S, Clarke DL, Risling M, Lendahl U & Frisen J. (1999). Identification of a neural stem cell in the adult mammalian central nervous system. Cell 96(1):25-34.

Kaneko Y, Sakakibara S, Imai T, Suzuki A, Nakamura Y, Sawamoto K, Ogawa Y, Toyama Y, Miyata T & Okano H. (2000). Musashi1: an evolutionarily conserved marker for CNS progenitor cells including neural stem cells. Dev Neurosci 22(1-2):139-53.

Kawai T, Takagi N, Miyake-Takagi K, Okuyama N, Mochizuki N & Takeo S. (2004). Characterization of BrdU-positive neurons induced by transient global ischemia in adult hippocampus. J Cereb Blood Flow Metab 24(5):548-55.

Kempermann G, Kuhn HG & Gage FH. (1997). More hippocampal neurons in adult mice living in an enriched environment. Nature 386(6624):493-5.

Kempermann G & Gage FH. (2000). Neurogenesis in the adult hippocampus. Novartis Found Symp 231:220-35; discussion 235-41, 302-6.

Kempermann G, Gast D & Gage FH. (2002). Neuroplasticity in old age: sustained fivefold induction of hippocampal neurogenesis by long-term environmental enrichment. Ann Neurol 52(2):135-43.

Kempermann G, Gast D, Kronenberg G, Yamaguchi M & Gage FH. (2003). Early determination and long-term persistence of adult-generated new neurons in the hippocampus of mice. Development 130(2):391-9.

Kempermann G, Jessberger S, Steiner B & Kronenberg G. (2004). Milestones of neuronal development in the adult hippocampus. Trends Neurosci 27(8):447-52.

Kim EH, Kim YJ, Lee HJ, Huh Y, Chung JH, Seo JC, Kang JE, Lee HJ, Yim SV & Kim CJ. (2001). Acupuncture increases cell proliferation in dentate gyrus after transient global ischemia in gerbils. Neurosci Lett 297(1):21-4.

Kim EH, Jang MH, Shin MC, Lim BV, Kim HB, Kim YJ, Chung JH & Kim CJ. (2002). Acupuncture increases cell proliferation and neuropeptide Y expression in dentate gyrus of streptozotocin-induced diabetic rats. Neurosci Lett 327(1):33-6.

Kim EJ, Battiste J, Nakagawa Y & Johnson JE. (2008). Ascl1 (Mash1) lineage cells contribute to discrete cell populations in CNS architecture. Mol Cell Neurosci 38(4):595-606.

Kim JS, Chang MY, Yu IT, Kim JH, Lee SH, Lee YS & Son H. (2004). Lithium selectively increases neuronal differentiation of hippocampal neural progenitor cells both in vitro and in vivo. J Neurochem 89(2):324-36.

Kitamura Y, Doi M, Kuwatsuka K, Onoue Y, Miyazaki I, Shinomiya K, Koyama T, Sendo T, Kawasaki H, Asanuma M and others. (2011). Chronic treatment with imipramine and lithium increases cell proliferation in the hippocampus in adrenocorticotropic hormone-treated rats. Biol Pharm Bull 34(1):77-81.

Kobayashi K, Ikeda Y, Sakai A, Yamasaki N, Haneda E, Miyakawa T & Suzuki H. (2010). Reversal of hippocampal neuronal maturation by serotonergic antidepressants. Proc Natl Acad Sci U S A 107(18):8434-9.

Kohl Z, Kuhn HG, Cooper-Kuhn CM, Winkler J, Aigner L & Kempermann G. (2002). Preweaning enrichment has no lasting effects on adult hippocampal neurogenesis in four-month-old mice. Genes Brain Behav 1(1):46-54.

Kralic JE, Ledergerber DA & Fritschy JM. (2005). Disruption of the neurogenic potential of the dentate gyrus in a mouse model of temporal lobe epilepsy with focal seizures. Eur J Neurosci 22(8):1916-27.

Kronenberg G, Reuter K, Steiner B, Brandt MD, Jessberger S, Yamaguchi M & Kempermann G. (2003). Subpopulations of proliferating cells of the adult hippocampus respond differently to physiologic neurogenic stimuli. J Comp Neurol 467(4):455-63.

Lai K, Kaspar BK, Gage FH & Schaffer DV. (2003). Sonic hedgehog regulates adult neural progenitor proliferation in vitro and in vivo. Nat Neurosci 6(1):21-7.

Lanz TA, Himes CS, Pallante G, Adams L, Yamazaki S, Amore B & Merchant KM. (2003). The gamma-secretase inhibitor N-[N-(3,5-difluorophenacetyl)-L-alanyl]-S-phenylglycine t-butyl ester reduces A beta levels in vivo in plasma and cerebrospinal fluid in young (plaque-free) and aged (plaque-bearing) Tg2576 mice. J Pharmacol Exp Ther 305(3):864-71.

Leanza G. (1998). Chronic elevation of amyloid precursor protein expression in the neocortex and hippocampus of rats with selective cholinergic lesions. Neurosci Lett 257(1):53-6.

Lee BH & Kim YK. (2010). The roles of BDNF in the pathophysiology of major depression and in antidepressant treatment. Psychiatry Investig 7(4):231-5.

Lee JE, Hollenberg SM, Snider L, Turner DL, Lipnick N & Weintraub H. (1995). Conversion of Xenopus ectoderm into neurons by NeuroD, a basic helix-loop-helix protein. Science 268(5212):836-44.

Leuner B, Glasper ER & Gould E. (2010). Sexual experience promotes adult neurogenesis in the hippocampus despite an initial elevation in stress hormones. PLoS One 5(7):e11597.

Li Z, Gao C, Huang H, Sun W, Yi H, Fan X & Xu H. (2010). Neurotransmitter phenotype differentiation and synapse formation of neural precursors engrafting in amyloid-beta injured rat hippocampus. J Alzheimers Dis 21(4):1233-47.

Lie DC, Colamarino SA, Song HJ, Desire L, Mira H, Consiglio A, Lein ES, Jessberger S, Lansford H, Dearie AR and others. (2005). Wnt signalling regulates adult hippocampal neurogenesis. Nature 437(7063):1370-5.

Lin L, LeBlanc CJ, Deacon TW & Isacson O. (1998). Chronic cognitive deficits and amyloid precursor protein elevation after selective immunotoxin lesions of the basal forebrain cholinergic system. Neuroreport 9(3):547-52.

Liu CZ, Yu JC, Zhang XZ, Fu WW, Wang T & Han JX. (2006). Acupuncture prevents cognitive deficits and oxidative stress in cerebral multi-infarction rats. Neurosci Lett 393(1):45-50.

Liu L, Ikonen S, Heikkinen T, Heikkila M, Puolivali J, van Groen T & Tanila H. (2002). Effects of fimbria-fornix lesion and amyloid pathology on spatial learning and memory in transgenic APP+PS1 mice. Behav Brain Res 134(1-2):433-45.

Liu M, Pleasure SJ, Collins AE, Noebels JL, Naya FJ, Tsai MJ & Lowenstein DH. (2000). Loss of BETA2/NeuroD leads to malformation of the dentate gyrus and epilepsy. Proc Natl Acad Sci U S A 97(2):865-70.

Liu Q, Yu J, Mi WL, Mao-Ying QL, Yang R, Wang YQ & Wu GC. (2007). Electroacupuncture attenuates the decrease of hippocampal progenitor cell proliferation in the adult rats exposed to chronic unpredictable stress. Life Sci 81(21-22):1489-95.

Liu Y, Namba T, Liu J, Suzuki R, Shioda S & Seki T. (2010). Glial fibrillary acidic protein-expressing neural progenitors give rise to immature neurons via early intermediate progenitors expressing both glial fibrillary acidic protein and neuronal markers in the adult hippocampus. Neuroscience 166(1):241-51.

Llorens-Martin M, Tejeda GS & Trejo JL. (2010). Differential regulation of the variations induced by environmental richness in adult neurogenesis as a function of time: a dual birthdating analysis. PLoS One 5(8):e12188.

Lois C & Alvarez-Buylla A. (1994). Long-distance neuronal migration in the adult mammalian brain. Science 264(5162):1145-8.

Lois C, Garcia-Verdugo JM & Alvarez-Buylla A. (1996). Chain migration of neuronal precursors. Science 271(5251):978-81.

Lugert S, Basak O, Knuckles P, Haussler U, Fabel K, Gotz M, Haas CA, Kempermann G, Taylor V & Giachino C. (2010). Quiescent and active hippocampal neural stem cells with distinct morphologies respond selectively to physiological and pathological stimuli and aging. Cell Stem Cell 6(5):445-56.

Machold R, Hayashi S, Rutlin M, Muzumdar MD, Nery S, Corbin JG, Gritli-Linde A, Dellovade T, Porter JA, Rubin LL and others. (2003). Sonic hedgehog is required for progenitor cell maintenance in telencephalic stem cell niches. Neuron 39(6):937-50.

Maekawa M, Takashima N, Arai Y, Nomura T, Inokuchi K, Yuasa S & Osumi N. (2005). Pax6 is required for production and maintenance of progenitor cells in postnatal hippocampal neurogenesis. Genes Cells 10(10):1001-14.

Magavi SS & Macklis JD. (2002). Induction of neuronal type-specific neurogenesis in the cerebral cortex of adult mice: manipulation of neural precursors in situ. Brain Res Dev Brain Res 134(1-2):57-76.

Malberg JE, Eisch AJ, Nestler EJ & Duman RS. (2000). Chronic antidepressant treatment increases neurogenesis in adult rat hippocampus. J Neurosci 20(24):9104-10.

Markakis EA & Gage FH. (1999). Adult-generated neurons in the dentate gyrus send axonal projections to field CA3 and are surrounded by synaptic vesicles. J Comp Neurol 406(4):449-60.

Martino G & Pluchino S. (2006). The therapeutic potential of neural stem cells. Nat Rev Neurosci 7(5):395-406.

Mason HA, Rakowiecki SM, Gridley T & Fishell G. (2006). Loss of notch activity in the developing central nervous system leads to increased cell death. Dev Neurosci 28(1-2):49-57.

McDonald HY & Wojtowicz JM. (2005). Dynamics of neurogenesis in the dentate gyrus of adult rats. Neurosci Lett 385(1):70-5.

Mehler MF, Mabie PC, Zhu G, Gokhan S & Kessler JA. (2000). Developmental changes in progenitor cell responsiveness to bone morphogenetic proteins differentially modulate progressive CNS lineage fate. Dev Neurosci 22(1-2):74-85.

Miles DK & Kernie SG. (2008). Hypoxic-ischemic brain injury activates early hippocampal stem/progenitor cells to replace vulnerable neuroblasts. Hippocampus 18(8):793-806.

Ming GL & Song H. (2005). Adult neurogenesis in the mammalian central nervous system. Annu Rev Neurosci 28:223-50.

Miyata T, Maeda T & Lee JE. (1999). NeuroD is required for differentiation of the granule cells in the cerebellum and hippocampus. Genes Dev 13(13):1647-52.

Murakami S, Imbe H, Morikawa Y, Kubo C & Senba E. (2005). Chronic stress, as well as acute stress, reduces BDNF mRNA expression in the rat hippocampus but less robustly. Neurosci Res 53(2):129-39.

Muroyama Y, Fujihara M, Ikeya M, Kondoh H & Takada S. (2002). Wnt signaling plays an essential role in neuronal specification of the dorsal spinal cord. Genes Dev 16(5):548-53.

Nacher J, Varea E, Blasco-Ibanez JM, Castillo-Gomez E, Crespo C, Martinez-Guijarro FJ & McEwen BS. (2005). Expression of the transcription factor Pax 6 in the adult rat dentate gyrus. J Neurosci Res 81(6):753-61.

Nakatomi H, Kuriu T, Okabe S, Yamamoto S, Hatano O, Kawahara N, Tamura A, Kirino T & Nakafuku M. (2002). Regeneration of hippocampal pyramidal neurons after ischemic brain injury by recruitment of endogenous neural progenitors. Cell 110(4):429-41.

Nasrallah HA, Hopkins T & Pixley SK. (2011). Differential effects of antipsychotic and antidepressant drugs on neurogenic regions in rats. Brain Res 1354:23-9.

Olson AK, Eadie BD, Ernst C & Christie BR. (2006). Environmental enrichment and voluntary exercise massively increase neurogenesis in the adult hippocampus via dissociable pathways. Hippocampus 16(3):250-60.

Palma V, Lim DA, Dahmane N, Sanchez P, Brionne TC, Herzberg CD, Gitton Y, Carleton A, Alvarez-Buylla A & Ruiz i Altaba A. (2005). Sonic hedgehog controls stem cell behavior in the postnatal and adult brain. Development 132(2):335-44.

Palmer TD, Willhoite AR & Gage FH. (2000). Vascular niche for adult hippocampal neurogenesis. J Comp Neurol 425(4):479-94.

Parent JM, Yu TW, Leibowitz RT, Geschwind DH, Sloviter RS & Lowenstein DH. (1997). Dentate granule cell neurogenesis is increased by seizures and contributes to aberrant network reorganization in the adult rat hippocampus. J Neurosci 17(10):3727-38.

Parent JM, Vexler ZS, Gong C, Derugin N & Ferriero DM. (2002). Rat forebrain neurogenesis and striatal neuron replacement after focal stroke. Ann Neurol 52(6):802-13.

Parent JM & Murphy GG. (2008). Mechanisms and functional significance of aberrant seizure-induced hippocampal neurogenesis. Epilepsia 49 Suppl 5:19-25.

Pilar-Cuellar F, Vidal R & Pazos A. (2011). Subchronic treatment with fluoxetine and the 5-HT(2A) antagonist ketanserin upregulates hippocampal BDNF and beta-catenin in parallel with antidepressant-like effect. Br J Pharmacol.

Pluchino S, Zanotti L, Rossi B, Brambilla E, Ottoboni L, Salani G, Martinello M, Cattalini A, Bergami A, Furlan R and others. (2005). Neurosphere-derived multipotent precursors promote neuroprotection by an immunomodulatory mechanism. Nature 436(7048):266-71.

Reus GZ, Stringari RB, Ribeiro KF, Ferraro AK, Vitto MF, Cesconetto P, Souza CT & Quevedo J. (2011). Ketamine plus imipramine treatment induces antidepressant-like behavior and increases CREB and BDNF protein levels and PKA and PKC phosphorylation in rat brain. Behav Brain Res 221(1):166-71.

Rogoz Z, Skuza G & Legutko B. (2008). Repeated co-treatment with fluoxetine and amantadine induces brain-derived neurotrophic factor gene expression in rats. Pharmacol Rep 60(6):817-26.

Russo-Neustadt A, Beard RC & Cotman CW. (1999). Exercise, antidepressant medications, and enhanced brain derived neurotrophic factor expression. Neuropsychopharmacology 21(5):679-82.

Sakakibara S, Imai T, Hamaguchi K, Okabe M, Aruga J, Nakajima K, Yasutomi D, Nagata T, Kurihara Y, Uesugi S and others. (1996). Mouse-Musashi-1, a neural RNA-binding protein highly enriched in the mammalian CNS stem cell. Dev Biol 176(2):230-42.

Sakurai K & Osumi N. (2008). The neurogenesis-controlling factor, Pax6, inhibits proliferation and promotes maturation in murine astrocytes. J Neurosci 28(18):4604-12.

Santarelli L, Saxe M, Gross C, Surget A, Battaglia F, Dulawa S, Weisstaub N, Lee J, Duman R, Arancio O and others. (2003). Requirement of hippocampal neurogenesis for the behavioral effects of antidepressants. Science 301(5634):805-9.

Saper CB. (1984). Organization of cerebral cortical afferent systems in the rat. II. Magnocellular basal nucleus. J Comp Neurol 222(3):313-42.

Schliebs R & Arendt T. (2006). The significance of the cholinergic system in the brain during aging and in Alzheimer's disease. J Neural Transm 113(11):1625-44.

Schmidt RH, Scholten KJ & Maughan PH. (1999). Time course for recovery of water maze performance and central cholinergic innervation after fluid percussion injury. J Neurotrauma 16(12):1139-47.

Seri B, Garcia-Verdugo JM, McEwen BS & Alvarez-Buylla A. (2001). Astrocytes give rise to new neurons in the adult mammalian hippocampus. J Neurosci 21(18):7153-60.

Seri B, Garcia-Verdugo JM, Collado-Morente L, McEwen BS & Alvarez-Buylla A. (2004). Cell types, lineage, and architecture of the germinal zone in the adult dentate gyrus. J Comp Neurol 478(4):359-78.

Silva R, Mesquita AR, Bessa J, Sousa JC, Sotiropoulos I, Leao P, Almeida OF & Sousa N. (2008). Lithium blocks stress-induced changes in depressive-like behavior and hippocampal cell fate: the role of glycogen-synthase-kinase-3beta. Neuroscience 152(3):656-69.

Son H, Yu IT, Hwang SJ, Kim JS, Lee SH, Lee YS & Kaang BK. (2003). Lithium enhances long-term potentiation independently of hippocampal neurogenesis in the rat dentate gyrus. J Neurochem 85(4):872-81.

Song H, Kempermann G, Overstreet Wadiche L, Zhao C, Schinder AF & Bischofberger J. (2005). New neurons in the adult mammalian brain: synaptogenesis and functional integration. J Neurosci 25(45):10366-8.

Stanfield BB & Trice JE. (1988). Evidence that granule cells generated in the dentate gyrus of adult rats extend axonal projections. Exp Brain Res 72(2):399-406.

Steiner B, Kronenberg G, Jessberger S, Brandt MD, Reuter K & Kempermann G. (2004). Differential regulation of gliogenesis in the context of adult hippocampal neurogenesis in mice. Glia 46(1):41-52.

Steiner B, Klempin F, Wang L, Kott M, Kettenmann H & Kempermann G. (2006). Type-2 cells as link between glial and neuronal lineage in adult hippocampal neurogenesis. Glia 54(8):805-14.

Steiner B, Zurborg S, Horster H, Fabel K & Kempermann G. (2008). Differential 24 h responsiveness of Prox1-expressing precursor cells in adult hippocampal neurogenesis to physical activity, environmental enrichment, and kainic acid-induced seizures. Neuroscience 154(2):521-9.

Su XW, Li XY, Banasr M & Duman RS. (2009). Eszopiclone and fluoxetine enhance the survival of newborn neurons in the adult rat hippocampus. Int J Neuropsychopharmacol 12(10):1421-8.

Suh H, Consiglio A, Ray J, Sawai T, D'Amour KA & Gage FH. (2007). In vivo fate analysis reveals the multipotent and self-renewal capacities of Sox2+ neural stem cells in the adult hippocampus. Cell Stem Cell 1(5):515-28.

Sui Y, Zhang Z, Guo Y, Sun Y, Zhang X, Xie C, Li Y & Xi G. (2009). The function of Notch1 signaling was increased in parallel with neurogenesis in rat hippocampus after chronic fluoxetine administration. Biol Pharm Bull 32(10):1776-82.

Szenborn M. (1993). Neuropathological study on the nucleus basalis of Meynert in mature and old age. Patol Pol 44(4):211-6.

Traiffort E, Charytoniuk DA, Faure H & Ruat M. (1998). Regional distribution of Sonic Hedgehog, patched, and smoothened mRNA in the adult rat brain. J Neurochem 70(3):1327-30.

Urrea C, Castellanos DA, Sagen J, Tsoulfas P, Bramlett HM & Dietrich WD. (2007). Widespread cellular proliferation and focal neurogenesis after traumatic brain injury in the rat. Restor Neurol Neurosci 25(1):65-76.

van Praag H, Christie BR, Sejnowski TJ & Gage FH. (1999a). Running enhances neurogenesis, learning, and long-term potentiation in mice. Proc Natl Acad Sci U S A 96(23):13427-31.

van Praag H, Kempermann G & Gage FH. (1999b). Running increases cell proliferation and neurogenesis in the adult mouse dentate gyrus. Nat Neurosci 2(3):266-70.

van Praag H, Schinder AF, Christie BR, Toni N, Palmer TD & Gage FH. (2002). Functional neurogenesis in the adult hippocampus. Nature 415(6875):1030-4.

Wang C, Zhang M, Sun C, Cai Y, You Y, Huang L & Liu F. (2011). Sustained increase in adult neurogenesis in the rat hippocampal dentate gyrus after transient brain ischemia. Neurosci Lett 488(1):70-5.

Wang JW, David DJ, Monckton JE, Battaglia F & Hen R. (2008). Chronic fluoxetine stimulates maturation and synaptic plasticity of adult-born hippocampal granule cells. J Neurosci 28(6):1374-84.

Wexler EM, Geschwind DH & Palmer TD. (2008). Lithium regulates adult hippocampal progenitor development through canonical Wnt pathway activation. Mol Psychiatry 13(3):285-92.

Willert K, Brown JD, Danenberg E, Duncan AW, Weissman IL, Reya T, Yates JR, 3rd & Nusse R. (2003). Wnt proteins are lipid-modified and can act as stem cell growth factors. Nature 423(6938):448-52.

Xuan AG, Luo M, Ji WD & Long DH. (2009). Effects of engrafted neural stem cells in Alzheimer's disease rats. Neurosci Lett 450(2):167-71.

Yagita Y, Kitagawa K, Ohtsuki T, Takasawa K, Miyata T, Okano H, Hori M & Matsumoto M. (2001). Neurogenesis by progenitor cells in the ischemic adult rat hippocampus. Stroke 32(8):1890-6.

Yamamoto T, Hirayama A, Hosoe N, Furube M & Hirano S. (2009). Soft-diet feeding inhibits adult neurogenesis in hippocampus of mice. Bull Tokyo Dent Coll 50(3):117-24.

Yap JJ, Takase LF, Kochman LJ, Fornal CA, Miczek KA & Jacobs BL. (2006). Repeated brief social defeat episodes in mice: effects on cell proliferation in the dentate gyrus. Behav Brain Res 172(2):344-50.

Yoshimura S, Takagi Y, Harada J, Teramoto T, Thomas SS, Waeber C, Bakowska JC, Breakefield XO & Moskowitz MA. (2001). FGF-2 regulation of neurogenesis in adult hippocampus after brain injury. Proc Natl Acad Sci U S A 98(10):5874-9.

Yu J, Liu C, Zhang X & Han J. (2005). Acupuncture improved cognitive impairment caused by multi-infarct dementia in rats. Physiol Behav 86(4):434-41.

Yu TS, Zhang G, Liebl DJ & Kernie SG. (2008). Traumatic brain injury-induced hippocampal neurogenesis requires activation of early nestin-expressing progenitors. J Neurosci 28(48):12901-12.

Zhang X, Jin G, Tian M, Qin J & Huang Z. (2007). The denervated hippocampus provides proper microenvironment for the survival and differentiation of neural progenitors. Neurosci Lett 414(2):115-20.

Zhao C, Teng EM, Summers RG, Jr., Ming GL & Gage FH. (2006). Distinct morphological stages of dentate granule neuron maturation in the adult mouse hippocampus. J Neurosci 26(1):3-11.

Zigova T, Pencea V, Wiegand SJ & Luskin MB. (1998). Intraventricular administration of BDNF increases the number of newly generated neurons in the adult olfactory bulb. Mol Cell Neurosci 11(4):234-45.

3

The Spinal Cord
Neural Stem Cell Niche

Jean-Philippe Hugnot
University of Montpellier 2, INSERM U1051,
Institute for Neurosciences of Montpellier
France

1. Introduction

The spinal cord is the caudal portion of the central nervous system (CNS) that extends from the lower part of the brain stem (the medulla) to the cauda equina. It receives several types of sensory information from the joints, muscles, organs and skin and contains the motoneurons responsible for voluntary/reflex movements and for the function of the autonomic nervous system. The spinal cord is divided into i) gray matter, which notably contains motoneurons and interneurons that form the spinal cord circuitry; ii) white matter, which surrounds the gray matter and is made up of ascending and descending longitudinal tracts; and iii) the central canal or ependymal region, which is organized as an oval or round-shaped epithelium whose apical pole abuts the cerebral spinal fluid. The spinal cord is not simply a relay that carries information between the brain and body, but it also contains a complex circuitry that is implicated in the generation and coordination of reflexive responses to sensory inputs. Furthermore, the spinal cord is involved in the formation of rhythmic movements, such as locomotion and swimming in animals. One emerging field of research concerns spinal cord plasticity, as this structure should not be considered a static and hard-wired system. Instead, the spinal cord displays considerable activity-dependent adaptation and, similar to other CNS regions, can learn and remember throughout life (Guertin 2008; Wolpaw 2010; Wolpaw and Tennissen 2001). Plasticity plays an important role in the acquisition and maintenance of motor skills. In pathology, it could be manipulated to alleviate spinal cord lesions that originate from traumas or degenerative diseases.

In parallel with spinal cord plasticity, one field of research that is rapidly growing concerns the presence of neural stem cells and progenitor cells in the adult spinal cord. In this review, I will describe recent findings regarding stem cells and attempt to formulate hypotheses concerning their role in spinal cord physiology and plasticity. The presence of stem cells in the spinal of lower vertebrates, such as salamanders and newts, has been reported for decades. These stem cells are at the basis of the phenomenal regeneration capacity of these animals that is observed when the spinal cord is transected. There are excellent reviews on this topic (for instance, see (Tanaka 2003)), and I will thus focus on the adult spinal cord stem cells in mammals.

2. Discovery and properties of mouse spinal cord neural stem cells

2.1 Spinal cord neurospheres

Definite proof of the presence of neural stem cells in the adult CNS using in vitro assays dates back to the early nineties (Gage, Ray, and Fisher 1995; Reynolds, W., and Weiss 1992). Since then, much attention has been given to stem and progenitor cells in the brain, whereas little is known about these cells in the spinal cord. The persistence of stem cells in this caudal region of the CNS was reported using adherent and non-adherent culture conditions in the late nineties (Shihabuddin, Ray, and Gage 1997; Weiss et al. 1996). The neurosphere assay (Deleyrolle and Reynolds 2009) was instrumental in their discovery, as this assay is particularly suited to demonstrate, at the clonal level, the cardinal properties of stem cells, i.e., multipotentiality, self-renewal and extended proliferation capabilities. Indeed, in 1996 Weiss et al. reported that in mice, 0.1 and 0.6% of isolated thoracic and lumbar spinal cord cells, respectively, that were grown in the presence of FGF2 and EGF, were able to form multipotent and passageable neurospheres (Weiss et al. 1996). Using microdissection and cytometric analysis, these cells were located primarily in the central canal region (Martens, Seaberg, and van der Kooy 2002; Meletis et al. 2008; Sabourin et al. 2009). Progenitor cells with a more limited proliferation potential are also present in the parenchyma (Horner et al. 2000; Kulbatski et al. 2007; Sabourin et al. 2009; Martens, Seaberg, and van der Kooy 2002; Yamamoto et al. 2001). More recently, we were able to show that the dorsal part of the central canal region is enriched in neurosphere-forming cells (Sabourin et al. 2009). Even when clonally-expanded, these neurospheres appear to be heterogeneous entities that are composed of different types of Nestin+ cells, which express various levels of stem cell (CD133), astrocytic (GFAP, Adhl1l1), radial glial cell (CD15, Blbp, Glast, RC2) and oligodendrocytic-lineage (NG2, A2B5, PDGFRα) markers (Fig. 1).

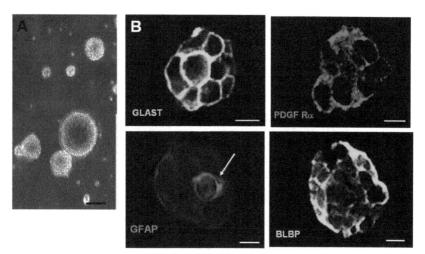

Fig. 1. A) Examples of adult spinal cord-derived neurospheres that were clonally expanded. Note the differences in the sizes of the neurospheres. Scale bar=500 μm. B) Examples of markers that were detected by immunofluorescence in the neurospheres. The white arrow shows a unique GFAP+ cell in a neurosphere. Scale bars=10 μm.

The widespread expression of the latter coincides with the higher propensity of the neurospheres to differentiate into oligodendrocytes vs. neurons in vitro and in vivo after spinal cord injury (SCI) (Kulbatski et al. 2007; Meletis et al. 2008). A few cells that express so-called neuronal markers, such as Map2 and Dcx, are also observed in some neurospheres (Fig. 2).

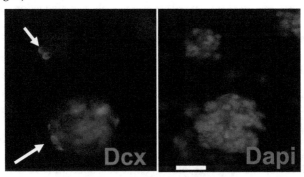

Fig. 2. Example of Dcx+ cells detected in spinal cord-derived neurospheres. Scale bar= 100 µm.

Often, several of these markers are coexpressed in the same cells, which may reflect the presence of intermediates and uncommitted states of differentiation. GFAP[+] cells in these spheres (Fig. 1) should not be considered to be astrocytic-differentiated cells but rather, as they frequently co-express immature markers (CD133, CD15), these cells likely represent GFAP[+] neural stem cells. Within neurospheres, only a fraction of the cells, typically between 1 to 10%, are able to generate new neurospheres and are considered to be bona fide neural stem cells. Other cells are considered to be progenitors because they give rise to small neurospheres with limited proliferative and self-renewal capabilities (Louis et al. 2008). The prospective isolation of stem vs. progenitor cells in neurospheres remains challenging, as no definitive cell surface marker has been clearly identified to distinguish these two types of cells.

Notably, as observed for neurospheres that were derived from different brain regions (Armando et al. 2007; Conti and Cattaneo 2010), neurospheres derived from different parts of the spinal cord have different growth and differentiation properties (Kulbatski and Tator 2009; Sabourin et al. 2009). We showed that neurospheres that were derived from the cervical, thoracic and lumbar regions maintained their expression of specific and different rostro-caudal combinations of developmental homeogenes of the Hox family. These data indicate that even after several passages in vitro, these cells maintain molecular cues from their original position. This phenomenon might affect considerations regarding cellular therapy with adult neural stem cells because not all cells might have equivalent capacities to replenish cell loss and to integrate into the adult host tissue. In addition to Hox genes, the adult spinal cord neurospheres express high levels of a set of transcription factors, including Dlx2, Nkx2.2, Nkx6.1, Olig2, Pax6, Sox2, Sox4 and Sox9 (Moreno-Manzano et al. 2009; Sabourin et al. 2009; Yamamoto et al. 2001) which are involved in spinal cord embryonic development. This expression likely reflects the maintenance, in adult stem cells, of embryonic transcriptional programs and active signaling pathways. Yet, these neurospheres appear to express only a limited range of developmental gene networks, as the transcription factors that are involved in motoneuron development, such as Islet1, Lim1 and HB9, are not expressed (Yamamoto et al. 2001), which illustrates a somewhat restricted fate for these cells. Indeed, upon differentiation in vitro, these cells primarily generate GABAergic neurons, oligodendrocytes and astrocytes (Moreno-Manzano et al. 2009; Sabourin et al. 2009). Importantly, these cells appear to remain competent to respond to morphogens to redirect their differentiation into other neuronal cell subtypes. Indeed, treatment with embryonic morphogens that are involved in spinal cord caudal regionalization and motoneuron development, i.e., retinoic acid and sonic hedgehog, was able to drive their differentiation toward electrophysiological active motoneurons (Moreno-Manzano et al. 2009).

2.2 Neurosphere differentiation

The differentiation of adult spinal cord neurospheres into neuronal and glial cells is generally achieved by plating them onto an adhesive substrate and by removing growth factors. This differentiation occurs even without the addition of serum, suggesting that endogenous cytokines are implicated in the differentiation process. Indeed, we found that undifferentiated and differentiated neurospheres expressed at a high level, a wide range of endogenous cytokines (Deleyrolle et al. 2005). The expression of several of them is controlled by the FGF2 and EGF which are present in the medium. Notably, upon differentiation, a striking upregulation of astrocytic differentiating factors, such as BMP4, BMP6 and CNTF, are observed. The active role of these endogenous cytokines is illustrated by inhibition experiments that impair neurosphere differentiation (Deleyrolle et al. 2005). This production of endogenous cytokines by adult spinal cord stem cells could be considered to be beneficial in the context of cellular therapy because these cytokines have been shown to actively participate in the therapeutic effects observed following neural precursor cell transplantation (Pluchino et al. 2003; Redmond et al. 2007). In contrast, these endogenous factors, together with host factors, might also contribute to the absence or the low rate of neuronal formation, which is frequently observed in grafting experiments. Further investigations of the neurosphere differentiation process would yield important insights on how to direct the fate of endogenous and exogenous neural stem cells into the most appropriate cell type to achieve rational and effective spinal cord cellular therapy.

3. The central canal niche and identity of adult spinal cord stem cells

Many adult organs harbor a pool of stem cells in specialized structures called niches. These act as a nest and a barrier to protect, nourish and regulate the fate of stem cells. They do so by providing, in highly organized structures, cellular and molecular cues suitable for the strict control of stem cell properties (e.g., self-renewal, differentiation, quiescence). Typically, these niches contain a high level of canonical developmental signaling pathways, notably, BMP, SHH, Wnt and Notch (Li and Clevers 2010). These signaling pathways precisely regulate the proliferation/quiescence, differentiation/self-renewal and migratory/stationary balances of the stem cell pool. In addition, their particular architecture favors interactions between stem cells and specific cells, such as vascular cells. Historically, the best-characterized niches in mammals are the hematopoietic and intestinal niches, and more recently, the CNS niches have been studied. In the brain, the hippocampus, the recently discovered sub-callosal zone and the subcortical white matter contain neural progenitors, whereas bona fide stem cells that are capable of sustained proliferation are preferentially found in the subventricular zone (SVZ) (Seaberg, Smukler, and van der Kooy

2005). In the latter, contacts with the cerebral spinal fluid (CSF) located in the ventricles appear to be essential for the maintenance of SVZ stem cells (Lehtinen et al. 2010). Stem and progenitor cells have also been identified in the peripheral nervous system, i.e., in the carotid body, the enteric nervous system and the adult dorsal root ganglia (Pardal et al. 2007; Schafer, Van Ginneken, and Copray 2009; Singh et al. 2009). Whereas there have been a tremendous number of publications on the brain niches, few have addressed this issue in the spinal cord.

3.1 Cellular diversity in the central canal region

The central canal region is composed of several cell types, which are located either in direct contact with the lumen or in a subependymal position, evoking a pseudo-stratified epithelium (Fig. 3). However, a distinct subependymal layer, as observed in the SVZ, is not present. Ependymocytes are the primary cell type found around the central canal. A second frequently observed cell type is the tanycyte (also referred to as radial ependymocytes) (Seitz, Lohler, and Schwendemann 1981), which is mostly observed on the lateral sides of the central canal region. This ependymal cell type sends a long basal process that terminates at the blood vessels (Horstmann 1954). Tanycytes are in contact with the lumen, but their soma can either be subependymally or ependymally located (Meletis et al. 2008; Rafols and Goshgarian 1985). As in the brain, they bridge the CSF to the capillaries, thereby providing a potential link between the CSF and the blood.

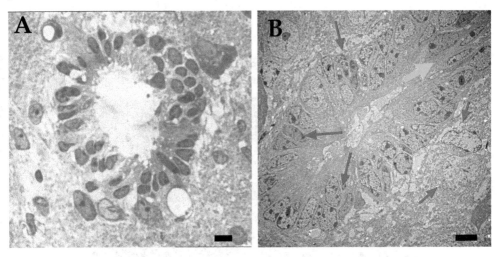

Fig. 3. A) Semi-thin section in the adult mouse thoracic spinal cord ependymal region (toluidine blue staining). Note the diversity of the cell types in contact with the lumen or in a subependymal position. B) An electron micrograph showing different types of cells around the central canal (red arrows). The green arrow indicates the dorsal region of the canal, which contains densely packed cells.

The central canal region contains also neuronal-like cells which contact the CSF. These are very common and well-described in several lower vertebrates especially fishes and amphibians (see for review (Vigh et al. 2004)). In mammals, their presence has been reported in several species including primates and rodents (Hugnot and Franzen 2010). These cells are sporadically distributed around the canal with a soma in an ependymal or subependymal position and they send a single thick dendritic-like process terminated by a large bulge in the lumen (Sabourin et al. 2009). Even in adults, these cells continue to express PSA-NCAM (Marichal et al. 2009; Seki and Arai 1993), Dcx (Marichal et al. 2009; Sabourin et al. 2009) and GAP43 (Stoeckel et al. 2003), three proteins that are involved in plasticity and migration, suggesting that they are endowed with some degree of immaturity. In rodents, these neuronal cells appear to be mainly GABAergic, and their function remains elusive. The expression of acidic pH-activated channels suggests that these cells might be implicated in CSF homeostasis (Huang et al. 2006; Marichal et al. 2009). They could also act as mechanoreceptors, which are sensitive to CSF pressure or flow or to spinal cord flexion. Importantly, these cells are not produced from continuous adult spinal cord neurogenesis, and a study performed in rats demonstrated that they are in fact produced during embryogenesis (Marichal et al. 2009).

The dorsal and ventral regions of the central canal display a divergent organization of a higher density of cells with a radial morphology, which are situated in ependymal and subependymal positions (Hamilton et al. 2009; Meletis et al. 2008; Sabourin et al. 2009). GFAP+ cells are frequently observed in these regions. Particularly in the dorsal region, some of these GFAP+ cells have long basal processes that extend along the dorsal midline up to the dorsal column white matter or pial surface (Bodega et al. 1994; Hamilton et al. 2009; Sabourin et al. 2009). GFAP+ cells can also be observed in the lateral region of the canal. These GFAP+ cells can lie in the ependymal layer adjacent to the canal lumen but are often located in a subependymal position, where they send a process toward the canal. Transgenic mice expressing a hGFAP promoter-GFP construct are particularly suited to visualize these cells (Fig. 4). Interestingly, some cells that express radial glia markers, such as CD15 or BLBP (some of which are GFAP+), are also occasionally detected in the dorsal region (Fig. 5).

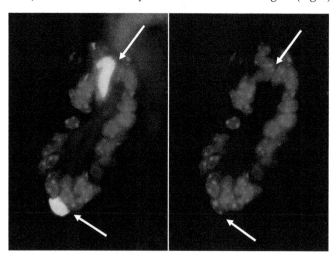

Fig. 4. Examples of GFP+ cells detected in the dorsal and ventral regions of the central canal region of hGFAP-GFP mice (Nolte et al. 2001). The dorsal GFP+ cell is located in the ependymal layer, whereas the ventral cell is located in the subependymal layer.

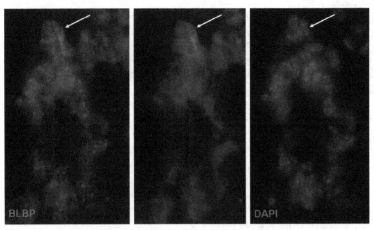

Fig. 5. Example of a subependymal BLBP+ cell detected in the dorsal part of the central canal of the mouse lumbar spinal cord (arrow).

The central canal region is surrounded by an abundant vasculature, and cellular proliferation within the niche occurs in close proximity to the vessels (Hamilton et al. 2009). This observation is consistent with the recently well-described interactions between neural stem/progenitor cells and endothelial cells (the so-called neurovascular niche (Palmer, Willhoite, and Gage 2000)).

Collectively, it appears that the central canal region is composed of several cell types that are localized at specific locations and express characteristic markers with different morphologies and potentially different functions. A schematic drawing of the lumbar central canal region is presented in Fig. 6.

3.2 Signaling within the niche

The persistence of stem cells within the central canal region implies that specific pathways are active or readily activated in the niche. These pathways will maintain the proliferation potential and multipotency of stem cells. Equally, the niche may contain molecules that act in a passive mode to protect stem cells from local or circulating growth and differentiation factors. Our lab used two approaches to identify important cues in the mouse spinal cord niche. First, we used immunofluorescence to screen for the presence of receptors, ligands and transcription factors that are associated with the Notch, SHH, Wnt and epithelial-mesenchymal transition (EMT) pathways. Second, we extensively screened online gene expression databases (notably, Allen Brain and the Gensat Atlas) for genes that are specifically expressed in the spinal cord central canal region. These approaches allowed us to identify the expression, at the transcript and/or the protein level, of several molecules involved in the Notch (Jagged, Hes1), Wnt (Wnt7a, Fzd3), BMP (DAN, BMP6) and Hedgehog (SHH) pathways (Hugnot and Franzen 2010; Sabourin et al. 2009). These genes are expressed by most of the cells in the central canal region or by restricted subpopulations. Unexpectedly, we also found that cells in this region highly expressed Zeb1 (Sabourin et al. 2009) (also known as δ-EF1, TCF8, AREB6), a zinc finger-homeodomain transcription factor, which has been described as an important regulator of EMT (Liu et al. 2008). Zeb1 protein is detected in the majority of cells surrounding the lumen but is present at higher levels in the cells that are located in the medial dorsal region, notably, the previously mentioned GFAP+ cells. Zeb1 is also detected in subpopulations of cells in the white and grey matter. Zeb1 is involved in the regulation of several cellular processes, such as migration, senescence and apoptosis. It exerts control by acting as a repressor for a number of genes, such as P15Ink4b, P21 Cdkn1, E-cadherin, CRB3 and myogenic transcription factors (Browne, Sayan, and Tulchinsky 2010). Conversely, it also acts as an activator for a group of genes that are typically expressed in mesenchymal cells, such as collagens, vimentin and smooth muscle actin (acta2) (Nishimura et al. 2006). As the two latter proteins are expressed in the central canal and SVZ cells (Sabourin et al, 2009), their expression might be under the control of Zeb1. Consistent with a role in adult precursor cells, Zeb1 and 2 are expressed by neurosphere cells derived from the adult spinal cord. These transcription factors are required for neurosphere formation and expansion because we demonstrated that the transfection of a dominant-negative form of Zeb1 and 2 induced massive apoptosis in vitro. In Drosophila, the Zeb1 orthologous protein Zfh-1 was recently shown to have a critical role in the maintenance of the somatic stem cell compartment in the testis stem cell niche (Leatherman and Dinardo 2008). These data suggest that the role of this family of transcription factors in the maintenance of immature properties has been conserved throughout evolution.

3.3 Identity of stem cells in the niche

Considering the diversity of cell types in the central canal region, the precise identity of the cells that are able to generate passageable neurospheres needed to be addressed by methods based on cell purification. A common and powerful technique is based on the cytometry of cells isolated from GFP transgenic animals, where a specific cell type is tagged using a cell-specific promoter. Alternatively, specific membranous markers and antibodies can be exploited for purification; however, this method can be challenging for studies of the adult spinal cord, as enzymes required for cellular dissociation could damage membrane-bound markers and lead to erroneous conclusions. To explore whether the GFAP+ cells we observed in the central canal region were endowed with stem cell properties, we used the hGFAP-GFP transgenic line established by Dr Kettenmann's group (Nolte et al. 2001). Sorting GFP+ cells by cytometry revealed that compared with GFP-, the vast majority of neurospheres (>80%) are derived from GFP+ cells (Sabourin et al. 2009). In total, 0.2% of GFP+ cells were able to generate neurospheres. This frequency might appear low, but one must consider that the purification of GFP+ cells from these animals cannot discriminate GFP+ cells located in the central canal region from those of the parenchyma, which are much more numerous. Consistent with our hypothesis that central canal GFAP+ cells are endowed with stem cells properties, we found that most primary neurospheres derived from these transgenic animals contained one or several GFAP+/GFP+ cells. This result supports the notion that as observed in the SVZ, the central canal cells with astrocytic features have neural stem cell properties. Another team conducted a second transgenic mouse approach with FoxJ1-GFP animals (Meletis et al. 2008). FoxJ1 expression is restricted to the central canal region, and it was assumed that there was no expression in GFAP+ cells. Using this line, Meletis et al. reported that the majority of spheres are derived from the GFP+ fraction with an approximate frequency of 0.2% of GFP+ cells giving rise to neurospheres. As no GFAP+ cell was observed around the canal in this study, it was concluded that adult spinal cord neural stem cells are

GFAP- ependymal cells. Yet, in contrast with the GFP+ population purified from hGFAP-GFP animals that contain GFP+ cells from both the central canal region and the parenchyma, the cells obtained from the FoxJ1-GFP mice appear to be exclusively derived from the cells in the central canal region. Thus, the obtained frequency of 0.2% for neurosphere formation in FoxJ1+ cells signifies that only a small subpopulation of undefined ependymal cells (1/5000) would be endowed with neural stem cell properties. Moreover, a recent elegant transcriptome analysis from Beckervordersandforth, et al. clearly indicated that in the SVZ, GFAP+ neural stem cells highly expressed FoxJ1 (Beckervordersandforth et al. 2010).

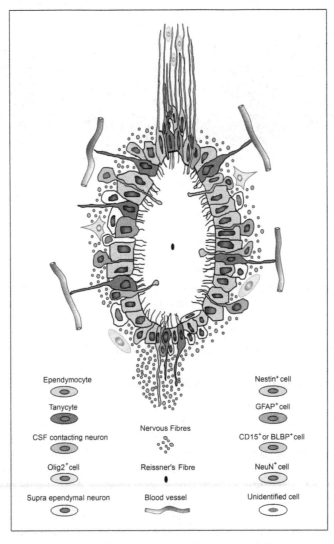

Fig. 6. Schematic drawing of the adult mouse ependymal region. Reproduced from (Sabourin et al. 2009)

Using immunofluorescence for FoxJ1 on hGFAP-GFP sections, we could readily observe double-labeled cells (Fig. 7, unpublished data). This indicated that in addition to the ependymocytes, the FoxJ1 transcription factor is also present in neural stem cells as also suggested by the study reported by Jacquet, BV et al (Jacquet et al. 2009).

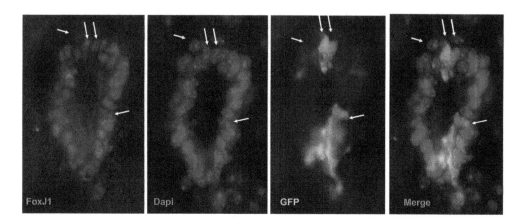

Fig. 7. Immunodetection of FoxJ1 in the cells around the central canal of the hGFAP-GFP adult mouse. The white arrows point to two GFP+ cells expressing FoxJ1. The yellow arrow indicates a subependymal FoxJ1-negative cell.

In the SVZ, neural stem cells are currently primarily considered to be CD133+ GFAP+ cells, whereas ependymocytes are endowed with a more restricted proliferative potential. In the spinal cord, most of the cells around the canal are CD133+ (Sabourin et al. 2009), and in primary neurospheres, CD133+ GFAP+ cells are frequently observed. Thus, it is likely that GFAP+ CD133+ cells in the adult spinal cord represent all or at least a substantial fraction of neural stem cells. Considering that in the SVZ, GFAP- transit amplifying cells can be converted into stem cells with EGF (Doetsch et al. 2002), the possibility still exists that a fraction of neurospheres could be derived from central canal GFAP- cells.

3.4 Developmental origin of the central canal region

Neurospheres derived from the mouse adult lumbar spinal cord express the Nkx6.1 transcription factor (Sabourin et al. 2009). In vivo, most cells around the central lumen also express this factor; however, there was a variable level of expression and the CSF-contacting neurons displayed the highest staining in our studies. During spinal cord development, Nkx6.1 is expressed in the ventral neural tube, which contains progenitor cells of three main neuronal classes: V2, MN and V3 interneurons (Briscoe et al. 2000). Using marker analysis, Fu et al. concluded that the central canal region in mice and chicks is derived from the Nkx6.1+ Nkx2.2- domain, which expresses the Olig2 transcription factor (Fu et al. 2003). The potential role of Nkx6.1 in the formation of the central canal niche might be to maintain adult stem cells, as suggested by its highly conserved expression in the chick, rodent and human (Fig. 9).

4. Neural precursor cells in the adult human spinal cord

Much of our knowledge of adult neural stem cells is derived from studies performed in rodents, but much less is known about these stem cells in humans. Adult neural stem and progenitor cells have been isolated from different parts of the human brain, i.e., the olfactory bulb, the SVZ, the hippocampus and the cortex, using the neurosphere assay (Arsenijevic et al. 2001; Roy et al. 1999; Roy et al. 2000; Nunes et al. 2003; Kukekov et al. 1999; Pagano et al. 2000; Scolding, Rayner, and Compston 1999; Sanai et al. 2004; Akiyama et al. 2001). There are major differences between the rodent and primate brain, not only concerning size and organization but also for the cell diversity and SVZ organization. Consequently, we set out to explore the organization of the central canal region and the presence of neural stem cells in the adult human spinal cord (Dromard et al. 2008). For this purpose, we used lumbar spinal cords from brain-dead organ-donor patients (24–70 years old) (Fig. 8) and cervical spinal cords from autopsy tissues.

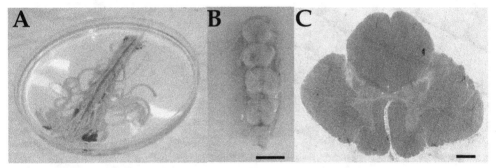

Fig. 8. A) Dissected human spinal cord (T9 thoracic region to caudal end). B) Thoracic, lumbar and sacral spinal cord fragments. Scale bar= 10 mm. C) Luxol staining of a thoraco-lumbar section. Scale bar=1 mm.

Histology and immunohistology studies revealed both similarities and dissimilarities between rodents and man. First, in contrast to mice, the central canal of the human spinal cord is often occluded (Dromard et al. 2008), as previously reported by (Fuller and Burger 1997; Milhorat, Kotzen, and Anzil 1994), and the ependymal region appeared disorganized, with the frequent presence of rosettes or microcanals. Reminiscent of the reported difference between the SVZ in rodents and humans (Quinones-Hinojosa et al. 2006), the human central canal is surrounded by a hypocellular region containing a high density of GFAP filaments and nerve fibers (Dromard et al. 2008). Equally contrasting with rodents, a cluster of Nestin+ subependymal cells was repeatedly observed in the ventral regions of cervical and lumbar spinal cords. Immunolabeling for CD15, Nestin, Nkx6.1, PSA-NCAM and Sox2 revealed, as observed in rodents, that this region retains immature features and is composed of several cell types in contact with the canal or in a subependymal position (Fig. 9).

Whereas most central canal cells expressed Nkx6.1 and Sox2, Nestin, GFAP and CD15 expression was restricted to cell subpopulations (Fig. 9). Nestin is only expressed by a fraction of cells in direct contact with the lumen or in a subependymal position. In contrast, to rodents, GFAP+ cells are numerous and more frequently located in direct contact with the lumen. Strikingly, CD15 expression is most often observed in cells in the dorsal region of the canal. In one lumbar spinal cord, we observed the expression of PSA-NCAM by a subpopulation of cells primarily localized on the ventral side of the central canal region. Taken together, these results represent the first analysis and reveal the complexity of this region in humans; however, further characterization, notably with new markers for neural stem cells, such as Bmi1, is required.

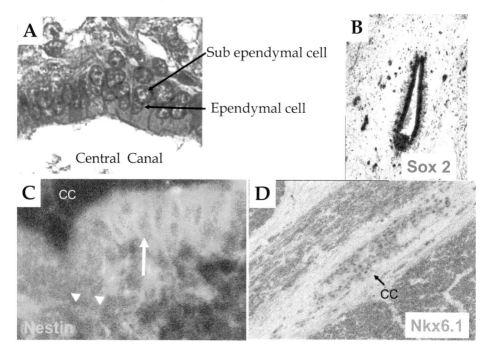

Fig. 9. A) Hematoxylin and eosin staining of a lumbar spinal cord section demonstrating the presence of several layers of cells in the central canal region. B, C, D) Immunodetection of the indicated protein. Note the intense Sox2 staining around the lumen (B), the presence of Nestin+ (arrows) and Nestin- (arrowheads) cells (C) and the expression of Nkx6.1 by central canal cells (D). In D, the central canal region is disorganized without a well-delimited lumen. These data may represent the actual organization or an artifact that occurred as a consequence of tissue processing for histology.

To explore the presence of neural stem or progenitor cells in the human spinal cord, we used the classical neurosphere assay. As compared with rodents, the frequency of neurosphere formation was at least 10 times lower (0.01-0.03 % of isolated cells). These neurospheres were Nestin+ Sox2+ and contained proliferative cells, as evidenced by Ki67 labeling and BrdU incorporation. In one sample, we were able to separate the central region from the surrounding tissue and observed that most of the spheres were derived from the central region. Upon differentiation (Fig. 10), these spheres generated glial (predominantly GFAP+ cells) and neuronal cells. These cells were mostly GABAergic, but some 5-HT neurons could be observed.

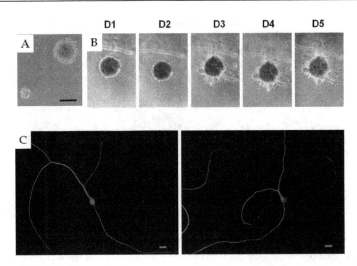

Fig. 10. A) Example of primary neurospheres derived from culturing dissociated human spinal cord cells (two weeks of culture). Scale bar= 500 μm. B) Neurosphere differentiation obtained by plating on an adhesive substrate for 5 days (D1-D5). C) Example of long Map2+ cells observed in differentiated neurospheres. Scale bars= 20 μm.

Importantly, despite intense attempts, we were not able to passage these neurospheres. This suggests that either these cells were progenitors with a limited proliferation potential or that the culture conditions were not adequate to sustain human neural stem cells self-renewal. As previously reported the long-term propagation of human neural stem cell culture is more challenging than that of rodents and might require specific techniques, such the absence of complete dissociation during the passaging process (Svendsen et al. 1998).

In addition to the neurosphere method, adherent conditions and a specific media containing serum could be used to isolate and propagate neural stem cells from the human temporal cortex and the hippocampus (Walton et al. 2006). We recently used these conditions as an attempt to isolate stem cells from the adult human spinal cord (Mamaeva et al. 2011). This attempt resulted in the isolation of a proliferating Nkx6.1+ Nestin+ cell population, which could be maintained for up to 9 passages. However, an in depth cellular characterization showed that these cells were acta2+ caldesmon+ calponin+ smooth muscle cells. These cells also displayed mesenchymal cell features, as evidenced by the high level of expression of the two transcription factors Snai2 and Twist1. We also observed that in vivo, Nkx6.1 was expressed by a subset of spinal cord vascular cells in addition to the central canal cells. Attempts to differentiate these cells into glial cells, neurons, chondrocytes and adipocytes were unproductive; however, these cells could readily become mineralized (formation of CaPO4) when placed under osteogenic conditions. The calcification of CNS muscular cell vessels has been observed since 1884 (Compston 2007; Obersteiner 1884) in pathological situations or as part of the aging process in the brain (Makariou and Patsalides 2009). These cells constitute a useful model for studying CNS vessel calcification in vitro.

Finally, preliminary work from our lab suggests that in addition to the central canal niche, neural precursor cells might also reside in the parenchyma. For instance, Dcx+ cells can be observed in the white matter, whereas scattered Sox2+ are notably present in the gray matter (Fig. 11). These results indicate that immature neural cells might represent a significant population of spinal cord cells with a completely unknown function.

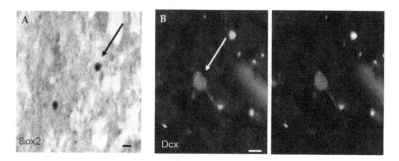

Fig. 11. A) Example of Sox2+ cells detected in the gray matter of the adult human spinal cord. B) Example of one Dcx+ cell detected in the white matter of the adult human spinal cord. Scale bars= 10 µm.

5. Role of the niche in spinal cord physiology and plasticity

5.1 Proliferation in the niche

The spinal cord elongates extensively during the post-natal period, and its size increases 2.5-fold in mice from birth to 13 weeks (Sabourin et al. 2009). In parallel with this extension, active proliferation is detected postnatally in the central canal region, notably in the ependymocytes, and subsequently declines at 12-13 weeks, which corresponds to the end of spinal cord elongation (Fu et al. 2003; Sabourin et al. 2009). This production of new cells is likely to be necessary for extending the length of the central canal. In addition, as observed postnatally in the brain SVZ (Suzuki and Goldman 2003), it is likely that cells are produced from the central region for myelination or for integration into the developing spinal cord circuitries. In contrast to young animals, in adult rodents and humans, proliferation is low or absent in the ependymal region. Thus, it appears that in adults, most central canal cells are quiescent, meaning that they are in an arrested but reversible state. Consistent with the proliferative decline observed in the postnatal period, we also noted that several markers, such as nestin, cadherin-13, and Sox4, are more highly expressed in young animals than in adults (Sabourin et al. 2009).

The central canal cells could, however, readily re-initiate proliferation in spinal cord traumas (Vaquero et al. 1981) and in several models for neurodegenerative diseases, such as in multiple sclerosis (Danilov et al. 2006) and amyotrophic lateral sclerosis (Chi et al. 2006). In these situations, cells migrate from the central canal region toward the lesion sites by a mechanism that may involve the SDF1/CXCR4 pathway which is present in these cells (Hugnot and Franzen 2010; Shechter, Ziv, and Schwartz 2007). Their fate appear to become mostly macroglial cells and not neurons, despite an increased expression of the transcription factor Pax-6 (Yamamoto et al. 2001; Johansson et al. 1999; Coksaygan et al. 2006). Indeed, they preferentially differentiate into GFAP+ astrocytes contributing to scar formation (Meletis et al. 2008; Johansson et al. 1999; Takahashi et al. 2003; Mothe and Tator 2005) and to some extent into myelinating Olig2 oligodendrocytes (Meletis et al. 2008) making them interesting candidates for myelin degeneration diseases like multiple sclerosis.

Collectively, these data emphasize an important postnatal role for the cells of the central canal region. In adults, these cells enter a dormant state, which could be reactivated in specific physiological situations or under pathological conditions.

5.2 Spinal cord central canal niche, physical exercise and spinal plasticity

Whereas the role of forebrain stem cell niches in memory and learning is being elucidated, the functions of the spinal cord niche, if there are any, remain elusive in adults. One important observation reported by (Cizkova et al. 2009; Foret et al. 2009; Krityakiarana et al. 2010) is that physical exercise (treadmill training and wheel running) can reactivate proliferation within the niche and increase nestin expression. The identity and fate of newly formed cells needs to be fully addressed using reliable labeling techniques, such as permanent genetic lineage tracing with Cre recombinase. One possibility is that the cells in the niche generate new CSF-contacting neurons upon training. Work by Marichal et al. showed that the latter are at different stages of maturation, which raises the possibility that they are in "standby mode" and, under some circumstances (e.g., injury or training), might complete maturation to integrate spinal circuits (Marichal et al. 2009). Another exciting possibility would be that newly formed cells contribute to spinal cord activity-dependent plasticity. For instance, in addition to the hippocampus, long-term potentiation (LTP) has recently been detected in the spinal cord dorsal horn following natural noxious stimulation (Randic, Jiang, and Cerne 1993; Rygh et al. 1999). In the brain, the experimental modification of neurogenesis alters hippocampal LTP (Snyder, Kee, and Wojtowicz 2001; Saxe et al. 2006). Similarly, one could consider the implication of cells generated in the central canal niche for dorsal horn LTP. Along this line, Shechter et al. reported the presence of newly formed GABAergic Dcx+ in the dorsal spinal cord region (Shechter, Ziv, and Schwartz 2007). Further investigations are needed to understand the origin and role of these cells.

The capacity of the spinal cord to learn and memorize is now acknowledged (Guertin 2008; Wolpaw 2010; Wolpaw and Tennissen 2001). For instance, basic spinal cord functions, such as stretch reflexes, can be conditioned even after complete spine transection. Locomotion is another flexible function. It is largely generated by spinal cord circuits localized, notably, in the lumbar region and called central pattern generators (Guertin and Steuer 2009). These circuits generate basic signals for walking. After spinal cord transection, these networks do not die and can be modified and reactivated by several days of specific training sessions. This learning allows rats and cats to display involuntary but structured walking on a treadmill (Rossignol et al. 2009). Whereas these examples of plasticity are largely mediated by synaptic modulations, one could also envision that long-term adaptation would involve the recruitment of new glial and potentially neuronal cells. By harboring cells with a high proliferation and differentiation potential, the central canal niche would be a particularly suited source for providing such new cells.

6. Conclusion

In addition to SVZ and hippocampus, the spinal cord central canal region constitutes a-third adult neural stem cell niche (Hugnot and Franzen 2010). In contrast with the brain, a sustained cell production is not observed in adults in which the niche appears to be largely dormant. In several spinal cord pathologies, the niche reactivates promptly to generate new astrocytes and oligodendrocytes, which participate in repopulating the damaged tissue in addition to forming the glial scar. It appears, therefore, that cells in the niche are in a stand-by but ready-to-go mode. This outstanding capacity is associated with the presence of fetal features in the niche that is well illustrated by the maintenance of activated developmental pathways and genes. These pathways will maintain cells at a high potential for proliferation, differentiation, delamination and migration. Far from being a simple layer of homogenous cells, both in man and in rodents, this region is highly organized and is composed of several cell types. Further work is required to exactly determine the different properties of these cells, which is particularly true for the Dcx+ CSF-contacting neuronal cells whose function is completely unknown. New cell-specific GFP transgenic mice together with fate mapping using Cre-Lox techniques will be valuable tools to address these issues.

Regarding spinal cord lesions, one important goal is to accurately control and redirect stem cell fate to endogenously repopulate the lesioned tissue with the appropriate cell type. This control and redirection would be an invaluable step for designing new therapeutic strategies against pathologies, such as amyotrophic lateral sclerosis or multiple sclerosis. It would require a detailed understanding of the molecular mechanisms involved in controlling spinal cord neural stem cell fate together with a broad knowledge of how stem cells generate specific neuronal cell subtypes during development. Thanks to intense developmental studies over the last 3 decades (Alaynick, Jessell, and Pfaff 2010), spinal cord development is particularly well described. These data are beginning to be exploited for redirecting adult stem cells into the appropriate cell types.

Investigating the presence and properties of neural precursor cells in humans is a prerequisite for designing regenerative strategies based on the endogenous cellular pool. However, work on adult human tissues is far more complicated than in rodents and raises important ethical, security, reproducibility, organizational and accessibility issues. These issues become exacerbated when research concerning non-pathological, non-fixed and well-preserved CNS is developed. The spinal cord is accessible in organ-donor patients, where thoracic and abdominal organs are removed for transplantation purposes (Dromard et al. 2008). Neurosurgeons could have access to this region of the CNS within hours after the patient is declared brain-dead. This access offers a unique opportunity to characterize the human spinal cord niche and to isolate different neural precursor cell types.

Finally, the spinal cord is an old (oldest ?) component of the CNS but is not just a simple bundle of fibers that connect the brain to the organs and the environment. Recent work has clearly revealed that this primitive CNS region harbors highly-organized internal circuits that are able to display short and long-term plasticity for adapting and memorizing. The spine cord possesses a well-described development and a relatively simple organization with a neural stem cell niche at the center. In addition, its activity can be easily and accurately manipulated by modulating different sensory components (e.g., nociception, temperature,...) and locomotor activity. Therefore, the spinal cord appears as a particularly interesting and simple model for studying the role of adult neural stem cells in CNS physiology. Further characterization of the niche in pathological situations will provide interesting clues on how to utilize this endogenous cell pool to treat spinal cord damage.

7. Acknowledgment

We would like to thank the Planiol foundation, the association Francaise contre les myopathies (AFM), the Rescue FP6 EU program, the Princess Grace de Monaco foundation and the Vertical Association for funding our work on spinal cord stem cells.

8. References

Akiyama, Y., O. Honmou, T. Kato, T. Uede, K. Hashi, and J. D. Kocsis. 2001. Transplantation of clonal neural precursor cells derived from adult human brain establishes functional peripheral myelin in the rat spinal cord. *Exp Neurol* 167 (1):27-39.

Alaynick, W. A., T. M. Jessell, and S. L. Pfaff. 2010. SnapShot: spinal cord development. *Cell* 146 (1):178-178 e1.

Armando, S., A. Lebrun, J. P. Hugnot, C. Ripoll, M. Saunier, and L. Simonneau. 2007. Neurosphere-derived neural cells show region-specific behaviour in vitro. *Neuroreport* 18 (15):1539-42.

Arsenijevic, Y., J. G. Villemure, J. F. Brunet, J. J. Bloch, N. Deglon, C. Kostic, A. Zurn, and P. Aebischer. 2001. Isolation of multipotent neural precursors residing in the cortex of the adult human brain. *Exp Neurol* 170 (1):48-62.

Beckervordersandforth, R., P. Tripathi, J. Ninkovic, E. Bayam, A. Lepier, B. Stempfhuber, F. Kirchhoff, J. Hirrlinger, A. Haslinger, D. C. Lie, J. Beckers, B. Yoder, M. Irmler, and M. Gotz. 2010. In vivo fate mapping and expression analysis reveals molecular hallmarks of prospectively isolated adult neural stem cells. *Cell Stem Cell* 7 (6):744-58.

Bodega, G., I. Suarez, M. Rubio, and B. Fernandez. 1994. Ependyma: phylogenetic evolution of glial fibrillary acidic protein (GFAP) and vimentin expression in vertebrate spinal cord. *Histochemistry* 102 (2):113-22.

Briscoe, J., A. Pierani, T. M. Jessell, and J. Ericson. 2000. A homeodomain protein code specifies progenitor cell identity and neuronal fate in the ventral neural tube. *Cell* 101 (4):435-45.

Browne, G., A. E. Sayan, and E. Tulchinsky. 2010. ZEB proteins link cell motility with cell cycle control and cell survival in cancer. *Cell Cycle* 9 (5):886-91.

Chi, L., Y. Ke, C. Luo, B. Li, D. Gozal, B. Kalyanaraman, and R. Liu. 2006. Motor neuron degeneration promotes neural progenitor cell proliferation, migration, and neurogenesis in the spinal cords of amyotrophic lateral sclerosis mice. *Stem Cells* 24 (1):34-43.

Cizkova, D., M. Nagyova, L. Slovinska, I. Novotna, J. Radonak, M. Cizek, E. Mechirova, Z. Tomori, J. Hlucilova, J. Motlik, I. Sulla, Jr., and I. Vanicky. 2009. Response of ependymal progenitors to spinal cord injury or enhanced physical activity in adult rat. *Cell Mol Neurobiol* 29 (6-7):999-1013.

Coksaygan, T., T. Magnus, J. Cai, M. Mughal, A. Lepore, H. Xue, I. Fischer, and M. S. Rao. 2006. Neurogenesis in Talpha-1 tubulin transgenic mice during development and after injury. *Exp Neurol* 197 (2):475-85.

Compston, A. 2007. From the archive "The cerebral blood-vessels in health and disease" by Pr H. Obersteiner. *Brain* 130:3057-3059.

Conti, L., and E. Cattaneo. 2010. Neural stem cell systems: physiological players or in vitro entities? *Nat Rev Neurosci* 11 (3):176-87.

Danilov, A. I., R. Covacu, M. C. Moe, I. A. Langmoen, C. B. Johansson, T. Olsson, and L. Brundin. 2006. Neurogenesis in the adult spinal cord in an experimental model of multiple sclerosis. *Eur J Neurosci* 23 (2):394-400.

Deleyrolle, L., S. Marchal-Victorion, C. Dromard, V. Fritz, M. Saunier, J. C. Sabourin, C. Tran Van Ba, A. Privat, and J. P. Hugnot. 2005. Exogenous and FGF2/EGF-regulated endogenous cytokines regulate neural precursor cell growth and differentiation. *Stem Cells.*

Deleyrolle, L. P., and B. A. Reynolds. 2009. Isolation, expansion, and differentiation of adult Mammalian neural stem and progenitor cells using the neurosphere assay. *Methods Mol Biol* 549:91-101.

Doetsch, F., L. Petreanu, I. Caille, J. M. Garcia-Verdugo, and A. Alvarez-Buylla. 2002. EGF converts transit-amplifying neurogenic precursors in the adult brain into multipotent stem cells. *Neuron* 36 (6):1021-34.

Dromard, C., H. Guillon, V. Rigau, C. Ripoll, J. C. Sabourin, F. E. Perrin, F. Scamps, S. Bozza, P. Sabatier, N. Lonjon, H. Duffau, F. Vachiery-Lahaye, M. Prieto, C. Tran Van Ba, L. Deleyrolle, A. Boularan, K. Langley, M. Gaviria, A. Privat, J. P. Hugnot, and L. Bauchet. 2008. Adult human spinal cord harbors neural precursor cells that generate neurons and glial cells in vitro. *J Neurosci Res* 86 (9):1916-26.

Foret, A., R. Quertainmont, O. Botman, D. Bouhy, P. Amabili, G. Brook, J. Schoenen, and R. Franzen. 2009. Stem cells in the adult rat spinal cord: plasticity after injury and treadmill training exercise. *J Neurochem* 112 (3):762-72.

Fu, H., Y. Qi, M. Tan, J. Cai, X. Hu, Z. Liu, J. Jensen, and M. Qiu. 2003. Molecular mapping of the origin of postnatal spinal cord ependymal cells: evidence that adult ependymal cells are derived from Nkx6.1+ ventral neural progenitor cells. *J Comp Neurol* 456 (3):237-44.

Fuller, G.N., and P.C. Burger. 1997. Central Nervous System. *Histology for Pathologists* Chapter 6:145-168.

Gage, F. H., J. Ray, and L. J. Fisher. 1995. Isolation, characterization, and use of stem cells from the CNS. *Annu Rev Neurosci* 18:159-92.

Guertin, P. 2008. Can the spinal cord learn and remember? *ScientificWorldJournal* 8:757-61.

Guertin, P. A., and I. Steuer. 2009. Key central pattern generators of the spinal cord. *J Neurosci Res* 87 (11):2399-405.

Hamilton, L. K., M. K. Truong, M. R. Bednarczyk, A. Aumont, and K. J. Fernandes. 2009. Cellular organization of the central canal ependymal zone, a niche of latent neural stem cells in the adult mammalian spinal cord. *Neuroscience* 164 (3):1044-56.

Horner, P. J., A. E. Power, G. Kempermann, H. G. Kuhn, T. D. Palmer, J. Winkler, L. J. Thal, and F. H. Gage. 2000. Proliferation and differentiation of progenitor cells throughout the intact adult rat spinal cord. *J Neurosci* 20 (6):2218-28.

Horstmann, E. 1954. [The fiber glia of selacean brain.]. *Z Zellforsch Mikrosk Anat* 39 (6):588-617.

Huang, A. L., X. Chen, M. A. Hoon, J. Chandrashekar, W. Guo, D. Trankner, N. J. Ryba, and C. S. Zuker. 2006. The cells and logic for mammalian sour taste detection. *Nature* 442 (7105):934-8.

Hugnot, J.P., and R. Franzen. 2010. The spinal cord ependymal region: A stem cell niche in the caudal central nervous system. *Frontiers in Bioscience* 16:1044-59.

Jacquet, B. V., R. Salinas-Mondragon, H. Liang, B. Therit, J. D. Buie, M. Dykstra, K. Campbell, L. E. Ostrowski, S. L. Brody, and H. T. Ghashghaei. 2009. FoxJ1-dependent gene expression is required for differentiation of radial glia into ependymal cells and a subset of astrocytes in the postnatal brain. *Development* 136 (23):4021-31.

Johansson, C. B., S. Momma, D. L. Clarke, M. Risling, U. Lendahl, and J. Frisen. 1999. Identification of a neural stem cell in the adult mammalian central nervous system. *Cell* 96 (1):25-34.

Krityakiarana, W., A. Espinosa-Jeffrey, C. A. Ghiani, P. M. Zhao, N. Topaldjikian, F. Gomez-Pinilla, M. Yamaguchi, N. Kotchabhakdi, and J. de Vellis. 2010. Voluntary exercise increases oligodendrogenesis in spinal cord. *Int J Neurosci* 120 (4):280-90.

Kukekov, V. G., E. D. Laywell, O. Suslov, K. Davies, B. Scheffler, L. B. Thomas, T. F. O'Brien, M. Kusakabe, and D. A. Steindler. 1999. Multipotent stem/progenitor cells with similar properties arise from two neurogenic regions of adult human brain. *Exp Neurol* 156 (2):333-44.

Kulbatski, I., A. J. Mothe, A. Keating, Y. Hakamata, E. Kobayashi, and C. H. Tator. 2007. Oligodendrocytes and radial glia derived from adult rat spinal cord progenitors: morphological and immunocytochemical characterization. *J Histochem Cytochem* 55 (3):209-22.

Kulbatski, I., and C. H. Tator. 2009. Region-specific differentiation potential of adult rat spinal cord neural stem/precursors and their plasticity in response to in vitro manipulation. *J Histochem Cytochem* 57 (5):405-23.

Leatherman, J. L., and S. Dinardo. 2008. Zfh-1 controls somatic stem cell self-renewal in the Drosophila testis and nonautonomously influences germline stem cell self-renewal. *Cell Stem Cell* 3 (1):44-54.

Lehtinen, M. K., M. W. Zappaterra, X. Chen, Y. J. Yang, A. D. Hill, M. Lun, T. Maynard, D. Gonzalez, S. Kim, P. Ye, A. J. D'Ercole, E. T. Wong, A. S. LaMantia, and C. A. Walsh. 2010. The cerebrospinal fluid provides a proliferative niche for neural progenitor cells. *Neuron* 69 (5):893-905.

Li, L., and H. Clevers. 2010. Coexistence of quiescent and active adult stem cells in mammals. *Science* 327 (5965):542-5.

Liu, Y., S. El-Naggar, D. S. Darling, Y. Higashi, and D. C. Dean. 2008. Zeb1 links epithelial-mesenchymal transition and cellular senescence. *Development* 135 (3):579-88.

Louis, S. A., R. L. Rietze, L. Deleyrolle, R. E. Wagey, T. E. Thomas, A. C. Eaves, and B. A. Reynolds. 2008. Enumeration of neural stem and progenitor cells in the neural colony-forming cell assay. *Stem Cells* 26 (4):988-96.

Makariou, E., and A.D. Patsalides. 2009. Intracranial calcifications. *Appl Radiol* 38 (11):48-50.

Mamaeva, D., C. Ripoll, C. Bony, M. Teigell, F. E. Perrin, B. Rothhut, I. Bieche, R. Lidereau, A. Privat, V. Rigau, H. Guillon, F. Vachiery-Lahaye, D. Noel, L. Bauchet, and J. P. Hugnot. Isolation of mineralizing Nestin+ Nkx6.1+ vascular muscular cells from the adult human spinal cord. *BMC Neurosci* 12 (1):99.

Marichal, N., G. Garcia, M. Radmilovich, O. Trujillo-Cenoz, and R. E. Russo. 2009. Enigmatic central canal contacting cells: immature neurons in "standby mode"? *J Neurosci* 29 (32):10010-24.

Martens, D. J., R. M. Seaberg, and D. van der Kooy. 2002. In vivo infusions of exogenous growth factors into the fourth ventricle of the adult mouse brain increase the proliferation of neural progenitors around the fourth ventricle and the central canal of the spinal cord. *Eur J Neurosci* 16 (6):1045-57.

Meletis, K., F. Barnabe-Heider, M. Carlen, E. Evergren, N. Tomilin, O. Shupliakov, and J. Frisen. 2008. Spinal cord injury reveals multilineage differentiation of ependymal cells. *PLoS Biol* 6 (7):e182.

Milhorat, T. H., R. M. Kotzen, and A. P. Anzil. 1994. Stenosis of central canal of spinal cord in man: incidence and pathological findings in 232 autopsy cases. *J Neurosurg* 80 (4):716-22.

Moreno-Manzano, V., F. J. Rodriguez-Jimenez, M. Garcia-Rosello, S. Lainez, S. Erceg, M. T. Calvo, M. Ronaghi, M. Lloret, R. Planells-Cases, J. M. Sanchez-Puelles, and M. Stojkovic. 2009. Activated spinal cord ependymal stem cells rescue neurological function. *Stem Cells* 27 (3):733-43.

Mothe, A. J., and C. H. Tator. 2005. Proliferation, migration, and differentiation of endogenous ependymal region stem/progenitor cells following minimal spinal cord injury in the adult rat. *Neuroscience* 131 (1):177-87.

Nishimura, G., I. Manabe, K. Tsushima, K. Fujiu, Y. Oishi, Y. Imai, K. Maemura, M. Miyagishi, Y. Higashi, H. Kondoh, and R. Nagai. 2006. DeltaEF1 mediates TGF-beta signaling in vascular smooth muscle cell differentiation. *Dev Cell* 11 (1):93-104.

Nolte, C., M. Matyash, T. Pivneva, C. G. Schipke, C. Ohlemeyer, U. K. Hanisch, F. Kirchhoff, and H. Kettenmann. 2001. GFAP promoter-controlled EGFP-expressing transgenic mice: a tool to visualize astrocytes and astrogliosis in living brain tissue. *Glia* 33 (1):72-86.

Nunes, M. C., N. S. Roy, H. M. Keyoung, R. R. Goodman, G. McKhann, 2nd, L. Jiang, J. Kang, M. Nedergaard, and S. A. Goldman. 2003. Identification and isolation of multipotential neural progenitor cells from the subcortical white matter of the adult human brain. *Nat Med* 9 (4):439-47.

Obersteiner, H. 1884. The cerebral blood-vessels in health and disease. *Brain* 7:289-389.

Pagano, S. F., F. Impagnatiello, M. Girelli, L. Cova, E. Grioni, M. Onofri, M. Cavallaro, S. Etteri, F. Vitello, S. Giombini, C. L. Solero, and E. A. Parati. 2000. Isolation and characterization of neural stem cells from the adult human olfactory bulb. *Stem Cells* 18 (4):295-300.

Palmer, T. D., A. R. Willhoite, and F. H. Gage. 2000. Vascular niche for adult hippocampal neurogenesis. *J Comp Neurol* 425 (4):479-94.

Pardal, R., P. , P. Ortega-Saenz, R. Duran, and J. Lopez-Barneo. 2007. Glia-like stem cells sustain physiologic neurogenesis in the adult mammalian carotid body. *Cell* 131 (2):364-77

Pluchino, S., A. Quattrini, E. Brambilla, A. Gritti, G. Salani, G. Dina, R. Galli, U. Del Carro, S. Amadio, A. Bergami, R. Furlan, G. Comi, A. L. Vescovi, and G. Martino. 2003. Injection of adult neurospheres induces recovery in a chronic model of multiple sclerosis. *Nature* 422 (6933):688-94.

Quinones-Hinojosa, A., N. Sanai, M. Soriano-Navarro, O. Gonzalez-Perez, Z. Mirzadeh, S. Gil-Perotin, R. Romero-Rodriguez, M. S. Berger, J. M. Garcia-Verdugo, and A. Alvarez-Buylla. 2006. Cellular composition and cytoarchitecture of the adult human subventricular zone: a niche of neural stem cells. *J Comp Neurol* 494 (3):415-34.

Rafols, J. A., and H. G. Goshgarian. 1985. Spinal tanycytes in the adult rat: a correlative Golgi gold-toning study. *Anat Rec* 211 (1):75-86.

Randic, M., M. C. Jiang, and R. Cerne. 1993. Long-term potentiation and long-term depression of primary afferent neurotransmission in the rat spinal cord. *J Neurosci* 13 (12):5228-41.

Redmond, D. E., Jr., K. B. Bjugstad, Y. D. Teng, V. Ourednik, J. Ourednik, D. R. Wakeman, X. H. Parsons, R. Gonzalez, B. C. Blanchard, S. U. Kim, Z. Gu, S. A. Lipton, E. A. Markakis, R. H. Roth, J. D. Elsworth, J. R. Sladek, Jr., R. L. Sidman, and E. Y. Snyder. 2007. Behavioral improvement in a primate Parkinson's model is associated with multiple homeostatic effects of human neural stem cells. *Proc Natl Acad Sci U S A* 104 (29):12175-80.

Reynolds, B. A., Tetzlaff W., and S. Weiss. 1992. A multipotent EGF-responsive striatal embryonic progenitor cell produces neurons and astrocytes. *J. Neurosci.* 12:4564-4574.

Rossignol, S., G. Barriere, O. Alluin, and A. Frigon. 2009. Re-expression of locomotor function after partial spinal cord injury. *Physiology (Bethesda)* 24:127-39.

Roy, N. S., S. Wang, C. Harrison-Restelli, A. Benraiss, R. A. Fraser, M. Gravel, P. E. Braun, and S. A. Goldman. 1999. Identification, isolation, and promoter-defined separation of mitotic oligodendrocyte progenitor cells from the adult human subcortical white matter. *J Neurosci* 19 (22):9986-95.

Roy, N. S., S. Wang, L. Jiang, J. Kang, A. Benraiss, C. Harrison-Restelli, R. A. Fraser, W. T. Couldwell, A. Kawaguchi, H. Okano, M. Nedergaard, and S. A. Goldman. 2000. In vitro neurogenesis by progenitor cells isolated from the adult human hippocampus. *Nat Med* 6 (3):271-7.

Rygh, L. J., F. Svendsen, K. Hole, and A. Tjolsen. 1999. Natural noxious stimulation can induce long-term increase of spinal nociceptive responses. *Pain* 82 (3):305-10.

Sabourin, J. C., K. B. Ackema, D. Ohayon, P. O. Guichet, F. E. Perrin, A. Garces, C. Ripoll, J. Charite, L. Simonneau, H. Kettenmann, A. Zine, A. Privat, J. Valmier, A. Pattyn, and J. P. Hugnot. 2009. A mesenchymal-like ZEB1(+) niche harbors dorsal radial glial fibrillary acidic protein-positive stem cells in the spinal cord. *Stem Cells* 27 (11):2722-33.

Sanai, N., A. D. Tramontin, A. Quinones-Hinojosa, N. M. Barbaro, N. Gupta, S. Kunwar, M. T. Lawton, M. W. McDermott, A. T. Parsa, J. Manuel-Garcia Verdugo, M. S. Berger, and A. Alvarez-Buylla. 2004. Unique astrocyte ribbon in adult human brain contains neural stem cells but lacks chain migration. *Nature* 427 (6976):740-4.

Saxe, M. D., F. Battaglia, J. W. Wang, G. Malleret, D. J. David, J. E. Monckton, A. D. Garcia, M. V. Sofroniew, E. R. Kandel, L. Santarelli, R. Hen, and M. R. Drew. 2006. Ablation of hippocampal neurogenesis impairs contextual fear conditioning and synaptic plasticity in the dentate gyrus. *Proc Natl Acad Sci U S A* 103 (46):17501-6.

Schafer, K. H., C. Van Ginneken, and S. Copray. 2009. Plasticity and neural stem cells in the enteric nervous system. *Anat Rec (Hoboken)* 292 (12):1940-52.

Scolding, N. J., P. J. Rayner, and D. A. Compston. 1999. Identification of A2B5-positive putative oligodendrocyte progenitor cells and A2B5-positive astrocytes in adult human white matter. *Neuroscience* 89 (1):1-4.

Seaberg, R. M., S. R. Smukler, and D. van der Kooy. 2005. Intrinsic differences distinguish transiently neurogenic progenitors from neural stem cells in the early postnatal brain. *Dev Biol* 278 (1):71-85.

Seitz, R., J. Lohler, and G. Schwendemann. 1981. Ependyma and meninges of the spinal cord of the mouse. A light-and electron-microscopic study. *Cell Tissue Res* 220 (1):61-72.

Seki, T., and Y. Arai. 1993. Highly polysialylated NCAM expression in the developing and adult rat spinal cord. *Brain Res Dev Brain Res* 73 (1):141-5.

Shechter, R., Y. Ziv, and M. Schwartz. 2007. New GABAergic interneurons supported by myelin-specific T cells are formed in intact adult spinal cord. *Stem Cells* 25 (9):2277-82.

Shihabuddin, L. S., J. Ray, and F. H. Gage. 1997. FGF-2 is sufficient to isolate progenitors found in the adult mammalian spinal cord. *Exp Neurol* 148 (2):577-86.

Singh, R. P. , Y. H. Cheng, P. Nelson, and F. C. Zhou. 2009. Retentive multipotency of adult dorsal root ganglia stem cells. *Cell Transplant* 18 (1):55-68

Snyder, J. S., N. Kee, and J. M. Wojtowicz. 2001. Effects of adult neurogenesis on synaptic plasticity in the rat dentate gyrus. *J Neurophysiol* 85 (6):2423-31.

Stoeckel, M. E., S. Uhl-Bronner, S. Hugel, P. Veinante, M. J. Klein, J. Mutterer, M. J. Freund-Mercier, and R. Schlichter. 2003. Cerebrospinal fluid-contacting neurons in the rat spinal cord, a gamma-aminobutyric acidergic system expressing the P2X2 subunit of purinergic receptors, PSA-NCAM, and GAP-43 immunoreactivities: light and electron microscopic study. *J Comp Neurol* 457 (2):159-74.

Suzuki, S. O., and J. E. Goldman. 2003. Multiple cell populations in the early postnatal subventricular zone take distinct migratory pathways: a dynamic study of glial and neuronal progenitor migration. *J Neurosci* 23 (10):4240-50.

Svendsen, C. N., M. G. ter Borg, R. J. Armstrong, A. E. Rosser, S. Chandran, T. Ostenfeld, and M. A. Caldwell. 1998. A new method for the rapid and long term growth of human neural precursor cells. *J Neurosci Methods* 85 (2):141-52.

Takahashi, M., Y. Arai, H. Kurosawa, N. Sueyoshi, and S. Shirai. 2003. Ependymal cell reactions in spinal cord segments after compression injury in adult rat. *J Neuropathol Exp Neurol* 62 (2):185-94.

Tanaka, E. M. 2003. Cell differentiation and cell fate during urodele tail and limb regeneration. *Curr Opin Genet Dev* 13 (5):497-501.

Vaquero, J., M. J. Ramiro, S. Oya, and J. M. Cabezudo. 1981. Ependymal reaction after experimental spinal cord injury. *Acta Neurochir (Wien)* 55 (3-4):295-302.

Vigh, B., M. J. Manzano e Silva, C. L. Frank, C. Vincze, S. J. Czirok, A. Szabo, A. Lukats, and A. Szel. 2004. The system of cerebrospinal fluid-contacting neurons. Its supposed role in the nonsynaptic signal transmission of the brain. *Histol Histopathol* 19 (2):607-28.

Walton, N. M., B. M. Sutter, H. X. Chen, L. J. Chang, S. N. Roper, B. Scheffler, and D. A. Steindler. 2006. Derivation and large-scale expansion of multipotent astroglial neural progenitors from adult human brain. *Development* 133 (18):3671-81.

Weiss, S., C. Dunne, J. Hewson, C. Wohl, M. Wheatley, A. C. Peterson, and B. A. Reynolds. 1996. Multipotent CNS stem cells are present in the adult mammalian spinal cord and ventricular neuroaxis. *J Neurosci* 16 (23):7599-609.

Wolpaw, J. R. 2010. What can the spinal cord teach us about learning and memory? *Neuroscientist* 16 (5):532-49.

Wolpaw, J. R., and A. M. Tennissen. 2001. Activity-dependent spinal cord plasticity in health and disease. *Annu Rev Neurosci* 24:807-43.

Yamamoto, S., M. Nagao, M. Sugimori, H. Kosako, H. Nakatomi, N. Yamamoto, H. Takebayashi, Y. Nabeshima, T. Kitamura, G. Weinmaster, K. Nakamura, and M. Nakafuku. 2001. Transcription factor expression and Notch-dependent regulation of neural progenitors in the adult rat spinal cord. *J Neurosci* 21 (24):9814-23.

4

Cellular Organization of the Subventricular Zone in the Adult Human Brain: A Niche of Neural Stem Cells

Oscar Gonzalez-Perez

Laboratory of Neuroscience, Facultad de Psicología, Universidad de Colima,
Department of Neuroscience,
Centro Universitario de Ciencias de la Salud,
Universidad de Guadalajara
Mexico

1. Introduction

The dogma that the brain is a quiescent organ incapable of postnatal neuron generation was first challenged in the sixties by Joseph Altman (Altman, 1962). He described the presence of thymidine-labeled cells in the subependymal zone located along the ventricular walls, which suggested the presence of dividing neurons in this brain region (Altman and Gopal, 1965; Altman and Das, 1967). A decade after, these findings were confirmed by other group using electron microscopy analyses (Kaplan and Hinds, 1977). Later, further studies described ongoing neurogenesis in female canaries (Goldman and Nottebohm, 1983), lizards (Pérez-Cañellas and García-Verdugo, 1996) and the adult mammalian brain (McDermott and Lantos, 1990; McDermott and Lantos, 1991; Lois and Alvarez-Buylla, 1993; Kornack and Rakic, 1995; Huang et al., 1998; Garcia-Verdugo et al., 2002). This process is mainly confined to the subventricular zone (SVZ) of the forebrain and the subgranular zone (SGZ) of the dentate gyrus in the hippocampus (Reznikov, 1991; Luskin, 1993; Lois and Alvarez-Buylla, 1994). The SVZ is the largest neurogenic niche in the adult brain (Luskin, 1993; Alvarez-Buylla and Garcia-Verdugo, 2002). Within this region resides a subpopulation of astrocytes with stem-cell-like features (Doetsch et al., 1999; Laywell et al., 2000; Imura et al., 2003; Morshead et al., 2003; Garcia et al., 2004). Recently, it has been suggested that the SVZ may be not only a source of neural precursor for brain repair, but also a source of brain tumors (Ignatova et al., 2002; Galli et al., 2004; Sanai et al., 2005; Vescovi et al., 2006). These hypotheses highlight the importance of studying and understanding the organization and regulation of the SVZ precursors. This chapter discusses and analyzes the cytoarchitecture and cellular composition of the human SVZ, as well as, its potential implications on the clinical treatment of neurodegenerative diseases and brain tumors.

2. Human neural stem cells

The gold standard for determining the presence of neural stem cells is the neurosphere assay (Reynolds and Rietze, 2005). This assay consists in plating a suspension of cells under serum-free, growth-factor-supplemented, non-adherent conditions in-vitro; thus, stem-like cells are able to divide and form multipotent undifferentiated clones called neurospheres (Reynolds and Weiss, 1992). The neurospheres can be serially dissociated and their single-cell clones are able to generate further spheres, while cells not capable of self-renewal eventually die (Reynolds and Rietze, 2005). These neurospheres are multipotent and can generate neurons, astrocytes and/or oligodendrocytes after the removal of mitogens and transfer to adherent plates (Reynolds and Weiss, 1992; Doetsch et al., 2002).

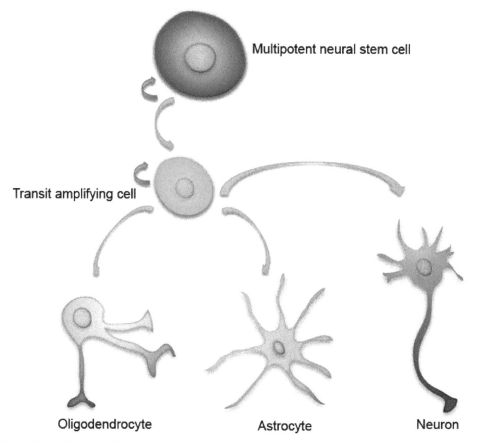

Fig. 1. Neural stem cells and their progeny in the adult SVZ. When a multipotent type B cell (on the top) divides, it generates to a type C cell, also known as transit-amplifying precursors, which can give rise to neurons and glial cells. The petite curved arrows represent the self-renewal capacity of type B and type C cells. *Figure reproduced with permission from: Alvarez-Palazuelos et al. Current Signal Transduction Therapy 2011;6(3) (Alvarez-Palazuelos et al., 2011). Copyright 2011 Bentham Science Publishers.*

Using neurosphere assays, neural stem cells have been isolated in human fetal cells (Chalmers-Redman et al., 1997). These multipotent human cells are also capable of self-renewal when maintained under serum-free conditions (Nunes et al., 2003). In the adult human brain, neural stem cells can be isolated from the SVZ and SGZ and give rise to neurons, oligodendrocytes and astrocytes in vitro (Figure 1) (Kukekov et al., 1999). Further evidence indicates that SVZ explants isolated from temporal lobectomies in patients with refractory epilepsy are capable of producing neurons in vitro (Kirschenbaum et al., 1994; Pincus et al., 1997). It has been suggested that new neurons are generated in the SGZ of the human hippocampus in vivo (Eriksson et al., 1998). This evidence has been obtained from postmortem brain tissue derived from patients with lung squamous cell carcinomas, who were diagnostically infused with bromodeoxyuridine to label mitotic cells. Nevertheless, despite this promising advances, none of these studies can demonstrate that the adult human brain possess neural stem cells per se, namely with self-renewal and multipotency properties (Vescovi et al., 2006).

2.1 The subventricular zone in the adult mammalian brain

The SVZ is the largest source of new neurons in the adult brain. This neurogenic region is located adjacent to the ependyma at the lateral wall of the lateral ventricles (Figure 2). The epithelial layer is composed by multiciliated non-mitotic ependymal cells, which contribute to the flow of cerebrospinal fluid and appear to play a role in the modulation of the stem cell niche (Lim et al., 2000; Spassky et al., 2005; Sawamoto et al., 2006; Mirzadeh et al., 2008). The SVZ contains a slowly dividing primary progeny (type B cells) and rapidly dividing cell precursors (type C cells) (Figure 2). Type B cells have been identified as the primary neural progenitors i.e., neural stem cells in the adult brain (Doetsch et al., 1999). Interestingly, based on differences in their location and morphology, type B progenitors are a subpopulation of astrocytes that can be categorized into two types: B1 and B2 astrocytes (Doetsch et al., 1997). At the ependymal side of the SVZ, type B1 astocytes are usually closely associated with the ependymal layer through adherens and gap junctions, and frequently extend a short apical process that reaches the ventricle (Mirzadeh et al., 2008). At the parenchymal side of the SVZ, type B1 astrocytes contact the basal lamina and blood vessels that underlie the SVZ (Shen et al., 2004; Mirzadeh et al., 2008). The ventricular end of the apical process of type B1 cells contains a non-motile primary cilium that contacts the cerebrospinal fluid (Mirzadeh et al., 2008). In contrast, type B2 astrocytes are located close to the brain parenchyma (Mirzadeh et al., 2008). It has been suggested that SVZ astrocytes play a dual role in neurogenesis, serving as both neural stem cells per se and supporting cells that promote neurogenesis (Lim and Alvarez-Buylla, 1999; Song et al., 2002).

The immediate progeny of type B1 astrocytes is known as transit amplifying progenitors or type C cells, which give rise to migrating neuroblasts (type A cells) (Figure 2)(Kriegstein and Alvarez-Buylla, 2009). These young neurons are surrounded by a glial sheath and migrate anteriorly toward the olfactory bulb (Jankovski and Sotelo, 1996; Lois et al., 1996; Doetsch et al., 1997). The adult SVZ also generates oligodendrocytes, although in much lower numbers than neuroblasts (Menn et al., 2006; Gonzalez-Perez et al., 2009; Gonzalez-Perez and Quinones-Hinojosa, 2010; Gonzalez-Perez et al., 2010b; Gonzalez-Perez and Alvarez-Buylla, 2011). The mechanisms that control the cell proliferation and renewal in the SVZ are not well-known, but increasing evidence indicates that neural stem cells are instructed via cell-cell contacts and extracellular signals from ependymal cells, immunological cells, the extracellular matrix, microglia, the local vasculature, neuronal inputs and the cerebrospinal fluid (Gonzalez-Perez et al., 2010a; Gonzalez-Perez and Alvarez-Buylla, 2011; Ihrie and Alvarez-Buylla, 2011).

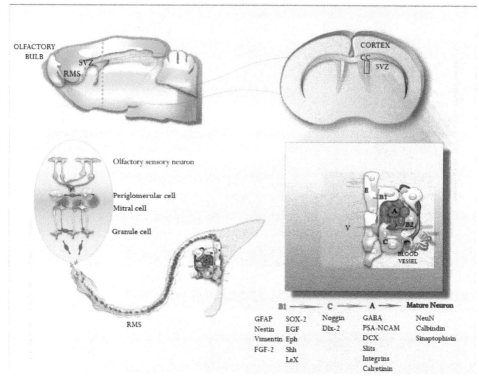

B1		C	A	Mature Neuron
GFAP	SOX-2	Noggin	GABA	NeuN
Nestin	EGF	Dlx-2	PSA-NCAM	Calbindin
Vimentin	Eph		DCX	Sinaptophisin
FGF-2	Shh		Slits	
	LeX		Integrins	
			Calretinin	

Fig. 2. Schematic representation of the localization and cellular composition of the adult subventricular zone (SVZ) in the rodent brain. Neuroblasts generated in the SVZ niche migrate to the olfactory bulb and, then, differentiate into granular and periglomerular GABAergic interneurons. Cell markers expressed by type B, type C, type A and mature neurons are listed under each cell label. V: Ventricle; E: Ependymal cell; CC: Corpus callosum; RMS: Rostral migratory stream. *Figure reproduced with permission from: Gonzalez-Perez et al. Current Immunology Reviews 2010;6(3):167 (Gonzalez-Perez et al., 2010b). Copyright 2010 Bentham Science Publishers.*

2.2 Cell type markers of the SVZ progenitors

As mentioned above, type B1 cells have astrocytic morphology and ultrastructure and express molecular markers that have been usually associated with astroglia, such as: the glial fibrillary acidic protein (GFAP), nestin, vimentin, connexin 30, the astrocyte-specific glutamate transporter (GLAST) and the brain-lipid-binding protein (BLBP) (Doetsch et al., 1999; Hartfuss et al., 2001; Kriegstein and Alvarez-Buylla, 2009). Type B1 astrocytes also express the cell surface carbohydrate Lewis X (LeX)/CD15/SSEA-, which has been proposed as a marker of neural stem cells in the SVZ (Capela and Temple, 2002). In addition, type B1 cells express prominin-1, also known as CD133, a protein commonly used as a stem-cell marker (Coskun et al., 2008; Shmelkov et al., 2008; Beckervordersandforth et al., 2010). However, prominin-1 expression at the apical endings of type B1 cells appears to be dynamically regulated (Mirzadeh et al., 2008). Therefore, given that Type B1 cells have many astroglial characteristics, finding potential markers to distinguish the B1 cell progeny from other non-multipotent astrocytes would be very useful in future studies. Some markers generally used to identify type-C cells are the epidermal growth factor receptor (EGFR), Dlx2 and Ascl1 (also known as Mash1) transcription factors (Doetsch et al., 2002; Parras et al., 2004), while doublecortin and the polysialylated neural cell adhesion molecule are useful to identify A-cell progeny (SVZ neuroblasts) (Lois and Alvarez-Buylla, 1994; Rousselot et al., 1995; Francis et al., 1999). Ependymal cells express S100beta and CD24 (Raponi et al., 2007; Mirzadeh et al., 2008).

Longitudinal analysis of molecular markers within the SVZ progenitor cells indicates that many of these proteins are expressed at particular points along the cell differentiation of neural stem cells. For instance, while GFAP expression is restricted to B cell progeny, GLAST and the orphan nuclear receptor Tlx is also present in a subpopulation of type C cells (Pastrana et al., 2009). Similarly, EGFR and Mash1are expressed in a limited number of type B cells, and they possibly may be useful to label "activated" type B cells (Doetsch et al., 2002; Gonzalez-Perez et al., 2010a; Gonzalez-Perez and Alvarez-Buylla, 2011). In addition, nestin expression that was thought to be exclusive to adult neural stem cells has been found broadly expressed within the brain (Hendrickson et al., 2011). Taken together, this evidence indicates that marker for stem and/or progenitor cells are likely to identify overlapping, but not identical subpopulations of SVZ cells. Therefore, researchers should be cautious when assigning biological characteristics to a subset of SVZ cells (Chojnacki et al., 2009).

2.3 The cell composition and architecture of the human subventricular zone

The human SVZ is located within the lateral wall of the lateral ventricles and consist of four layers with very particular cell compositions (Figure 3) (Quinones-Hinojosa et al., 2006). The layer adjacent to the lateral ventricle (Layer I) is formed by a monolayer of multiciliated ependymal cells with basal cytoplasm expansions that are either tangential or perpendicular to the ventricular surface. The Layer II or hypocellular layer is comprised of some of ependymal cytoplasm expansions interconnected with a number of astrocyte processes and very rare astrocytic and neuronal cell bodies (Figure 3) (Quinones-Hinojosa et al., 2006). The biological relevance of this hypocellular gap, is unknown, but it may be a remnant of the brain development at embryonic stages, because from this region a number of new neurons born and migrate radially and tangentially toward cortical and subcortical structures (Guerrero-Cazares et al., 2011). Other hypotheses suggest that the astrocytic and ependymal interconnections within this layer regulate neuronal functions or preserve metabolic homeostasis in the SVZ (Ihrie and Alvarez-Buylla, 2011; Ihrie et al., 2011). Abutting the hypocellular layer is a ribbon of astrocyte somata (Layer III) (Figure 3), which shows some proliferative activity as indicated by postmortem Ki67 expression (Sanai et al., 2004; Quinones-Hinojosa et al., 2006). It is believed that a subpopulation of astrocytes within this ribbon can proliferate in vivo, as well as form multipotent neurospheres (Sanai et al., 2004; Quinones-Hinojosa et al., 2007). Based on differences in their location and morphology by electron microscopy, the SVZ astrocytes can be subdivided into three types (Quinones-Hinojosa et al., 2006): The small astrocytes that are predominantly found in the hypocellular layer, and possess long, tangential cytoplasm processes. These astrocytes contain scarce cytoplasm, very dense bundles of intermediate filaments and sparse organelles. The second type of astroglia is the large astrocyte that has large cytoplasm expansions, abundant organelles and is found at the interface between Layer II and III and within the ribbon itself. This type of astrocyte is primarily found in the medial wall at the level of the body of the lateral ventricle. The third type of astrocyte is also large, but it possesses few organelles and is primarily found in the ventral temporal horn overlying the hippocampus. To date, the physiological relevance n of these three types of astrocytes is unknown differences, but in vitro evidence sugests that neural stem cells may belong to one of these astrocytic subtypes (Sanai et al., 2004). On the other hand, small clusters of displaced ependymal ells can be occasionally found embedded within this ribbon. This type of cells has abundant cilia, junctional complexes and microvilli (Figure 3). Finally, a few oligodendrocytes that do not appear to be myelinating axons are also seen in the Layer III (Figure 3). The deepest layer, the Layer IV is comprised of a number of myelin tracts and is considered a transition zone between the astrocytic ribbon and the brain parenchyma (Quinones-Hinojosa et al., 2007).

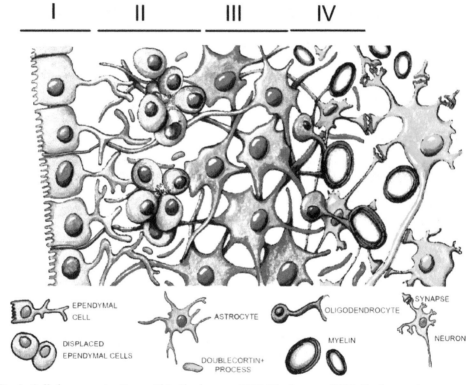

Fig. 3. Cellular organization within the human SVZ. The human SVZ displays unique characteristics as compared to the rodent or primate SVZ. Briefly, layer II devoid of cell bodies, type B cells (astrocytes) are organized as a ribbon of GFAP+ cells, which is not in close contact with the ependymal layer, no chains of migrating neuroblasts are found along the ventricular wall, and very few neuronal cell bodies as well as proliferating cells can be found within the human SVZ. *Figure reproduced with permission from: Alvarez-Palazuelos et al. Current Signal Transduction Therapy 2011;6(3) (Alvarez-Palazuelos et al., 2011). Copyright 2011 Bentham Science Publishers.*

As described above, many features of the human SVZ (Figure 3) are dissimilar to the well-studied rodent SVZ (Figure 2). Some of these fundamental differences are: First, the presence of a layer devoid of cell bodies (Layer II), which contrast with findings reported in the lizard, rodent, feline, canine or primate SVZ that show that all of them have type B cells in close contact to ependymal cells (Doetsch et al., 1997). The second dissimilarity is that the human SVZ lacks chains of migrating neuroblasts (Sanai et al., 2004; Quinones-Hinojosa et al., 2006; Sanai et al., 2007; Wang et al., 2011). Although some authors have suggested that other regions might have migrating cells in the human brain (Bernier et al., 2000; Curtis et al., 2007). Third, the number of proliferating cells (Ki-67 or PCNA expressing cells) in the human SVZ is significantly less than that reported in the rodent SVZ (Sanai et al., 2004; Quinones-Hinojosa et al., 2006; Sanai et al., 2007). Finally, the human SVZ has also very few neuronal cell bodies as compared to other species (Doetsch et al., 1997; Sanai et al., 2004; Quinones-Hinojosa et al., 2006; Sanai et al., 2007). In summary, all these obvious differences between the cell compositions of the human versus the rodent SVZ may also indicate functional differences that need to be studied in detail.

3. Conclusion

Until the end of the twenty century, the brain was perceived as a quiescent organ, with only glia able to have postnatal mitosis. This view was challenged with the isolation of neural stem cells within the adult brain. These multipotent and self-renewing cells are primary located within two germinal niches, the SVZ and SGZ of the hippocampus. The SVZ is the largest source of new cells in adult mammals; thus, a detailed understanding of this neurogenic region may have fundamental medical implications. Nevertheless, a number of questions remain to be elucidated, including the understanding of the role of SVZ neurogenesis in physiological processes such as learning, memory and cell migration. Moreover, SVZ neural stem cells might have some medical uses for a number of neurological disorders including Alzheimer's disease, multiple sclerosis, ischemia, Parkinson's disease, schizophrenia, depression and others. In contrast, since genetic alterations can be acquired through our life time, some groups have proposed that the SVZ may also represent a source of cells for the development of malignant brain tumors but, so far, there is no concluding evidence to support this hypothesis. In summary, the study of neural stem cells in the human SVZ, which is distinct region from those of other animal species, is a vital step with potential medical implications. Therefore new research on the human brain tissue is very important to elucidate these questions.

4. Acknowledgment

This work was supported by grants from the Consejo Nacional de Ciencia y Tecnologia (CONACyT; CB-2008-101476) and The National Institute of Health and the National Institute of Neurological Disorders and Stroke (NIH/NINDS; R01 NS070024-02).

5. References

Altman J (1962) Are new neurons formed in the brains of adult mammals? Science 135:1127-1128.

Altman J, Gopal DD (1965) Post-natal origin of microneurones in the rat brain. Nature 207:953-956.

Altman J, Das GD (1967) Autoradiographic and Histological Studies of Postnatal Neurogenesis. I. A Longitudinal Investigation of the Kinetics, Migration and Transformation of Cells Incorporating Tritiated Thymidine in Neonate Rats, with Special Reference to Postnatal Neurogenesis in Some Brain Regions. JCompNeurol 126:337-390.

Alvarez-Buylla A, Garcia-Verdugo JM (2002) Neurogenesis in adult subventricular zone. J Neurosci 22:629-634.

Alvarez-Palazuelos LE, Robles-Cervantes MS, Castillo-Velázquez G, Rivas-Souza M, Guzman-Muniz J, Moy-Lopez N, González-Castañeda RE, Luquín S, González-Pérez O (2011) Regulation of neural stem cell in the SVZ by thopic and morphogenic factors. Current Signal Transduction Therapy 6:in press.

Beckervordersandforth R, Tripathi P, Ninkovic J, Bayam E, Lepier A, Stempfhuber B, Kirchhoff F, Hirrlinger J, Haslinger A, Lie DC, Beckers J, Yoder B, Irmler M, Gotz M (2010) In vivo fate mapping and expression analysis reveals molecular hallmarks of prospectively isolated adult neural stem cells. Cell Stem Cell 7:744-758.

Bernier PJ, Vinet J, Cossette M, Parent A (2000) Characterization of the subventricular zone of the adult human brain: evidence for the involvement of Bcl-2. Neurosci Res 37:67-78.

Capela A, Temple S (2002) LeX/ssea-1 is expressed by adult mouse CNS stem cells, identifying them as nonependymal. Neuron 35:865-875.

Coskun V, Wu H, Blanchi B, Tsao S, Kim K, Zhao J, Biancotti JC, Hutnick L, Krueger RC, Jr., Fan G, de Vellis J, Sun YE (2008) CD133+ neural stem cells in the ependyma of mammalian postnatal forebrain. Proc Natl Acad Sci U S A 105:1026-1031.

Curtis MA, Kam M, Nannmark U, Anderson MF, Axell MZ, Wikkelso C, Holtas S, van Roon-Mom WM, Bjork-Eriksson T, Nordborg C, Frisen J, Dragunow M, Faull RL, Eriksson PS (2007) Human neuroblasts migrate to the olfactory bulb via a lateral ventricular extension. Science 315:1243-1249.

Chalmers-Redman RM, Priestley T, Kemp JA, Fine A (1997) In vitro propagation and inducible differentiation of multipotential progenitor cells from human fetal brain. Neuroscience 76:1121-1128.

Chojnacki AK, Mak GK, Weiss S (2009) Identity crisis for adult periventricular neural stem cells: subventricular zone astrocytes, ependymal cells or both? Nat Rev Neurosci 10:153-163.

Doetsch F, Garcia-Verdugo JM, Alvarez-Buylla A (1997) Cellular composition and three-dimensional organization of the subventricular germinal zone in the adult mammalian brain. JNeurosci 17:5046-5061.

Doetsch F, Caille I, Lim DA, Garcia-Verdugo JM, Alvarez-Buylla A (1999) Subventricular zone astrocytes are neural stem cells in the adult mammalian brain. Cell 97:703-716.

Doetsch F, Petreanu L, Caille I, Garcia-Verdugo JM, Alvarez-Buylla A (2002) EGF converts transit-amplifying neurogenic precursors in the adult brain into multipotent stem cells. Neuron 36:1021-1034.

Eriksson PS, Perfilieva E, Bjork-Eriksson T, Alborn A, Nordborg C, Peterson DA, Gage FH (1998) Neurogenesis in the adult human hippocampus. Nature Medicine 4:1313-1317.

Francis F, Koulakoff A, Boucher D, Chafey P, Schaar B, Vinet M-C, G., McDonnell N, Reiner O, Kahn A, McConnell SK, Berwald-Netter Y, Denoulet P, Chelly J (1999)

Doublecortin Is a Developmentally Regulated, Microtubule-Associated Protein Expressed in Migrating and Differentiating Neurons. Neuron 23:247-256.

Galli R, Binda E, Orfanelli U, Cipelletti B, Gritti A, De Vitis S, Fiocco R, Foroni C, Dimeco F, Vescovi A (2004) Isolation and characterization of tumorigenic, stem-like neural precursors from human glioblastoma. Cancer Res 64:7011-7021.

Garcia-Verdugo JM, Ferron S, Flames N, Collado L, Desfilis E, Font E (2002) The proliferative ventricular zone in adult vertebrates: a comparative study using reptiles, birds, and mammals. Brain Res Bull 57:765-775.

Garcia AD, Doan NB, Imura T, Bush TG, Sofroniew MV (2004) GFAP-expressing progenitors are the principal source of constitutive neurogenesis in adult mouse forebrain. Nat Neurosci 7:1233-1241.

Goldman SA, Nottebohm F (1983) Neuronal production, migration, and differentiation in a vocal control nucleus of the adult female canary brain. ProcNatlAcadSciUSA 80:2390-2394.

Gonzalez-Perez O, Quinones-Hinojosa A (2010) Dose-dependent effect of EGF on migration and differentiation of adult subventricular zone astrocytes. Glia 58:975-983.

Gonzalez-Perez O, Alvarez-Buylla A (2011) Oligodendrogenesis in the subventricular zone and the role of epidermal growth factor. Brain Res Rev 67:147-156.

Gonzalez-Perez O, Quinones-Hinojosa A, Garcia-Verdugo JM (2010a) Immunological control of adult neural stem cells. J Stem Cells 5:23-31.

Gonzalez-Perez O, Jauregui-Huerta F, Galvez-Contreras AY (2010b) Immune system modulates the function of adult neural stem cells. Curr Immunol Rev 6:167-173.

Gonzalez-Perez O, Romero-Rodriguez R, Soriano-Navarro M, Garcia-Verdugo JM, Alvarez-Buylla A (2009) Epidermal growth factor induces the progeny of subventricular zone type B cells to migrate and differentiate into oligodendrocytes. Stem Cells 27:2032-2043.

Guerrero-Cazares H, Gonzalez-Perez O, Soriano-Navarro M, Zamora-Berridi G, Garcia-Verdugo JM, Quinones-Hinojosa A (2011) Cytoarchitecture of the lateral ganglionic eminence and rostral extension of the lateral ventricle in the human fetal brain. J Comp Neurol 519:1165-1180.

Hartfuss E, Galli R, Heins N, Gotz M (2001) Characterization of CNS precursor subtypes and radial glia. Dev Biol 229:15-30.

Hendrickson ML, Rao AJ, Demerdash ON, Kalil RE (2011) Expression of nestin by neural cells in the adult rat and human brain. PLoS One 6:e18535.

Huang L, DeVries GJ, Bittman EL (1998) Photoperiod Regulates Neuronal Bromodeoxyuridine Labeling in the Brain of a Seasonally Breeding Mammal. JNeurobiol 36:410-420.

Ignatova TN, Kukekov VG, Laywell ED, Suslov ON, Vrionis FD, Steindler DA (2002) Human cortical glial tumors contain neural stem-like cells expressing astroglial and neuronal markers in vitro. Glia 39:193-206.

Ihrie RA, Alvarez-Buylla A (2011) Lake-front property: a unique germinal niche by the lateral ventricles of the adult brain. Neuron 70:674-686.

Ihrie RA, Shah JK, Harwell CC, Levine JH, Guinto CD, Lezameta M, Kriegstein AR, Alvarez-Buylla A (2011) Persistent sonic hedgehog signaling in adult brain determines neural stem cell positional identity. Neuron 71:250-262.

Imura T, Kornblum HI, Sofroniew MV (2003) The Predominant Neural Stem Cell Isolated from Postnatal and Adult Forebrain But Not Early Embryonic Forebrain Expresses GFAP. J Neurosci 23:2824-2832.

Jankovski A, Sotelo C (1996) Subventricular zone-olfactory bulb migratory pathway in the adult mouse: cellular composition and specificity as determined by heterochronic and heterotopic transplantation. J Comp Neurol 371:376-396.

Kaplan MS, Hinds JW (1977) Neurogenesis in the adult rat: Electron microscopic analysis of light radioautographs. Science 197:1092-1094.

Kirschenbaum B, Nedergaard M, Preuss A, Barami K, Fraser RAR, Goldman SA (1994) In vitro Neuronal Production and Differentiation by Precursor Cells Derived from the Adult Human Forebrain. CerebCortex 6:576-589.

Kornack DR, Rakic P (1995) Radial and horizontal deployment of clonally related cells in the primate neocortex: Relationship to distinct mitotic lineages. Neuron 15:311-321.

Kriegstein A, Alvarez-Buylla A (2009) The glial nature of embryonic and adult neural stem cells. Annu Rev Neurosci 32:149-184.

Kukekov VG, Laywell ED, Suslov O, Davies K, Scheffler B, Thomas LB, O'Brien TF, Kusakabe M, Steindler DA (1999) Multipotent stem/progenitor cells with similar properties arise from two neurogenic regions of adult human brain. Exp Neurol 156:333-344.

Laywell ED, Rakic P, Kukekov VG, Holland EC, Steindler DA (2000) Identification of a multipotent astrocytic stem cell in the immature and adult mouse brain. Proc Natl Acad Sci U S A 97:13883-13888.

Lim DA, Alvarez-Buylla A (1999) Interaction between astrocytes and adult subventricular zone precursors stimulates neurogenesis. Proc Natl Acad Sci U S A 96. 96:7526-7531.

Lim DA, D. TA, Trevejo JM, Herrera DG, García-Verdugo JM, Alvarez-Buylla A (2000) Noggin Antagonizes BMP Signaling to Create a Niche for Adult Neurogenesis. Neuron 28:713-726.

Lois C, Alvarez-Buylla A (1993) Proliferating subventricular zone cells in the adult mammalian forebrain can differentiate into neurons and glia. ProcNatlAcadSciUSA 90:2074-2077.

Lois C, Alvarez-Buylla A (1994) Long-distance neuronal migration in the adult mammalian brain. Science 264:1145-1148.

Lois C, Garcia-Verdugo JM, Alvarez-Buylla A (1996) Chain migration of neuronal precursors. Science 271:978-981.

Luskin MB (1993) Restricted proliferation and migration of postnatally generated neurons derived from the forebrain subventricular zone. Neuron 11:173-189.

McDermott KW, Lantos PL (1991) Distribution and fine structural analysis of undifferentiated cells in the primate subependymal layer. JAnat 178:45-63.

McDermott KWG, Lantos PL (1990) Cell proliferation in the subependymal layer of the postnatal marmoset, Callithrix jacchus. DevBrain Res 57:269-277.

Menn B, Garcia-Verdugo JM, Yaschine C, Gonzalez-Perez O, Rowitch D, Alvarez-Buylla A (2006) Origin of oligodendrocytes in the subventricular zone of the adult brain. J Neurosci 26:7907-7918.

Mirzadeh Z, Merkle FT, Soriano-Navarro M, Garcia-Verdugo JM, Alvarez-Buylla A (2008) Neural stem cells confer unique pinwheel architecture to the ventricular surface in neurogenic regions of the adult brain. Cell Stem Cell 3:265-278.

Morshead CM, Garcia AD, Sofroniew MV, van Der Kooy D (2003) The ablation of glial fibrillary acidic protein-positive cells from the adult central nervous system results in the loss of forebrain neural stem cells but not retinal stem cells. Eur J Neurosci 18:76-84.

Nunes MC, Roy NS, Keyoung HM, Goodman RR, McKhann G, 2nd, Jiang L, Kang J, Nedergaard M, Goldman SA (2003) Identification and isolation of multipotential neural progenitor cells from the subcortical white matter of the adult human brain. Nat Med 9:439-447.

Parras CM, Galli R, Britz O, Soares S, Galichet C, Battiste J, Johnson JE, Nakafuku M, Vescovi A, Guillemot F (2004) Mash1 specifies neurons and oligodendrocytes in the postnatal brain. Embo J 23:4495-4505.

Pastrana E, Cheng LC, Doetsch F (2009) Simultaneous prospective purification of adult subventricular zone neural stem cells and their progeny. Proc Natl Acad Sci U S A 106:6387-6392.

Pérez-Cañellas MR, García-Verdugo JM (1996) Adult neurogenesis in the telencephalon of a lizard: A [3H]thymidine autoradiographic and bromodeoxyuridine immunocytochemical study. DevBrain Res 93:49-61.

Pincus DW, Harrison-Restelli C, Barry J, Goodman RR, Fraser RA, Nedergaard M, Goldman SA (1997) In vitro neurogenesis by adult human epileptic temporal neocortex. Clin Neurosurg 44:17-25.

Quinones-Hinojosa A, Sanai N, Gonzalez-Perez O, Garcia-Verdugo JM (2007) The human brain subventricular zone: stem cells in this niche and its organization. Neurosurg Clin N Am 18:15-20, vii.

Quinones-Hinojosa A, Sanai N, Soriano-Navarro M, Gonzalez-Perez O, Mirzadeh Z, Gil-Perotin S, Romero-Rodriguez R, Berger MS, Garcia-Verdugo JM, Alvarez-Buylla A (2006) Cellular composition and cytoarchitecture of the adult human subventricular zone: a niche of neural stem cells. J Comp Neurol 494:415-434.

Raponi E, Agenes F, Delphin C, Assard N, Baudier J, Legraverend C, Deloulme JC (2007) S100B expression defines a state in which GFAP-expressing cells lose their neural stem cell potential and acquire a more mature developmental stage. Glia 55:165-177.

Reynolds B, Weiss S (1992) Generation of neurons and astrocytes from isolated cells of the adult mammalian central nervous system. Science 255:1707-1710.

Reynolds BA, Rietze RL (2005) Neural stem cells and neurospheres--re-evaluating the relationship. Nat Methods 2:333-336.

Reznikov KY (1991) Cell proliferation and cytogenesis in the mouse hippocampus. Adv Anat Embryol Cell Biol 122:1-74.

Rousselot P, Lois C, Alvarez-Buylla A (1995) Embryonic (PSA) N-CAM reveals chains of migrating neuroblasts between the lateral ventricle and the olfactory bulb of adult mice. JCompNeurol 351:51-61.

Sanai N, Alvarez-Buylla A, Berger MS (2005) Neural stem cells and the origin of gliomas. N Engl J Med 353:811-822.

Sanai N, Berger MS, Garcia-Verdugo JM, Alvarez-Buylla A (2007) Comment on "Human neuroblasts migrate to the olfactory bulb via a lateral ventricular extension". Science 318:393; author reply 393.

Sanai N, Tramontin AD, Quinones-Hinojosa A, Barbaro NM, Gupta N, Kunwar S, Lawton MT, McDermott MW, Parsa AT, Manuel-Garcia Verdugo J, Berger MS, Alvarez-Buylla A (2004) Unique astrocyte ribbon in adult human brain contains neural stem cells but lacks chain migration. Nature 427:740-744.

Sawamoto K, Wichterle H, Gonzalez-Perez O, Cholfin JA, Yamada M, Spassky N, Murcia NS, Garcia-Verdugo JM, Marin O, Rubenstein JL, Tessier-Lavigne M, Okano H, Alvarez-Buylla A (2006) New neurons follow the flow of cerebrospinal fluid in the adult brain. Science 311:629-632.

Shen Q, Goderie SK, Jin L, Karanth N, Sun Y, Abramova N, Vincent P, Pumiglia K, Temple S (2004) Endothelial cells stimulate self-renewal and expand neurogenesis of neural stem cells. Science 304:1338-1340.

Shmelkov SV, Butler JM, Hooper AT, Hormigo A, Kushner J, Milde T, St Clair R, Baljevic M, White I, Jin DK, Chadburn A, Murphy AJ, Valenzuela DM, Gale NW, Thurston G, Yancopoulos GD, D'Angelica M, Kemeny N, Lyden D, Rafii S (2008) CD133 expression is not restricted to stem cells, and both CD133+ and CD133- metastatic colon cancer cells initiate tumors. J Clin Invest 118:2111-2120.

Song H, Stevens CF, Gage FH (2002) Astroglia induce neurogenesis from adult neural stem cells. Nature 417:39-44.

Spassky N, Merkle FT, Flames N, Tramontin AD, Garcia-Verdugo JM, Alvarez-Buylla A (2005) Adult ependymal cells are postmitotic and are derived from radial glial cells during embryogenesis. J Neurosci 25:10-18.

Vescovi AL, Galli R, Reynolds BA (2006) Brain tumour stem cells. Nat Rev Cancer 6:425-436.

Wang C, Liu F, Liu YY, Zhao CH, You Y, Wang L, Zhang J, Wei B, Ma T, Zhang Q, Zhang Y, Chen R, Song H, Yang Z (2011) Identification and characterization of neuroblasts in the subventricular zone and rostral migratory stream of the adult human brain. Cell Res.

5

Development of New Monoclonal Antibodies for Immunocytochemical Characterization of Neural Stem and Differentiated Cells

Aavo-Valdur Mikelsaar[1], Alar Sünter[2], Peeter Toomik[3],
Kalmer Karpson[4] and Erkki Juronen[5]

[1]Institute of General and Molecular Pathology, University of Tartu and LabAs Ltd., Tartu
[2]Institute of General and Molecular Pathology, University of Tartu
[3]Department of Food Science and Hygiene, Estonian University of Life Sciences, Tartu
[4]LabAs Ltd., Tartu
[5]Institute of General and Molecular Pathology, University of Tartu
Estonia

1. Introduction

Neural stem cells are present in both the developing and adult nervous system of all mammals, including humans. Due to their therapeutic promise, considerable attention has been focused on identifying the sources of stem cells, the signals that regulate their proliferation and the specification of neural stem cells towards more differentiated cell lineages (Bauer et al., 2006). Presently, neural stem cells are often identified based upon the presence of molecular markers that are correlated with the stem and/or progenitor state along with the absence of a more differentiated phenotype as assessed through marker analysis. Nevertheless, from the very beginning of NSC research the frame was set by the search for such markers and some have been identified, which, at least, allow for the identification of NSC clonal cells in cell culture. Still, the task proves to be difficult because of the changing identity that NSC can undergo and the demands that are imposed on markers. A reliable marker should identify NSC not only in the embryonic brain but also in the adult brain. Generally, markers may either be selected for cell function or for some phenotypic differences. There exist several commonly used immunomarkers for the identification of cells of neural lineages. CD 15 (SSEA1), CD133 (Prominin-1), CD184 (CXCR4) , CD271 (p75-NTR), CDw338 (ABCG2), Ki67, Musashi-1, Musashi-2, nestin, Notch-1, PAX-6, SOX-1, SOX-2 are known as neural stem cell markers; PSA-NCAM and CD271(p75-NTR) as neuronal restricted progenitor markers; CD56 (N-CAM), MAP2, DCX, β-III- A2B5 and NG2. GFAP, FGFR3, Ran-2, S100B and CD44 (H-CAM) are known as Type 1 astrocyte, and GFAP, A2B5, CD44 and S100B as Type 2 astrocyte markers. The tubulin and neurofilament NF-H are used as neuron markers. Glial restricted progenitor markers are differentiation of glial restricted progenitors to oligodendrocyte progenitors has been marked by A2B5, NG2, Olig2 and CD140a (PDGFRα). GalC, MBP, CD140a (PDGFRα), O1, O4, Olig1, Olig2 and Olig3 have been used as mature oligodendrocyte markers. In addition CD57, CD271 (p75-NTR), MASH1, Neurogenin 3 and Notch-1 have been used as neural crest stem cell markers (Kennea & Mehmet, 2002; Schwartz et al., 2008; Yuan et al., 2011). The expression overlap of markers requires a use of different immunomarkers for the identification of specific cells in neural lineages. The most problematic point, however, is the potential pitfall in identifying the phenotype of any newborn cell by a single marker. There exists a great need for more and specific monoclonal antibodies as immunomarkers for the characterization of both normal and malignant neural cells.

2. Aim of the study

The main aim of the study is the development of new monoclonal antibodies (MAbs) against neuronal tissue cells to investigate the differentiation and malignization of human nerve cells. The antibody producing hybridomas were obtained by immunizing Balb/c mice with the native fragments of human glioblastoma and foetal neural stem/progenitor cells (see Fig. 1).

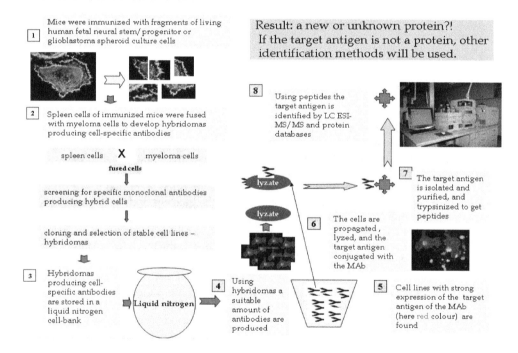

Fig. 1. Flow chart of developing hybridomas and monoclonal antibodies.

In this way it is possible to obtain MAbs against all kinds of antigenic determinants (proteins, glycans and lipids and conformational complex epitopes) that are co-expressed in the living cell, also including those determinants that are expressed on the cell surface. Used immunization scheme allows to obtain MAb panels which characterise the given cell type, including tumour cells. It is possible to obtain MAbs, differentiating between normal and tumour cells. Such specific antibodies against cell surface antigens may be the primary candidates for therapeutic antibodies and/or diagnostic purposes.

3. Methods

3.1 The isolation of human fetal neural stem/progenitor and glioblastoma spheroid cells

Human fetal neural stem/progenitor and glioblastoma spheroid cell lines were developed as described earlier (Kalev et al., 2006). In a greater detail, stem cells were isolated from the brains of 18-21-weeks old fetuses aborted due to medical indications (pregnancy problems). The study was approved by the Ethics Review Committe on Human Research of the University of Tartu. The tissue was mechanically dispersed into a cell suspension in the DMEM/F12 medium, containing gentamicin as antibiotic (Gibco BRL, Gaithersburg, USA). The cell suspension was centrifuged and washed once with the same medium and seeded into 6-well tissue culture plates with a density of 5000-10000 living cells per ml in the medium composed of DMEM/F12, B27 supplement (Gibco BRL) and growth factors bFGF (20 ng/ml; Peprotech), EGF (20 ng/ml; Peprotech), LIF (20 ng/ml, Chemicon) and gentamicin (Gibco BRL). The stem/progenitor cells were grown as neurospheres, the medium was changed every three days, the spheres were dissociated by mechanical trituration after every 12-15 days. Glioblastoma biopsy materials (obtained from Dr E.Jõeste, Department of Pathology, North-Estonian Regional Hospital, Tallinn) were from patients who had signed a consent form. Materials were manipulated by the same method as in the isolation of CNS stem/progenitor cells. The isolation of both CNS stem/progenitor cells and neurosphere-like growing cells from glioblastoma biopsies were performed earlier in LabAs Ltd. In this study five neural stem/progenitor cell lines (hBrSc003, hBrSc004, hBrSc005, hBrSc006 and hBrSc009) and two glioblastoma spheric cell lines (glioblastoma TiVi M-cells and glioblastoma OtAi M-cells) were used for the development and characterization of new monoclonal antibodies (Fig. 2). During differentiation all these cell lines produced three main neural cell types: neurons, astrocytes and oligodendrocytes as it was shown by staining cells with β-III-tubulin, GFAP and GalC (Fig. 3) although in glioblastoma spheroid cultures the cellular and nuclear heterogeneity was significantly higher than in fetal neural stem cell cultures (unpublished). Differentiation of fetal neurospheres and neurosphere-like growing glioblastoma cells (spheroids) was initiated by plating cells onto laminin-coated cover-glasses in the growth media containing all-trans retinoic acid (RA; 10-6 M) and dibutyryl cyclic AMP (dBcAMP; 1mM) and the cells were fixed on different days after the initiation of differentiation.

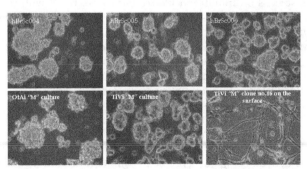

Fig. 2. Neurospheres in fetal neural stem/progenitor cell lines (hBrSc004, hBrSc005 and hBrSc006) and spheroids in glioblastoma OtAi "M" and TiVi "M" cell lines. The last picture shows a clone of TiVi M culture, adapted to grow on surface (Inverted microscope, obj. LWD A20PL 0.40 160/1.2).

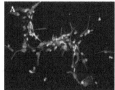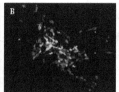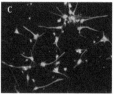

Fig. 3. Expression of different neural immunomarkers in fetal neural stem/progenitor cell line hBrSc006. Neurospheres were differentiated for 7 days. Cells were fixed with 4% PFA and permeabilized with Tritone X-100. (A) Double staining for β-III-tubulin (green – Alexa 488) and GFAP (red – Alexa 594); (B) Double staining for β-III-tubulin (green – Alexa 488) and GalC (red – Alexa 594); (C) Double staining for GFAP (green – Alexa 488) and GalC (red – Alexa 594), note co-location of GFAP and GalC – yellow staining. Obj. 40x. DAPI is used for nuclei staining (blue).

3.2 Development of new mouse monoclonal antibodies

3.2.1 Preparation of immunogen

The three neural stem/progenitor cell lines (hBrSc003, hBrSc004 and hBrSc005) and one glioblastoma spheric cell line (glioblastoma TiVi M-cells) were used as immunogens in this study. The stem/progenitor cells were grown as neurospheres, the DMEM/F12 medium with B27 supplement (Gibco BRL) and growth factors bFGF (20 ng/ml; Pepro Tech, Princeton, USA), EGF (20 ng/ml; Pepro Tech, LIF (20 ng/ml, Chemicon, Temecula, USA) and gentamicin (Gibco BRL) was changed every 3 days. Two-three-week old neurospheres from one 25cm^2 cell culture flask were mechanically dispersed into cell suspension and thereafter repeatedly frozen and thawn to get cell fragments.

3.2.2 Development of mouse hybridoma cells

About 100 µl of the disrupted cell suspension were injected intraperitoneally into 6-week-old normal female Balb/c mice. The injections were repeated 4 times at 4-week intervals.

The cells from the spleens of immunized Balb/c mice were fused with the Sp2/0 myeloma cells by standard procedure (Mikelsaar et al., 2009). Hybridomas were grown in the RPMI 1640/HAT medium containing 10% FCS (Gibco BRL) and gentamicin. Primary screening of supernatants from hybridomas was performed starting from the 10th day of growth. Both unfixed and/or non-permeabilized paraformaldehyde (PFA) fixed human fetal stem/progenitor cells were tested immunocytochemically for the reaction with MAbs. The unfixed cells were incubated with hybridoma supernatants for 1 h at 37°C or overnight at 4°C, washed three times with PBS and a specific reaction of the MAb was revealed by incubating cells with fluorochrome ALEXA 594® - conjugated secondary goat anti-mouse IgG antibody (Molecular Probes, Eugene, USA) for 1 h. The cell fixation without permeabilization was performed with 8% PFA in PBS for 15 min at room temperature (RT), washed three times with PBS, the excess of aldehyde being quenched with 50mM NH$_4$Cl in PBS (10 min) and blocked (0.3% casein, 0.01% Tween 20 in PBS) for 1 h at RT or overnight at 4°C. Ice-cold 100% methanol producing permeabilization was used for a further characterization of MAbs. The cells were incubated for 15 min at RT, washed three times with PBS and blocked. From plenty of MAb-producing clones, only those that revealed heterogeneity of reaction with stem/progenitor cells, and glioblastoma spheroid cultures, were further investigated. The expression of antigens of selected monoclonal antibodies was further characterized besides neural stem/progenitor cells also on other living and/or fixed cells of different origin. It is important to find the cells where the target antigen of MAbs has the strongest expression in order to use these cells for molecular characterization of the antigen.

3.2.3 MAb cloning and isotyping

Selected hybridomas were cloned by limiting dilution and isotypes of the MAbs were determined by using goat anti-mouse Ig isotype specific antibodies developed in LabAs Ltd Cloned hybridomas are stored in a liquid nitrogen cell bank.

3.3 Immunocytochemical characterization of monoclonal antibodies

3.3.1 Cells and cell lines used to characterize monoclonal antibodies

Besides the cells used as immunogens (fetal neural stem/progenitor and glioblastoma spheroid cells) other types of cells and cell lines were used to characterize monoclonal antibodies. This was necessary to study the specificity of antibodies and is also useful to find out the positive cell lines with shorter duplication time. These cell lines were often used for getting more cellular material in shorter time for the identification of target antigens of MAbs (see also 3.4.2). The following additional cells and cell lines were used for the characterization of monoclonal antibodies: normal human cells - human blood thrombocytes, human sperms, normal fetal and adult skin fibroblast cell lines NL011 (LabAs Ltd) and SA-54, respectively, human normal amniotic epithelial cell line KM (LabAs Ltd.); malignant cell lines - human glioblastoma TiViMNBFCS10 cell line, glioblastoma TiVi M clone 16, glioblastoma OjArMNBFCS and OjFeMNBFCS cell lines (all developed in LabAs Ltd), Bowes melanoma cell line; cells of other species - COS-1 cell line (simian origin), rat granulare cell culture (kindly provided by Prof. A. Žarkovsky).

3.3.2 Fixation methods

Paraformaldehyde or methanol fixation methods were used. In PFA fixation the coverslips were transferred without any previous washing into dishes containing prewarmed 4% PFA in PBS and left for 5 min at RT. Then the coverslips were washed for 3x 5 min with PBS and the excess of aldehyde was quenched with 50mM of NH_4Cl in PBS (10 min). After washing twice with PBS, the cells were permeabilized for 10 min with 0.1% Tritone X-100 in PBS, washed with PBS and blocked. (In methanol fixation the coverslips were treated for 5 min with ice cold methanol and washed with PBS). The coverslips were then transferred into a blocking solution (0.3% casein, 0.01% Tween 20 in PBS) for 1 h at RT or overnight at 4°C.

3.3.3 Staining methods

The blocking solution was removed by aspiration and the cells were stained as follows: they were incubated for 1 hour at RT with the MAb supernatant. The coverslips were washed at least for 3x5 min with PBS and immunolabeling was visualized by incubating the cells with the goat anti-mouse IgG antibody conjugated with fluorochrome Alexa 594 (Molecular Probes) for 1 h at RT. In all cases, the coverslips were washed at least for 3x5 min with PBS, 10 μl of DAPI solution 1μg/ml was added into the last PBS and then the coverslips were incubated for 5 minutes at RT. After quick rinsing in distilled water, the coverslips were mounted in the anti-fading mounting medium Prolong Gold Antifade (Molecular Probes). The cells were checked by a visual microscoping system (Olympus BX, using objectives UplanFI 20x/0.50, 40x/0.75, or 100x/1.30 Oil Iris and the Olympus DP50-CU Photographing System).

3.4 Characterization and identification of target antigens of new monoclonal antibodies

3.4.1 Strategy for target antigen identification

Our strategy for the identification of target antigens of monoclonal antibodies was the following: (1) lysing , electrophoresis and the immunoblotting of suitable cellular material were performed to identify where the bands reacting with specific monoclonal antibodies are located; (2) for immunoprecipitation antibodies were caught to protein-G-conjugated Sepharose beads from the culture medium or used DVS-activated beads for purified antibodies; (3) the immunoprecipitated antigen was separated from the antibody and nonspecifically associated material by using electrophoresis in the SDS-PAGE gel; (4) the bands containing antigen were identified by using immunoblotting from the same gel; (5) the bands containing the antigen were cut out from the gel and trypsinized; (6) tryptic peptides and target antigens were identified with aid of mass-spectroscopy (LC ESI-MS-MS) and protein databases.

3.4.2 Cells and cell lines used for identification of target antigenes

For molecular identification of the target antigens of MAbs different cells and cell lines were used (see also 3.3.1). However, in this study mainly the Bowes melanoma cell line (neural crest origin) and glioblastoma cell line TiViMNBFCS10 (glioblastoma TiVi M spheroid culture, but adapted to growing on the surface) were used. Both the cell lines were propagated in medium DMEM/F12 with 10% FCS and gentamicin (Gibco BRL).

3.4.3 Purification of antigens

3.4.3.1 Purification of antigens from cells growing on surface

The cells of the human Bowes melanoma or TiViMNBFCS10 cell lines were lysed in 8M urea, 3% SDS, 50mM Tris-HCL, pH 6.8 and diluted with 30 volumes of TBS. About 50 μl of Sepharose-bound MAbs were added to 30 ml of the diluted sample solution and incubated overnight at 4°C. The beads were washed, incubated in an electrophoresis sample buffer for 10 min at 95°C and loaded onto the top of the 10% SDS-PAGE gel. After electrophoresis immunopositive bands were located by immunoblotting an one part of the gel, whereas the rest of the gel was stained with colloidal Coomassie G-250 for the confirmation of protein location. This electrophoresis step was absolutely necessary to avoid interferences with non-specifically bound proteins. The immunopositive band was cut out, minced, washed and dried (about 15 min at RT) by CentriVac. The dried pieces of the gel were rehydrated and the proteins trypsinized overnight at 37°C with sequencing grade trypsin (Promega, Madison WI, USA).

3.4.3.2 Purification of human blood thrombocytes

Purification of platelets was performed essentially according to the method of P.J. Canvar and co-workers (Canvar et al., 2007). Shortly, human platelet-rich plasma from the blood center of Tartu University Clinicum was further purified by centrifuging at 1400g for 15 min to pellet any remaining white or red blood cells and the platelet-rich plasma was decanted. Protease inhibitors (Roche Complete, Roche Diagnostics GmbH, Mannheim, Germany) were added as recommended by manufacturer and incubated 10 min at RT. Platelets were pelleted by centrifuging in at 4°C and washed once in Tyrode's buffer by centrifuging at 2400g for 15 min at 4°C. The pellets were stored in Tyrode's buffer at -80°C until used.

3.4.3.3 Cell lysis

Radioimmunoprecipitation assay buffer (RIPA) was used containing 50 mM of Tris/HCl pH 7.4 (ultrapure, AppliChem, Darmstadt, Germany); 0.1% SDS (ultrapure, AppliChem, Darmstadt, Germany); 1% NP40 (Octylphenoxy polyethoxy ethanol, reagent grade, AMRESCO, Solon Ind. Ohio, USA); 1% Tritone X-100 (Schuchardt, München, Germany); 0.5% DOC (Natriumdeoxycholat, AppliChem, Darmstadt, Germany); 500 mM NaCl (AppliChem, Darmstadt, Germany); protease inhibitor tablets (Roche Complete, Roche Diagnostics GmbH, Mannheim, Germany). For more gently lysis of the cells simply 1%NP40 solution in PBS (AppliChem, Darmstadt, Germany) was used.

3.4.3.4 SDS-polyacrylamid gel electrophoresis (SDS-PAGE)

Cells for electrophoresis were lysed in the RIPA buffer or with 1% NP-40 in PBS and centrifuged at maximum speed in Eppendorf centrifuge 5415C for 10 min at 4°C. The supernatant was diluted 1:1 in the SDS-electrophoresis sample buffer with DTT (AppliChem, Darmstadt, Germany) and heated for 10 min at 95°C or at 60°C for sensitive antigenes. Before electrophoresis 8M of urea was added to the sample solution until 2M of the end concentration. Electrophoresis was run in a mighty small Hoefer electrophoresis system (Hoefer Scientific Instruments, CA, USA) with the glasses of 10 x 12 cm and the spacers of 0.75 mm. The end concentration of the gel buffer was 0.43 M and pH 8.4. Usually the samples were separated in the gradient (8-24%) SDS-PAGE gel for achieving sharper bands, yet the concentrating gel was not used. The parameters for prerunning electrophoresis were 60 V and 30 min. Electrophoresis was run for 4 hours at max 210V and 16mA.

3.4.3.5 Colloid Coomassie G250 staining

Colloid Coomassie G250 staining was performed essentially according to the D.Kang and co-workers (Kang et al., 2002). Shortly, the SDS-PAGE gel was fixed in a mixture of 30% ethanol and 2% phosphoric acid for 15 min and washed in distilled water 3x for 15 minutes. Staining was performed in a solution containing 5% w/v aluminium sulphate (Applichem, Darmstadt, Germany), 0.02% Coomassie G-250 (Serva Electrophoresis GmbH, Heidelberg, Germany), 2% phosphoric acid and 10% ethanol for 1 hour. Destaining was performed in distilled water until the bands became clearly visible.

3.4.3.6 Western blot

The method described in the Millipore manual for immunoblotting to the PVDF membrane was used. Buffer components and the stain were from AppliChem, Darmstadt, Germany. The procedure was as follows: the membrane was wetted in methanol for 1 to 3 seconds.

Methanol was eluted incubating the membrane for 5 min in distilled water on a shaker. Thereafter the membrane was equilibrated in the transfer buffer for 2 to 3 min. SDS-PAGE gel was equilibrated in the cathode buffer for 15 min on the shaker. GEHealthcare electrophoresis unit Multiphor II and a semidry immunoblotting kit for electroblotting were used. The anode buffers were Tris 0.3 M (no.1) and Tris 15 mM (no.2); the cathode buffer contained 40 mM of glycine and 25 mM of Tris. Two sheets of chromatography papers (Whatman CHR17, Mainstone, England) were soaked in anode buffer no.1 and one sheet in the anode buffer no.2. The wetted PVDF membrane was placed on the top of the soaked anode sheets and then equilibrated SDS-PAGE gel was placed on the top of them. After that three chromatography papers with the cathode buffer were located on the top of the gel and immunoblotting was performed at 0.8 mA /cm^2 for 2 hours. After electroblotting nonspecific binding of antibodies was blocked by incubating the membrane in TBS with 0.1% Tween 20 (Sigma, MO, USA). For vimentin-specific antibody GB26 10G3 a mixture of 1% horse serum and 0.1% Tween 20 in TBS was used as a blocking solution. The membrane was incubated with monoclonal antibody in the blocking buffer for overnight at 4°C. After washing 3 x for 10 min in PBS 0.1% Tween 20 the membrane was incubated with a secondary antibody (goat anti-mouse IgG polyclonal antibody conjugated with horseradish peroxidase) in PBS 0.1% Tween 20 for one hour at RT. After that the membrane was washed with 0.1% Tween 20 in PBS 3 times for 10 min and then 1 x for 10 min in PBS. The membrane was incubated for 10 minutes in the staining solution containing 50 mg of DAB (diaminobenzidin trihydrochloride, AppliChem, Darmstadt, Germany), 6 ml chloronaphtole (Sigma, MO,USA) solution (3 mg/ml) in ethanol and 20 µl of 30% H_2O_2 in PBS and washed 3 times for 5 minutes in distilled water. After drying the membrane can be saved in the archive.

3.4.3.7 Conjugation of antibody with horseradish peroxidase

Antibodies were conjugated to HRP as described previously (Tjissen, 1985). Shortly, 1 mg of horseradish peroxidase (Boehringer Mannheim, Germany) was solubilized in the Eppendorf tube in 0.1 ml of the freshly prepared 0.1M $NaHCO_3$ solution and 0.1 ml of 8-16 mM $NaIO_4$ (Merck, Darmstadt, Germany) was added and incubated for 2 hours in the dark room at RT. 3 mg of antibody was solubilized in 1 ml of the sodium carbonate buffer pH 9.2 and dry Sephadex G-25 (GE Healthcare, Sweden) was added of about 1/6 from the total amount of the solution and the mix was incubated for 3 hours in the dark room at RT. The conjugate was eluted from Sephadex and mixed (1/20 from the total volume) with the freshly prepared $NaBH_4$ (Sigma, MO, USA) solution in 0.1M of NaOH (5 mg/ml) on a shaker. After 30 min an additional amount of the $NaBH_4$ solution (1/10 from the total volume) was added and the mix was incubated for 1 hour at 4°C. Then 50% of glycerol (AppliChem, Darmstadt, Germany) was added and the conjugate was stored at -20°C. For immunoblotting HRP-conjugated antibodies were diluted from 1:500 to 1:1500.

3.4.3.8 Activating of Sepharose granules with divinylsulphone (DVS) and binding of antibodies to activated granules

Sepharose CL-4B granules (Pharmacia, Uppsala, Sweden) were washed with distilled water of 4 to 5 gel volumes. The granules were equilibrated with 4 to 5 gel volumes of 0.5 M carbonate buffer (pH 11), 10 ml of the 0.5 M carbonate buffer (pH 11) containing 1 ml of divinylsulphone (Sigma, MO, USA) were added to 10 ml of the gel and incubated on a shaker for 1.5 hr. The activated granules were washed once with the carbonate buffer, then 2

Development of New Monoclonal Antibodies for Immunocytochemical Characterization of Neural Stem and
Differentiated Cells

101

x with distilled water and stored in PBS with 0.01% NaN_3 at 4°C. Activated granules are useable during about 1 year. For the binding of antibodies the granules were washed with 4 to 5 volumes of distilled water and then equilibrated in 0.1 M carbonate buffer pH 9.0. The buffer for antibodies was changed to the carbonate buffer pH 9.0 using the PD 10 column (GE Healthcare, Sweden). DVS-activated Sepharose CL-4B granules (200 μl) were added to antibody solution (1-2 mg in 3.5 ml) in the carbonate buffer and incubated for 10 min at RT. Then 5% PEG 20,000 was added and the granules were incubated overnight at RT on a shaker. Afterwards the granules with conjugated antibodies were washed and blocked in TBS buffer and stored in TBS at 4°C with 0.01% NaN_3 until used.

3.4.3.9 Immunoprecipitation

For immunoprecipitation the lysates in RIPA buffer, PBS with 1%NP40 or PBS/TBS diluted 1:30 electrophoresis sample buffer were used. Before immunoprecipitation MAbs from 1.5 ml of the hybridoma medium (sometimes more) were conjugated to 50 μl of Protein-G Sepharose 4 Fast Flow granules (GE Healthcare, Sweden). The granules were washed 3 times in the immunoprecipitation buffer and incubated with cell lysate at 4°C overnight. Then the granules were washed in one of the immunoprecipitation buffers 4 times and once with distilled water. The washed granules (50 μl) were diluted in 150 μl of the SDS-PAGE sample buffer and incubated for 5 min at 95°C or in case of sensitive antigenes for 10 min at 60°C. Then 50 μl of 8M urea were added and the granules were incubated for 15 min at RT on a shaker and thereafter put on the top of the electrophoresis gel. When purified monoclonal antibodies not hybridoma supernatants were used for immunoprecipitation, MAbs were directly conjugated to the divinyl-sulphone-activated granules.

3.4.3.10 Trypsinization of isolated antigenes

After electrophoresis, immunopositive bands were located by immunoblotting a part of the gel, whereas the rest of the gel was stained with colloidal Coomassie G-250 for the confirmation of protein location. This electrophoresis step is necessary to avoid interferences with non-specifically bound proteins. The immunopositive band was cut out from the gel and minced to pieces of about 1 x 1 mm using a scalpel. Pieces of the gel were washed once with methanol on a shaker for 1-2 minutes, then with 10 mM $(NH_4)_2CO_3$ 2 times for 5 min and thereafter with 50% acetonitrile in 10 mM $(NH_4)_2CO_3$. The gel pieces were dried with the CentriVac for 15 min and treated for 10 min with the solution containing 2μg of trypsine in 1 ml of 50 mM $(NH_4)_2CO_3$ with 0.05% ProteasMax surfactant (Promega, USA). 10 mM of $(NH_4)_2CO_3$ was added to fully coated gel pieces and incubated at 37°C overnight. The solution from the top of the gel and the washing solutions were collected into one tube. The gel pieces were washed two times with 50% acetonitrile in 10 mM $(NH_4)_2CO_3$ and once in pure acetonitrile. The solution containing peptides was concentrated until the amount of 100 μl and analyzed using mass-spectroscopy. Sometimes for confirming the exact band location in the gel direct staining of proteins on the membrane is needed. To that end colloid Coomassie stain diluted 1:1 in distilled water was used. After that we destained the membrane washing with distilled water about ten times 10 min or until protein bands became visible. On the dry membrane we saw strongly stained black bands containing the antigen or antibody components and other blue-stained bands containing different co-immunoprecipitated nonantigenic proteins.

3.4.3.11 Peptide analysis by LC ESI-MS/MS and protein identification with Mascot and the Global Proteome Machine

The Agilent 1100 Series chromatograph with LC/MSD Trap XCT (Agilent, Santa Cruz, USA) was used for LC/MS experiments applying the 2.1 x 150 mm Agilent 300Extend C18 column of 3.5 μm particle size. 50 μl of the peptide mixture was injected into the column and eluted with a gradient from 0.1% HCOOH/5% acetonitrile to 75% acetonitrile during 120 minutes at 0.3 ml/min. The column was thermostated at 35°C. Positive ions were detected in a "smart mode" with the target mass set to 1000 m/z, whereas doubly charged ions were preferred. The data were analyzed with both Mascot www.matrixscience.com and GPM www.thegpm.org search engines (1000 most abundant ions). For the positive identification of the antigen the consent of both search engines was necessary.

4. Results

During our study we have developed several hundreds of new monoclonal antibodies. The characterization and identification of the target antigens of them are in progress. Some results of this work have been recently published (Mikelsaar et al., 2009). Here we present data on the five new monoclonal antibodies (see Table 1), which we have developed according to the strategy described in this chapter.

Name of monoclonal antibodies	Ig sub-class	Immunogen	Identified target antigen	Neural cell types identified by antibody
E14G2	IgG1	Mix of fetal neural cell lines hBrSc003/ hBrSc004/ hBrSc005	Annexin A1	Annexin A1- and + cells among differentiated fetal neural stem cells, glioblastoma spheroid cells and in glioblastomas; microglia; annexin A1+ glial cells and Purkinje (?) cells in rat granule cell culture
E15F10.B9	IgG1	Mix of fetal neural cell lines hBrSc003/ hBrSc004/ hBrSc005	Calnexin	Calnexin- and + cells among differentiated fetal neural stem cells and glioblastoma spheroid cells; shows cellular heterogeneity in glioblastomas
W4A8.F4	Ig2a	hBrSc003	14-3-3 ζ/δ	Both human and rat glial and neuronal cells
GB26 10G3	IgG1	Mix of different glioblas-toma cells	Vimetin	The precursors cells of both neuronal and glial lineages; shows cellular heterogeneity in glioblastomas
A3G2.B4	IgG1	hBrSc003	Lupus La protein	La protein- and + cells among differentiated fetal neural stem cells and glioblastoma spheroid cells; shows cellular heterogeneity in glioblastomas

Table 1. Summary of new monoclonal antibodies described in this chapter. All these antibodies may be useful for detailed analysis of the expression of target antigens in all types of neural cells .

4.1 New monoclonal antibodies

4.1.1 Monoclonal antibody E14G2 (MAb E14G2)

Here we describe the results of the immunocytochemical analysis of MAb E14G2 (Table 1)
with different cell types and the biochemical/molecular analysis for identifying the target
antigen of the antibody. In Fig. 4 we can see a distinct heterogenous expression of MAb
E14G2 antigen in differentiated fetal neural stem/progenitor (A,B,C,D), in glioblastoma
spheroid cells (E) and also in the rat granule primary culture (H). However, the expression
of the target antigen of MAb E14G2 was strong and homogenous in glioblastoma OjAr
secondary culture and in Bowes melanoma cell lines (F and G, respectively).

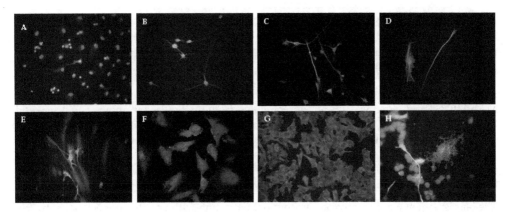

Fig. 4. Presence of MAb E14G2 target antigen (Annexin A1) in different cells. (A) Human
fetal hBrSc003 neurosphere cells differentiated for 11 days. Double immunofluorescent
staining, cells were fixed with 4% PFA and permeabilized. Annexin A1 expression was
revealed by red staining – Alexa 594, β-III-tubulin by green staining – Alexa 488, obj. 40x. (B-
D). Human fetal hBrSc005 neurosphere cells differentiated for 3 days (B,C) and 7 days (D).
Double immunofluorescent staining, cells were fixed with 4% PFA and permeabilized.
Annexin A1 expression was revealed by red staining – Alexa 594, β-III-tubulin by green
staining – Alexa 488, obj. 40x. (E) Human glioblastoma TiVi spheroid cell line differentiated
for 7 days. Double immunofluorescent staining, cells were fixed with 4% PFA and
permeabilized. Annexin A1 expression was revealed by red staining – Alexa 594, β-III-
tubulin by green staining – Alexa 488, obj. 40x. (F) Human glioblastoma OjAr secondary cell
culture on the 6th day of cultivation. Cells were fixed with 4% PFA and permeabilized.
Annexin A1 expression was revealed by red staining – Alexa 594, obj. 40x. (G) Bowes
melanoma cell line on the 2nd day of cultivation, fixed with 4%PFA, no permeabilization.
Specific Annexin A1 staining was revealed by red staining – Alexa 594, obj. 40x. (H) Rat
granulare cell culture. Double immunofluorescent staining, cells were fixed with 4% PFA
and permeabilized. Annexin A1 expression was revealed by red staining – Alexa 594, GFAP
by green staining – Alexa 488, obj. 100x. DAPI is used for nuclei staining (blue).

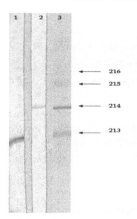

Fig. 5. Electrophoresis and Western blot of MAb E14G2 target antigen. (1) negative control, MAb Y1C7 directly conjugated with peroxidase; (2) MAb E14G2 directly conjugated with peroxidase; (3) gel stained with colloid Coomassie G-250. Arrows with numbers indicate bands analyzed by LC ESI-MS/MS.

In Fig. 5 we present the data on electrophoresis and immunoblot of the target antigen of MAb 14G2. The antigen was immunoprecipitated from the Bowes melanoma cell lysate and the precipitated cells (100 μl) were lysed in 10 ml of RIPA buffer. MAb E14G2 was conjugated directly to the divinylsulphone-activated Sepharose granules. Then 50 μl of the activated granules were incubated in 10 ml of the cleared Bowes melanoma cell lysate overnight at 4°C, washed 4x with the buffer and 1x with distilled water. Then 150 μl of SDS-PAGE sample buffer was added and the sample heated 5 min at 95°C before electrophoresis.

The bands, which were positive according to the reaction with specific monoclonal antibody MAb E14G2 (Fig. 4, arrows 213-216) were analyzed by LC ESI-MS/MS and the proteins were identified using Mascot and the GPM software databases (see Table 2).

Band	Identified proteins	Mass	Mascot score	Sequence coverage %
213	ANXA1 - Annexin A1	38690	41	8
	KV401 - Ig kappa chain V-IV region	13372	37	7
214	ANXA1 - Annexin A1	38690	2274	71
215	ANXA1 - Annexin A1	38690	198	34
	TBB5 - Tubulin beta chain	49639	113	24
	K2C1- Keratin, type II cytoskeletal 1	65999	84	6
216	DHSA- Succinate dehydrogenase [ubiquinone] flavoprotein subunit, mit	72645	103	26
	K2C1- Keratin, type II cytoskeletal 1	65999	82	7
	ANXA1 - Annexin A1	38690	65	18

Table 2. LC ESI-MS/MS and Mascot software analysis of immunoprecipitated with MAb 14G2 proteins in bands 213, 214, 215 and 216 (Fig. 4, arrows 213-216).

```
  1 MAMVSEFLKQ AWFIENEEQE YVQTVKSSKG GPGSAVSPYP TFNPSSDVAA
 51 LHKAIMVKGV DEATIIDILT KRNNAQRQQI KAAYLQETGK PLDETLKKAL
101 TGHLEEVVLA LLKTPAQFDA DELRAAMKGL GTDEDTLIEI LASRTNKEIR
151 DINRVYREEL KRDLAKDITS DTSGDFRNAL LSLAKGDRSE DFGVNEDLAD
201 SDARALYEAG ERRKGTDVNV FNTILTTRSY PQLRRVFQKY TKYSKHDMNK
251 VLDLELKGDI EKCLTAIVKC ATSKPAFFAE KLHQAMKGVG TRHKALIRIM
301 VSRSEIDMND IKAFYQKMYG ISLCQAILDE TKGDYEKILV ALCGGN
```

Fig. 6. Amino acid sequences of Annexin A1, ANXA1. In red are marked amino acids
sequences identified by mass-spectroscopy (band 214 in Fig. 5).

Conclusion

On the basis of data presented above we conclude that the target antigen of MAb E14G2 is
protein Annexin A1. According to UniProtKB/Swiss-Prot database Annexin A1 is a
calcium/phospholipid-binding protein which promotes membrane fusion and is involved
in exocytosis. This protein regulates phospholipase A2 activity.
(http://www.uniprot.org/uniprot/P04083#section_comments).

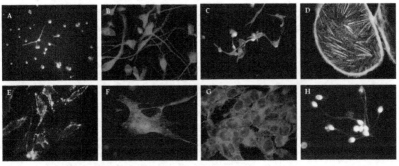

Fig. 7. Presence of MAb E15F10.B9 target antigen (calnexin) in different cells. (A) Human
fetal hBrSc003 neurosphere cells differentiated for 11 days. Double immunofluorescent
staining, cells were fixed with 4% PFA and permeabilized. Calnexin expression was
revealed by red staining – Alexa 594, β-III-tubulin by green staining – Alexa 488, obj. 40x. (B)
Human fetal hBrSc003 neurosphere cells differentiated for 7 days, cells were fixed with 4%
PFA and permeabilized. Calnexin expression was revealed by red staining – Alexa 594, obj.
100x. (C) Human glioblastoma TiVi spheroid cell line differentiated for 7 days. Double
immunofluorescent staining, cells were fixed with 4% PFA and permeabilized. Calnexin
expression was revealed by red staining – Alexa 594, β-III-tubulin by green staining – Alexa
488, obj. 40x. (D) Human normal amniotic epithelial cell line KM on the fifth days of
cultivation. Double immunofluorescent staining, cells were fixed with 4% PFA and
permeabilized. Calnexin expression was revealed by red staining – Alexa 594, actin by green
staining with Alexa 488 conjugated Phalloidin, obj. 100x. (E) Unfixed cells of adult skin
fibroblast cell line SA-54 on the 3rd day of cultivation. Specific calnexin staining revealed by
green staining – Alexa 488, obj. 20x. (F) Human glioblastoma TiViMNBFCS10 cells on the
3rd day of cultivation, fixed with 4%PFA, no permeabilization. Specific calnexin staining
revealed by red staining – Alexa 594, obj. 100x. (G) Bowes melanoma cell line on the 2nd day
of cultivation, fixed with 4%PFA, no permeabilization. Specific calnexin staining revealed by
red staining – Alexa 594, obj.100x. (H) Unfixed sperms of a normal human male. Specific
calnexin staining revealed by red staining – Alexa 488, obj. 100x (note a red staining between
the sperm head and tail). DAPI is used for nuclei staining (blue).

4.1.2 Monoclonal antibody E15F10.B9 (MAb E15F10.B9)

In Fig. 7 we can see different expression of MAb E15F10.B9 (Table 1) detected antigen in differentiated fetal neural stem/progenitor (A) and glioblastoma spheroid cells (C). In some regions of hBrSc003 cell line differentiated for 7 days there was a very strong expression of MAb E15F10.B9 target antigen (B). Strong expression of the antigen one can see also in unfixed adult skin fibroblasts and in fixed, but not permeabilized glioblastoma and Bowes melanoma cells. Interestly, in unfixed human sperms the staining of MAb E15F10.B9 was seen as two separate points between the head and neck of the sperm (H). Double staining with actin in normal amniotic epithelial cells (D) shows an independent staining of actin and target antigen of MAb E15F10.B9, whereas the last one shows nuclear membrane and punctate cytoplasma staining.

The LC ESI-MS/MS and Mascot database analysis of peptides from the immunoprecipitated band 208 (Fig. 8) identified two possible candidates for the target antigen of MAb E15F10.B9 – calnexin and Keratin, type II cytoskeletal 1. However, as immunocytochemical analysis on different cell types including normal epithelial amniotic cells (Fig. 7) showed no typical cytoskeletal staining for cytokeratin we consider the keratin to be in immunoprecipitate as a contaminant substance. In Fig. 8 and 9 and Table 3 the results of Western blot and molecular identification of the target antigen of MAb E15F10.B9 are shown.

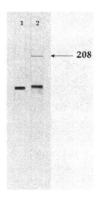

Fig. 8. Western blot of MAb E15F10.B9 target antigen (calnexin). MAb E15F10.B9 from hybridoma supernatant was conjugated to Protein G granules and thereafter target antigen immunoprecipitated from Bowes melanoma cell line lysed with RIPA buffer. Proteins were separated in SDS-PAGE 4-12% gradient gel. (1) negative control with HRP-conjugated goat anti-mouse IgG secondary antibody; (2) incubation with MAb E15F10.B9 and secondary antibody. Arrow indicates the band analyzed by ESI-MS/MS.

Band	Identified proteins	Mass	Mascot score	Sequence coverage %
208	CALX - Calnexin	67526	384	22
	K2C1- Keratin, type II cytoskeletal 1	65999	313	20

Table 3. LC ESI-MS/MS and Mascot software analysis of the proteins in the band which was immunoprecipitated with MAb E15F10.B9 proteins (Fig. 8).

```
  1 MEGKWLLCML LVLGTAIVEA HDGHDDDVID IEDDLDDVIE EVEDSKPDTT
 51 APPSSPKVTY KAPVPTGEVY FADSFDRGTL SGWILSKAKK DDTDDEIAKY
101 DGKWEVEEMK ESKLPGDKGL VLMSRAKHHA ISAKLNKPFL FDTKPLIVQY
151 EVNFQNGIEC GGAYVKLLSK TPELNLDQFH DKTPYTIMFG PDKCGEDYKL
201 HFIFRHKNPK TGIYEEKHAK RPDADLKTYF TDKKTHLYTL ILNPDNSFEI
251 LVDQSVVNSG NLLNDMTPPV NPSREIEDPE DRKPEDWDER PKIPDPEAVK
301 PDDWDEDAPA KIPDEEATKP EGWLDDEPEY VPDPDAEKPE DWDEDMDGEW
351 EAPQIANPRC ESAPGCGVWQ RPVIDNPNYK GKWKPPMIDN PSYQGIWKPR
401 KIPNPDFFED LEPFRMTPFS AIGLELWSMT SDIFFDNFII CADRRIVDDW
451 ANDGWGLKKA ADGAAEPGVV GQMIEAAEER PWLWVVYILT VALPVFLVIL
501 FCCSGKKQTS GMEYKKTDAP QPDVKEEEEE KEEEKDKGDE EEEGEEKLEE
551 KQKSDAEEDG GTVSQEEEDR KPKAEEDEIL NRSPRNRKPR RE
```

Fig. 9. Amino acid sequences of Calnexin. With red colour are marked amino acids
sequences identified by mass-spectroscopy (band 208 in Fig. 8).

Conclusion

On the basis of data presented above we conclude that the target antigen of MAb E15F10.B9
is protein Calnexin. According to UniProtKB/Swiss-Prot database Calnexin is a calcium-
binding protein that interacts with newly synthesized glycoproteins in the endoplasmic
reticulum. It may act in assisting protein assembly and/or in the retention within the ER of
unassembled protein subunits. It seems to play a major role in the quality control apparatus
of the ER by the retention of incorrectly folded proteins (http://www.uniprot.org/
uniprot/P27824).

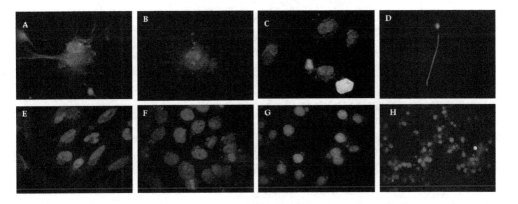

Fig. 10. Presence of MAb W4A8.F4 target antigen (protein 14-3-3) in different cells. Specifc
staining of MAb W4A8.F4 was revealed by red staining –Alexa 594. (A,B) Human fetal
hBrSc006 (A) and hBrSc009 (B) neurosphere cells differentiated for 3 days. Cells were fixed
with 4% PFA and permeabilized, obj. 100x. (C) Human fetal skin fibroblast culture on the
3rd day of cultivation. Cells were fixed with 4% PFA and permeabilized, obj. 100x. (D)
Unfixed sperms of a normal human male, obj. 100x. (E-F) Human glioblastoma cell line
TiViMNBFCS10 (E), Bowes melanoma cell line (F), COS-1 cell line and rat granulare cell
culture (H) on the 3rd day of cultivation. Cells were fixed with 4% PFA and permeabilized,
obj. 100x. DAPI is used for nuclei staining (blue).

4.1.3 Monoclonal antibody W4A8.F4 (MAb W4A8.F4)

In Fig. 10 we can see the expression of MAb W4A8.F4 (Table 1) in the fetal neural stem/progenitor cell lines hBrSc006 (A) and hBrSc009 (B). The strong staining was seen in the cytoplasm in Golgi region but also in cell projections and nuclei. In the fetal skin fibroblasts, glioblastoma, Bowes melanoma and COS-1 cell lines the cytoplasm, especially Golgi region was strongly stained (C,E,F and G respectively). In the rat granulare cell culture there was a heterogeneous staining of the cytoplasm and nuclei (H). Interestly, in the unfixed human sperms the entire tail, except the neck, was strongly and homogeneously stained (D).

In Fig. 11 and 12 and Table 4 the results of Western blot and molecular identification of the target antigen of MAb W4A8.F4 are shown.

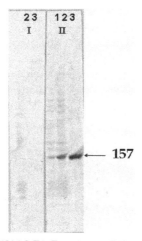

Fig. 11. Western blot with MAb W4A8.F4. Proteins in RIPA lysate were separated electrophoretically in SDS-PAGE gradient (8-25%) gel and transferred to PVDF membrane: (1) Bowes cell line, (2) glioblastoma TiViMNBFCS10 cell line and (3) human thromocytes. I – negative control with HRP-conjugated goat anti-mouse IgG secondary antibody; II – reaction with MAb W4A8.F4 and secondary antibody. Arrow indicates the band 157, analyzed by ESI-MS/MS.

Band	Identified proteins	Mass	Mascot score	Sequence coverage %
157	14-3-3 protein zeta/delta	27728	139	40
	14-3-3 protein gamma	28295	64	18
	14-3-3 protein eta	28201	64	19
	14-3-3 protein sigma	27757	64	12
	Chloride intracellular channel protein 1	26906	62	19

Table 4. LC ESI-MS/MS and Mascot software analysis of immunoprecipitated with MAb W4A8.F4 proteins in band 157 (Fig. 11).

```
  1 MDKNELVQKA KLAEQAERYD DMAACMKSVT EQGAELSNEE RNLLSVAYKN
 51 VVGARRSSWR VVSSIEQKTE GAEKKQQMAR EYREKIETEL RDICNDVLSL
101 LEKFLIPNAS QAESKVFYLK MKGDYYRYLA EVAAGDDKKG IVDQSQQAYQ
151 EAFEISKKEM QPTHPIRLGL ALNFSVFYYE ILNSPEKACS LAKTAFDEAI
201 AELDTLSEES YKDSTLIMQL LRDNLTLWTS DTQGDEAEAG EGGEN
```

Fig. 12. Amino acid sequences of protein 14-3-3 protein zeta/delta. With red colour are marked amino acids sequences identified by mass-spectroscopy (band 157 in Fig. 11).

Conclusion

On the basis of data presented above we conclude that most probably the target antigen of MAb W4A8.F4 is protein 14-3-3 zeta/delta. According to UniProtKB/ Swiss-Prot database protein 14-3-3 zeta/delta is an adapter protein implicated in the regulation of a large spectrum of both general and specialized signaling pathways. Binds to a large number of partners, usually by recognition of a phosphoserine or phosphothreonine motif. Binding generally results in the modulation of the activity of the binding partner (http://www.uniprot.org/uniprot/P63104).

4.1.4 Monoclonal antibody GB26 10G3 (MAb GB26 10G3)

In Fig. 13 we can see the filamentous staining of MAb GB26 10G3 (Table 1) antigen in human adult skin fibroblasts (A) and in glioblastoma cell line TiViMNBFCS10 (B). In glioblastoma cell lines the staining pattern was very heterogeneous, some cells did not show any signs of staining. Double staining for β-III-tubulin and the MAb GB26 10G3 (C) showed an independent staining pattern, some cells were double stained, some cells showed only β-III-tubulin staining and the majority of cells was only MAb GB26 10G3 positive. In D the double staining of target antigen of MAb GB26 10G3 and glial fibrillar acid protein (GFAP) is shown. Note that the both antigens are located in the same cells, but show an independent staining pattern.

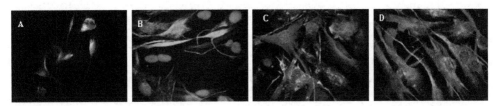

Fig. 13. Presence of MAb GB26 10G3 target antigen in different cells. (A,B) Human adult skin fibroblast cell line SA-54 (A) and human glioblastoma cell line TiViMNBFCS10 (B) on the 3rd day of cultivation. Cells were fixed with 4% PFA and permeabilized. The target antigen of MAb GB26 10G3 expression was revealed by green staining – Alexa 488, obj. 100x. (C) Human glioblastoma cell line TiViMNBFCS10 on the 3rd day of cultivation. Double immunofluorescent staining, cells were fixed with 4% PFA and permeabilized. The target antigen of MAb GB26 10G3 expression was revealed by green staining – Alexa 488, β-III-tubulin by red staining – Alexa 488, obj. 100x. (D) Human glioblastoma cell line TiViMNBFCS10 on the 3rd day of cultivation. Double immunofluorescent staining, cells were fixed with 4% PFA and permeabilized. The target antigen of MAb GB26 10G3 expression was revealed by green staining – Alexa 488, GFAP by red staining – Alexa 488, obj. 100x. DAPI is used for nuclei staining (blue).

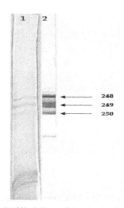

Fig. 14. SDS-PAGE gradient gel (8-24%) (1) and immunoblot (2) with MAb GB26 10G3. The sample was in RIPA buffer insoluble fraction of glioblastoma TiViNBFCS10 cells that was heated with SDS-PAGE sample buffer with DTT at 60°C for 10 min and 8M urea was added to 2M final concentration. Arrows with numbers indicate bands analyzed by ESI-MS/MS.

As molecular masses of antibody light chain and vimentin are similar and vimentin binds nonspecifically to the secondary antibody, we could not purify vimentin by immuno-precipitation as we did for other MAbs. Only gradient electrophoresis of lysate and immunoblotting were used to separate the target antigen of MAb GB26 10G3.

In Fig. 14 and 15 and Table 5 the results of electrophoresis, Western blot and molecular identification of the target antigen of MAb GB26 10G3 are shown.

Band	Identified proteins	Mass	Mascot score	Sequence coverage %
248	Vimentin	53619	198	39
249	Glial fibrillar acid protein - GFAP	49850	135	32
	Vimentin	53619	123	28
250	Actin, cytoplasmic 1	41710	43	14

Table 5. LC ESI-MS/MS and Mascot software analysis of proteins in bands 248- 250 (Fig. 14).

```
  1 MSTRSVSSSS YRRMFGGPGT ASRPSSSRSY VTTSTRTYSL GSALRPSTSR
 51 SLYASSPGGV YATRSSAVRL RSSVPGVRLL QDSVDFSLAD AINTEFKNTR
101 TNEKVELQEL NDRFANYIDK VRFLEQQNKI LLAELEQLKG QGKSRLGDLY
151 EEEMRELRRQ VDQLTNDKAR VEVERDNLAE DIMRLREKLQ EEMLQREEAE
201 NTLQSFRQDV DNASLARLDL ERKVESLQEE IAFLKKLHEE EIQELQAQIQ
251 EQHVQIDVDV SKPDLTAALR DVRQQYESVA AKNLQEAEEW YKSKFADLSE
301 AANRNNDALR QAKQESTEYR RQVQSLTCEV DALKGTNESL ERQMREMEEN
351 FAVEAANYQD TIGRLQDEIQ NMKEEMARHL REYQDLLNVK MALDIEIATY
401 RKLLEGEESR ISLPLPNFSS LNLRETNLDS LPLVDTHSKR TLLIKTVETR
451 DGQVINETSQ HHDDLE
```

Fig. 15. Amino acid sequences of Vimentin. With red colour are marked amino acids sequences identified by mass-spectroscopy (band 248 in Fig. 14.).

Conclusion

On the basis of data presented above we conclude that the target antigen of MAb GB26 10G3 is protein Vimentin. According to UniProtKB/Swiss-Prot database vimentins are class-III intermediate filaments found in various non-epithelial cells, especially mesenchymal cells (http://www.uniprot.org/uniprot/P08670).

4.1.5 Monoclonal antibody A3G2.B4 (MAb A3G2.B4)

In Fig. 16 we can see the expression of MAb A3G2.B4 antigen (Table 1) in differentiated fetal neural stem/progenitor cell lines hBrSc003 (A,B) and hBrSc005 (B). Note a clear heterogeneous staining of cell nuclei. In D, E,F and G the staining of glioblastoma spheroid cell line differentiated for 7 days, normal epithelial amniotic cells, adult skin fibroblasts and glioblastoma OjFe secondary cell culture are shown, respectively. Note the heterogeneous nuclear and nucleolar staining and a weak cytoplasma staining. However, in Bowes melanoma cell line both the nuclear and strong granular cytoplasmic staining was observed (H).

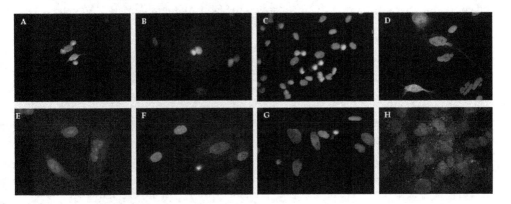

Fig. 16. Presence of MAb A3G2.B4 antigen in different cells. In all cases the cells were fixed with 4% PFA, permeabilized with Tritone X-100 and specifc staining of MAb A3G2.B4 revealed by red staining –Alexa 594. (A,B) Human fetal hBrSc003 neurosphere cells differentiated for 11 days. Double immunofluorescent staining. β-III-tubulin is revealed by green staining – Alexa 488, obj. 40x. (C) Human fetal hBrSc005 neurosphere cells differentiated for 7 days, obj. 40x. (D) Human glioblastoma TiVi spheroid cell line differentiated for 7 days. Double immunofluorescent staining. β-III-tubulin is revealed by green staining – Alexa 488obj. 100x. (E-H) Human normal amniotic epithelial cell line KM on the 2nd days of cultivation, human adult skin fibroblast cell line SA-54 on the 3rd day of cultivation, human glioblastoma OjFe secondary cell culture on the 3rd day of cultivation , and Bowes melanoma cell line on the 2nd day of cultivation, respectively, obj. 100x. DAPI is used for nuclei staining (blue).

In Fig. 17 and 18 the results of Western blot and molecular identification of the target antigen of MAb A3G2.B4 are shown.

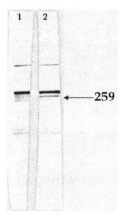

Fig. 17. Western blot with MAb A3G2.B4. Target antigen Lupus La antigen was first immunoprecipitated with MAb A3G4.B4 in 1% NP-40 PBS solution from the concentrated lysate of Bowes melanoma cells. Precipitate was heated at 60°C 15 min, added urea up to end concentration of 2M and proteins separated in SDS-PAGE gradient (8-24%) gel. 1 – negative control with HRP-conjugated goat anti-mouse IgG secondary antibody; 2 – reaction with MAb A3G2.B4 and secondary antibody.

```
  1 MAENGDNEKM AALEAKICHQ IEYYFGDFNL PRDKFLKEQI KLDEGWVPLE
 51 IMIKFNRLNR LTTDFNVIVE ALSKSKAELM EISEDKTKIR RSPSKPLPEV
101 TDEYKNDVKN RSVYIKGFPT DATLDDIKEW LEDKGQVLNI QMRRTLHKAF
151 KGSIFVVFDS IESAKKFVET PGQKYKETDL LILFKDDYFA KKNEERKQNK
201 VEAKLRAKQE QEAKQKLEED AEMKSLEEKI GCLLKFSGDL DDQTCREDLH
251 ILFSNHGEIK WIDFVRGAKE GIILFKEKAK EALGKAKDAN NGNLQLRNKE
301 VTWEVLEGEV EKEALKKIIE DQQESLNKWK SKGRRFKGKG KGNKAAQPGS
351 GKGKVQFQGK KTKFASDDEH DEHDENGATG PVKRAREETD KEEPASKQQK
401 TENGAGDQ
```

Fig. 18. Amino acid sequences of Lupus La protein. With red colour are marked amino acids sequences identified by mass-spectroscopy (band 259 in Fig. 17).

Conclusion
On the basis of data presented above we conclude that the target antigen of MAb A3G2.B4 is protein Lupus La protein. According to UniProtKB/Swiss-Prot database Lupus La protein binds to the 3' poly(U) terminii of nascent RNA polymerase III transcripts, protecting them from exonuclease digestion and facilitating their folding and maturation (http://www.uniprot.org/uniprot/P05455).

5. Discussion and conclusions

The main aim of present study is the development of new monoclonal antibodies against neuronal tissue cells to investigate the differentiation and malignization of human nerve cells. The antibody producing hybridomas were obtained by immunizing mice with the native fragments of human glioblastoma and foetal neural stem/progenitor cells to obtain MAbs against all kinds of antigenic determinants, that are expressed in the living cells, including those determinants, that are expressed on the cell surface. From plenty of MAb-

Development of New Monoclonal Antibodies for Immunocytochemical Characterization of Neural Stem and Differentiated Cells

113

producing clones only those that revealed heterogeneity of reaction with stem/progenitor cells and glioblastoma spheroid cultures were further characterize and the target antigens identified. In this way there is possible to obtain panels of MAbs, that characterizes the given cell types, including tumour cells. The spectrum of the monoclonal antibodies obtained using our method is quite large, including antibodies against proteins as well as against their different modifications. Previously, using described approach we have developed MAb F10H2.B3 specific to Ku80 (ATP-dependent DNA helicase 2 subunit 2). We suggest this antibody could be used in certain conditions as a proliferation marker for cells of different origin (Mikelsaar et al., 2009). In this chapter we present the data about development the five new monoclonal antibodies against neural antigens

Annexin A1 has been reported to take part in different functions as both inhibition of phospholipase A2, acute inflammation, pituitary hormone regulation, fever, neutrophil migration, cell proliferation, and stimulation of cell proliferation, differentiation, apoptosis, membrane repair, macrophage phagocytosis and neuroprotection (Solito et al., 2008). Less information is about annexin A1 expression in the developing brain. It seems to have limited neuronal distribution, but is strongly expressed in glia and ependymocytes (Fava et al., 1989). The studies have shown that annexin A1 (LC-1) positive cells carry other microglial markers and are quite distinct from astrocytes identified by S100B immunoreactivity (McKanna, 1993). It has been also proposed that LC1 can be a comprehensive and reliable marker for microglia (McKanna & Zhang, 1997). Annexins are generally cytosolic proteins, soluble or reversibly associated with components of the cytoskeleton or proteins that mediate interactions between the cell and the extracellular matrix (matricellular proteins) (Moss & Morgan, 2004). In certain cases, annexins may be expressed at the cell surface, despite the absence of any secretory signal peptide (Solito et al., 1994). In differentiated fetal neural stem/progenitor (Fig. 4, A,B,C,D) and glioblastoma spheroid cells (Fig.4, E) MAb E14G2 antigen (annexin A1) is expressed mainly in glial cells but not in β-III-tubulin positive neuronal cells.This observation is in accordance with data on the developing brain obtained by R.A.Fava and coworkers (Fava et al.,1989). Similar picture of expressing of annexin A1 only in limited cell types we have seen also in rat granule primary culture (Fig. 4, H). We propose that the cell expressing annexin A1 might be a Purkinje cell, which have been shown to be annexin A1 positive in adult rat cerebellum (Solito et al., 2008). In rat granule primary culture we have also seen a small amount of GFAP$^+$/annexin A1$^+$ double positive glial cells (data not shown here). The majority of glial cells were only GFAP positive. The expression of annexin A1 was strong and homogenous in glioblastoma OjAr secondary culture and in Bowes melanoma cell lines (Fig. 4, F and G respectively). We propose that MAb E14G2 may be a perspective marker for some distinct neural cell types..

Calnexin is a calcium-binding protein that interacts with newly synthesized glycoproteins in the endoplasmic reticulum (Ellgaard & Helenius, 2003; Ou et al, 1995). Like calreticulin, calnexin is predominantly located in the ER but it has also been identified at the cell surface of a number of cells. Okazaki Y. and co-workers (Okazaki et al., 2000) reported that a small fraction of calnexin is normally expressed on the surface of various cells. The results of these authors suggest that there is continuous exocytosis and endocytosis of calnexin, and the amount of calnexin on the plasma membrane results from the balance of the rates of these two events. The findings suggest that the surface expression of calnexin depends on the association with glycoproteins and that calnexin may play a certain role as a chaperone on the plasma membrane as well (Okazaki et al., 2000). Our observations are in good accordance with previous data. We observed the expression of of MAb E15F10.B9 detected calnexin on the surface of unfixed human adult skin fibroblasts and on fixed, but not permeabilized cells of glioblastoma TiViMNBFCS10 and Bowes melanoma cell line, respectively (Fig. 7, E-G). In Fig. 7 we can see a different expression of MAb E15F10.B9 detected calnexin in differentiated fetal neural stem/progenitor (A) and glioblastoma spheroid cells (C) in which β-III-tubulin-positive cells are negative or very weakly calnexin-positive. In the human fetal hBrSc003 neurosphere culture differentiated for 11 days we see at least three populations of cells, namely the calnexin+/β-III-tubulin-cells, calnexin-/β-III-tubulin+ cells and also cells which are negative for both antigens. It shows that MAb E15F10.B9 may be used for detection of some distinct population of neural cells (see also a strongly calnexin+ cell among other totally calnexin- cells in TiViMNBFCS10 glioblastoma cell culture, Fig.7, F). Interestingly, in the unfixed human sperms we see two separate points between the head and neck of the sperm (H). This phenomenon needs further investigation.

14-3-3 proteins. There are seven genes that encode 14-3-3s in most mammals (Takashi, 2003). 14-3-3 proteins are abundantly expressed in the brain and have been detected in the cerebrospinal fluid of patients with different neurological disorders. By their interaction with more than 100 bindingpartners, 14-3-3 proteins modulate the action of proteins that are involved in cell cycle and transcriptional control, signal transduction, intracellular trafficking and regulation of ion channels. The study of some of these interactions is sheding light on the role of 14-3-3 proteins in processes such as apoptosis and neurodegeneration (Berg et al., 2003). The immunohistological and subcellular location of the 14-3-3 proteins was studied using different isoform-specific antisera (Martin et al., 1994). The immunohistochemical examination using the specific antibody showed significant staining of the cytoplasm, including neuronal axons and dendrites. This result was confirmed by the ultracentrifugal cellular fractionation method, indicating that 14-3-3 is mainly localized in the neuronal cytoplasm and a portion of 14-3-3 may be bound to the plasma membrane, endoplasmic reticulum, and Golgi membrane. This is in good accordance with our *in vitro* study on different cell lines. In Fig. 10 we see the expression of the protein 14-3-3 in the fetal neural stem/progenitor cell lines hBrSc006 (A) and hBrSc009 (B). The strong staining was seen in the cytoplasm in Golgi region, but also in cell projections and nuclei in many cells. In the rat granulare cell culture there are two different 14-3-3 stained cell populations, detected by MAb W4A8.F4: negatively stained cells and cells with positively stained cytoplasm and nuclei (Fig.10, H). It shows that the MAb W4A8.F4 may work in certain conditions as a marker for some types of neural cells. In the fetal skin fibroblasts, glioblastoma, Bowes melanoma and COS-1 cell lines the cytoplasm, especially Golgi region was strongly stained (Fig.10, C,E,F and G respectively).

Interestingly, in the unfixed human sperms the entire tail, except the neck, was strongly and homogeneously stained (Fig.10, D). This is a very interesting fact and needs further investigation.

Vimentins are class-III intermediate filaments found in various non-epithelial cells, especially mesenchymal cells. During the development of the nervous system, vimentin is transiently expressed in virtually all the precursors cells of both neuronal and glial lineages. In the astroglial cell lineage, vimentin is the only IF protein expressed in radial glia and immature astrocytes in the embryonic nervous system (Alonso, 2001; Colluci-Guyon et al., 1999; Schnitzer et al., 1981). The expression of glial fibrillary acidic protein (GFAP), vimentin and fibronectin (Fn) was studied in cells cultured from human glioma and fetal brain by indirect immunofluorescence (IIF) microscopy and multiple labelling experiments (Paetau 1988). The results of the study demonstrate a general coexpression of GFAP and vimentin in cultured astroglial cells, in addition to cells expressing only vimentin. This is in good accordance with our data. In Fig. 13 we see the filamentous staining of the vimentin with MAb GB26 10G3 in human adult skin fibroblasts (A) and in glioblastoma cell line TiViMNBFCS10 (B). In glioblastoma cell lines the staining pattern was very heterogeneous, some cells did not show any signs of staining. Double staining for β-III-tubulin and vimentin (Fig. 13,C) showed an independent staining pattern, some cells were double stained (vimentin+/β-III-tubulin+), some cells showed only β-III-tubulin staining (vimentin- /β-III-tubulin+) and the majority of cells were only vimentin positive. The double staining of vimentin and glial fibrillar acid protein (GFAP) is shown in Fig. 13, D. Note that all the cells are vimentin+/GFAP+, but show an independent staining pattern. We propose that our MAb GB26 10G3 may be a good additional tool for detecting and characterization of expression of vimentin in different types of neural cells, including glioblastomas.

Lupus La protein (known also as Sjogren syndrome antigen B and autoantigen La) is ubiquitous in eukaryotic cells and associates with the 3′ termini of many newly synthesized small RNAs. The La protein protects the 3′ ends of these RNAs from exonucleases (Wolin & Cedervall, 2002). The immunohistochemical location of La antigen was shown to be the nucleus but an intense staining of the nucleolus was seen in human cerebral cortical neurons as well as a subset of neurons of rat brain (Graus et al., 1985). Further it was shown that La ribonucleoproteins (RNP) exist in distinct states that differ in subcellular localization (Intine et al., 2003). This is in good accordance with our results of the immunocytochemical study. In Fig. 16 we see the staining of La protein with MAb A3G2.B4 in nuclei of all cell lines studied. However, the staining of nuclei was very heterogeneous in differentiated fetal neural stem cells (A-C), clearly showing the existence of two cell population for MabA3G2.B4 detected La protein – La protein+ and La protein- cells. This may be a sign of real existence of two different cell populations and needs further investigation. A clear nucleolar staining was also seen in many cells, especially in normal amniocytes and glioblastoma cells (E-G). In the Bowes melanoma cell line both the nuclear and strong granular cytoplasmic staining was observed (H).

Further perspectives. The characterization of the target antigenes and epitopes of all other monoclonal antibodies obtained during our main project is in progress.

6. Acknowledgment

This work was partly supported by target financing SF018809s08 of the Estonian Ministry of Science and Education.

7. References

Alonso, G. (2001). Proliferation of Progenitor Cells in the Adult Rat Brain Correlates With the Presence of Vimentin-Expressing Astrocytes. *Glia*, 34, No.4 , (May), pp. 253-266, ISSN 1098-1136
Bauer, H.C.; Tempfer, H.; Bernroider, G. & Bauer, H. (2006). Neuronal Stem Cells in Adults. *Experimental Gerontology* , Vol.41, No.2, (February), pp. 111-116, ISSN 0531-5565

Bedard, K.; Szabo, E.; Michalak, M. & Opas, M. (2005). Cellular Functions of Endoplasmic Reticulum Chaperones Calreticulin, Calnexin and Erp57. *International Review of Cytology*, Vol.245, pp. 91-121, ISSN 0074-7696

Berg, D.; Holzmann, C. & Riess, O. (2003). 14-3-3 Proteins in the Nervous System. *Nature Reviews Neuroscience*, Vol.4, No.9, (September), pp. 752-762, ISSN 1471-0048

Bez, A.; Corsini, E.; Curti, D.; Biggiogera, M.; Colombo, A.; Nicosia, R.F.; Pagano, S.F. & Parati, E.A. (2003). Neurosphere and neurosphere-forming cells: morphological and ultrastructural characterization. *Brain Research*, Vol.993, No.1-2., (December), pp. 18-29, ISSN 0006-8993

Canvar, P.J.; Olenych, S.G.& Keller III, T.C.S. (2007). Molecular Identification and Localization of Cellular Titin, A Novel Titin Isoform in the Fibroblast Stress Fiber. *Cell Motility and the Cytosceleton*, Vol 64, No. 6, (June), pp. 418-433, ISSN 1097-0169

Colluci-Guyon, E.; Ribotta, M.G.Y.; Maurice, T.; Babinet, C. & Privat, A. (1999). Cerebellar Defect and Impaired Motor Coordination in Mica Lacking Vimentin. *Glia*, Vol.25, No.1, (January), pp. 33-43,ISSN 1098-1136

Ellgaard, L. & Helenius, A.(2003). Quality control in the endoplasmic reticulum. *Nature Reviews Molecular Cell Biology*, Vol. 4, No.3, (March), pp. 181–191, ISSN 1471-0072

Fava, R.A.; McKanna, J. & Cohen, S. (1989). Lipocortin I (p35) is abundant in a restricted number of differentiated cell types in adult organs. Journal of Cellular Physiology, Vol.141, No.2, (November), pp. 284-293, ISSN 0021-9541

Graus, F.; Cordon-Cardo, C.; Bonfa, E. & Elkon, K.B. (1985). Immunohistochemical Localization of La Nuclear Antigen in Brain. Selective Concentration of the La Protein in Neuronal Nucleoli. *Journal of Neuroimmunolgy*, Vol.9, No.5, (September), pp. 307-319, ISSN 0165-5728

Intine, R.V., Tenenbaum, S.A.; Sakulich, A.L,; Keene, J.D. & Maraia, R.J. (2003). Differential phosphorylation and subcellular localization of La RNPs associated with precursor tRNAs and translation-related mRNAs. *Molecular Cell*, Vol.12, No.5, (November), pp. 1301-1307, ISSN 1097-2765

Kalev, I.; Kaasik, A.; Žarkovski, A.& Mikelsaar, A.-V. (2006). Chemokine Receptor CCR5 Expression in *in vitro* Differentiating Human Fetal Neural Stem/Progenitor and Glioblastoma Cells. *Neuroscience Letters*, Vol.394, No.1, pp. 22-27, ISSN 0304-3940

Kang, D.; Gho, Y.S.; Suh, M.& Kang, C.(2002). Highly Sensitive and Fast Protein Detection with Coomassie Brilliant Blue in Sodium Dodecyl Sulfate-Polyacrylamide Gel Electrophoresis. *Bulletin of the Korean Chemical Society*, Vol.23, No.11, pp. 1511-1512, ISSN 0253-2964

Kennea, N.L. & Mehmet, H. (2002). Neural Stem Cells. *Journal of Pathology*, Vol.197, No.4, (July), pp. 536–550, ISSN 0022-3417

Kraus, A.; Groenendyk, J.; Bedard, K.; Baldwin, T.A., Krause, K.-H.; Dubois-Dauphin, M.; Dyck, J.; Rosenbaum, E.E.; Korngut, L.; Colley, N.J.; Gosgnach, S.; Zochodne, D.; Todd, K.; Agellon, L.B. & Michalak, M. (2010). Calnexin Deficiency Leads to Desmyelination. *Journal of Biological Chemistry*, Vol.285, No.24, (June), pp. 18928-18938, ISSN 0021-9258

Martin, H.; Rostas, J.; Patel, Y. & Aitken, A. (1994). Subcellular localization of 14-3-3 isoforms in rat brain using specific antibodies. *Journal of Neurochemistry*, Vol. 63, No. 6, (December), pp. 2259–2265, ISSN 0022-3042

McArthur, S.; Cristante, E.; Paterno, M.; Christian, H; Roncaroli, F.; Gillies, G.E. & Solito, E. (2010). Annexin A1: A Central Player in the Anti-Inflammatory and Neuroprotective Role of Microglia. *Journal of Immunology*, Vol.185, No.10, (November), pp. 6317-6328, ISSN 0022-1767

McKanna, J.A. (1993). Primitive glial compartments in the floor plate of mammalian embryos: distinct progenitors of adult astrocytes and microglia support the notoplate hypothesis. *Perspectives on Developmental Neurobiology*, Vol.1, No.4, pp. 245–255, ISSN 1064-0517

McKanna, J.A. & Zhang, M.-Z. (1997). Immunohistochemical Localization of Lipocortin 1 in Rat Brain is Sensitive to pH, Freezing and Dehydratation. *Journal of Histochemistry & Cytochemistry*, Vol.45, No.4, (April), pp. 527-538, ISSN 0022-1554

Mikelsaar, A.-V.; Sünter, A.; Toomik, P.; Karpson, K.& Juronen, E. (2009). New Anti-Ku80 Monoclonal Antibody F10H2.B3 As a Useful Marker for Dividing Cells in Culture. *Hybridoma*, Vol.28, No.2, (April), pp. 107-111, ISSN 1554-0014

Moss, S.E. & Morgan, R.O. (2004). The annexins. *Genome Biology*, Vol.5, No.4, (March), pp. 219-219.8, ISSN 1465-6906

Ou, W. J.; Cameron, P. H.; Thomas, D. Y. & Bergeron, J. J. (1993). Association of folding intermediates of glycoproteins with calnexin during protein maturation. *Nature*, Vol. 364, No.6440, (August), pp. 771–776, ISSN 0028-0836

Okazaki, Y.; Ohno, H.; Takase, K.; Ochiai, T. & Takashi, S. (2000). Cell Surface Expression of Calnexin, a Molecular Chaperone in the Endoplasmic Reticulum. *The Journal of Biological Chemistry*, Vol.275, No.46, (November), pp. 35751-35758, ISSN 0021-9258

Paetau, A. (1988). Glial fibrillary acidic protein, vimentin and fibronectin in primary cultures of human glioma and fetal brain. *Acta Neuropathologica (Berl.)*, Vol.75, 5, (May), pp. 448-455, ISSN 0001-6322

Perretti, M. & D'Acquisto, F. (2009). Annexin A1 and Glucocorticoid as Effectors of the Resolution of Inflammation. *Nature Reviews Immunology*, Vol.9, No.1, (January), pp. 62-70, ISSN 1474-1733

Riemekasten, G. & Hahn, B.H. (2005). Key Autoantigens in SLE. *Rheumatology*, Vol.44, No.8 , (August), pp. 975-982, ISSN 0315-162X

Schnitzer, J.; Franke, W.W. & Schachner, M. (1981). Immunocytochemical Demonstration of Vimentin in Astrocytes and Ependymal Cells of Developing and Adult Mouse Nervous System. *The Journal of Cell Biology*, Vol. 90, No.2, (August), pp. 435-447, ISSN 0021-9525

Schwartz, P.H.; Brick, D.J.; Alexander E. Stover, A.E.; Loring, J.F. & Müller, F.-J. (2008). Differentiation of Neural Lineage Cells from Human Pluripotent Stem Cells. *Methods*, Vol.45, No.2, (June), pp. 142–158, ISSN 1046-2023

Solito, E.; Nuti, S. & Parente, L. (1994). Dexamethasone-induced translocation of lipocortin (annexin) 1 to the cell membrane of U-937 cells. *British Journal of Pharmacology*, Vol.112, No.2, (June), pp. 347-348, ISSN 0007-1188

Solito, E.; McArthur, S.; Christian, H., Gavins, F.; Buckingham, J.C. & Gillies, G.E. Annexin A1 in the Brain – Undiscovered Roles? *Trends in Pharmacological Sciences*, Vol.29, No.3, (March), pp. 135-142, ISSN 0165-6147

Takahashi, Y. (2003). The 14-3-3 Proteins: Gene, Gene Expression and Function. Neurochemical Research. Vol. 28, No.8, (August), pp. 1265-1273, ISSN 0364-3190

Young, K.A.; Hirst, W.D.; Solito, E. & Wilkin, G.P. (1999). De Novo Expression of Lipocortin-1 in Reactive Microglia and Astrocytes in Kainic Acid Lesioned Rat Cerebellum. *Glia*, Vol.26, No.4, (June), pp. 333-343, ISSN 1098-1136

Tijssen P.,(1985) *Practice and theory of enzyme immunoassays*, in: Laboratory techniques in biochemistry and molecular biology, R.H.Burdon and P.H. van Knippenberg Elsevier pp. 221-278, Elsevier, ISBN 0-444-80633-4, Netherlands

Yuan, S.H.; Martin, J.; Elia, J.; Flippin, J.; Paramban, R.I.; Hefferan, M.P.; Vidal, J.G.; Mu, Y.; Killian, R.L.; Mason A. Israel, M.A.; Emre, N.; Marsala, S.; Marsala, M.; Gage, F.H.; Goldstein, L.S.B. & Carson, Ch.T. (2011). Cell-Surface Marker Signatures for the Isolation of Neural Stem Cells, Glia and Neurons Derived from Human Pluripotent Stem Cells. *PLoS ONE*, Vol.6, No.3, (March), pp. 1-16, ISSN 1932-6203

Zhang, X.; Szabo, E.; Michalak, M. & Opas, M. (2007). Endoplasmic Reticulum Stress During the Embryonic Development of the Central Nervous System in the Mouse. Intenational *Journal of Developmental Neuroscience*, Vol. 25, No.7 , (November), pp. 455-463, ISSN 0736-5748

Witusik-Perkowska, M.; Rieske, P.; Hulas-Bigoszewska, K.; Zakrzewska, M.; Stawski, R.; Kulczycka-Wojdala, D.; Bienkowski, M.; Stoczynska-Fidelus, E.; Grešner, S.M.; Piaskowski, S.; Jaskolski, D.J.; Papierz, W.; Zakrzewski, K.; Kolasa, M.; Ironside, J.W. & Liberski, P.P. (2011). Glioblastoma-Derived Spheroid Cultures as an Experimental Model for Analysis of EGFR Anomalies. *Journal of Neuro-Oncology*, Vol.102, No.3, (May), pp. 395-407, ISSN 0167-594X

Wolin, S.L. & Cedervall, T. (2002). The La Protein. *Annual Review of Biochemistry*, Vol. 71, No.1, pp. 375-403, ISSN 15454509, 0066-4154

Part 2

Neural Stem Cells in Invertebrates

6

Regeneration of Brain and Dopaminergic Neurons Utilizing Pluripotent Stem Cells: Lessons from Planarians

Kaneyasu Nishimura[1,3], Yoshihisa Kitamura[2] and Kiyokazu Agata[1]
[1]Department of Biophysics, Graduate School of Science, Kyoto University
[2]Department of Neurobiology, Kyoto Pharmaceutical University
[3]Department of Cell Growth and Differentiation,
Center for iPS Cell Research and Application (CiRA), Kyoto University
Japan

1. Introduction

Cell-transplantation therapy for Parkinson's disease is close to becoming a reality thanks to the recent development of methods for the differentiation of dopaminergic neurons and/or dopaminergic progenitor cells from embryonic stem cells (ESCs) and induced pluripotent stem cells (iPSCs) under *in vitro* conditions (Kawasaki et al., 2000, Perrier et al., 2004). There have been several reports concerning pre-clinical trial research for cell-transplantation therapy for Parkinson's disease with dopaminergic progenitor cells derived from either ESCs or iPSCs using rodent and non-human primate disease models before clinical trial (Björklund et al., 2002; Takagi et al., 2005; Wernig et al., 2008). Many researchers have contributed to improve the technology to create more efficient differentiation methods of donor cells for clinical applications (Chambers et al., 2009; Morizane et al., 2011). However, we still need to overcome many problems before such technology can be used in clinical settings. Even if we succeed in obtaining an optimized donor cell population for cell-transplantation, the rate of success of the transplantation may depend not only on the quality of donor cells but also on the host brain environment. One important issue is how to integrate dopaminergic neurons or dopaminergic progenitor cells into target regions after transplantation. However, we do not know what kind of donor cells will be efficiently integrated into the neural networks of the host brain. Also, we do not know whether fully differentiated neurons will really survive in the host brain. In addition, we need to know what state of the host brain environment will allow the participation of donor cells in the neural networks of the host brain. In order to solve such problems, planarians provide unique opportunities because they show robust regenerative ability based on their pluripotent stem cell system.

Planarians can regenerate lost tissues, including the nervous system, via their pluripotent stem cells (neoblasts) that are distributed throughout their body. In contrast, it is difficult for higher vertebrates to achieve the regeneration of the nervous system, in spite of their possession of neural stem cells. The success of tissue regeneration requires not only the presence of proliferating stem cells as a source but also the presence of the regulatory system for stem cells. Knowledge gained about the planarian stem cell system can provide hints about how to conduct cell-transplantation therapy for regenerative medicine in the future.

In this chapter, we focus on two different regenerative phenomena utilizing the stem cell system in planarians. The first one is brain regeneration after decapitation. The second is brain neurogenesis after selective neuronal degeneration (without decapitation). Both of them are achieved by regulation of the pluripotent stem cells distributed throughout the body. We address the following questions: (1) what type(s) of cells recognize the loss of the organs or cells? (2) What signal(s) initiate the regeneration or neurogenesis? (3) What signal(s) are necessary for recruitment of stem cells to defined type(s) of cells and the replacement in the proper positions.

2. Pluripotent stem cells of planarians

The flatworm *Dugesia japonica* is a common species of freshwater planarian in Japan, and has been extensively used as an experimental animal for regeneration and neuroscience studies. When planarians are artificially amputated, they can regenerate their whole body from even very small fragments (is the smallest competent fragment reported was 1/279th of the body; Morgan, 1898). This strong regenerative ability is supported by pluripotent stem cells called neoblasts. The neoblasts are the only mitotic cell population, and are distributed in the mesenchymal space throughout the body except for the region around the brain and the pharynx of *D. japonica* (Shibata et al., 1999; 2010) (Fig. 1). The neoblasts can differentiate in all types of cells and self-renew under both homeostatic and injured conditions. X-ray-irradiation induces selective elimination of proliferating stem cells in planarians, resulting in the loss of regenerative ability (Shibata et al., 1999; Hayashi et al., 2006). Therefore, X-ray irradiation is a powerful experimental tool for analyzing the stem cell system. We identified a *vasa*-like gene *(Djvlg)* as the first reported gene specifically expressed in neoblasts (Shibata et al., 1999). Recently, many reliable molecular markers for neoblasts, such as *piwi* homologue genes, have been identified (Fig. 1) (Salvetti et al., 2000, 2005, Orii et al., 2005; Reddien et al., 2005; Eisenfoffer et al., 2007; Shibata et al., 2010). Since pluripotent stem cells are the only proliferating and mitotic cell population, experimental methods using 5-bromo-2'-deoxyuridine (BrdU) (Newmark & Sánchez Alvarado, 1999), and immunostaining using anti-phosphohistone H3 (pH3) antibody (Hendzel et al., 1997; Newmark & Sánchez Alvarado, 1999) are also useful tools for staining neoblasts.Recently, the pluripotency of these cells was demonstrated by single Icell-transplantation experiments (Wagner et al., 2011). In addition, we found that pluripotent stem cells can be categorized into several cell populations by electromicroscopy analysis, suggesting that pluripotent stem cells are not a homogenous population, but may have heterogeneity like stem cell systems in higher animals (Higuchi et al., 2007). In addition, we recently developed single-cell PCR technology that is able to analyze the gene expression profile in individual cells at the single cell level (Hayashi et al., 2010). This method is a powerful tool for determining gene characteristics of not only pluripotent stem cells but also of tissues such as the nervous system.

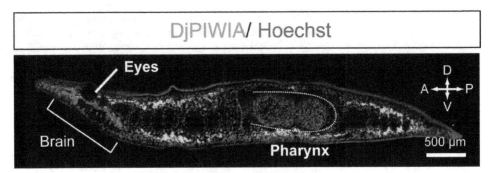

Fig. 1. Distribution of pluripotent stem cells of planarian *D. japonica*. Immunostaining using anti-DJPIWIA antibody (a marker of pluripotent stem cells) (Shibata et al., 2010) in a transverse section. Planarian stem cells are distributed in the mesenchymal space throughout the body.

3. Fundamental brain structure and function

Planarians have a simple body shape with cephalization, a dorso-ventral axis and bilateral symmetry, and are thought to be primitive animals, that acquired a central nervous system (CNS) at an early stage of evolution. The planarian CNS composed of a bilobed brain and a pair of ventral nerve cords (VNCs) (Agata et al., 1998; Tazaki et al., 1999). The brain is located in the anterior region of the body, and forms an inverted U-shaped structure (Fig. 2A). A pair of VNCs are located more ventral by relative to the brain, extending along the anterior-posterior (A-P) axis. The VNCs are a structure independent of the brain, although they are directly connected to it (Okamoto et al., 2005). The brain can be divided into several functional domains (Cebrià et al., 2002a; Nakazawa et al., 2003). The nine pairs of lateral branches of the brain project to the head margin, and function as the sensory system (Okamoto et al., 2005). A pair of eyes is located on the dorsal side of the brain, and the optic nerves forms the optic chiasm, and project to the dorso-medial position of the brain, which functions as the photosensory center (Sakai et al., 2000). The two main lobes of the brain consist of a mass of interneurons that function in the integration of multiple stimuli.

When planarians are exposed to some stimuli such as light-, chemo-, thermo- and mechano-stimulations, they can integrate different stimuli in the brain and decide on a response to these multiple stimuli. Planarians show light avoidance behavior known as negative phototaxis. We established a quantitative analytical method for this behavior that involves measuring the distance, direction, and speed of movement (Inoue et al., 2004). By using this method and RNA interference (RNAi), we showed that several molecules such as a planarian synaptosome-associated protein of 25 kDa (*Djsnap-25*) and a planarian glutamic acid decarboxylase (*DjGAD*) play important roles in photorecognition (Takano et al., 2007; Nishimura et al., 2008a). These results indicate that planarian behavior is regulated the molecular level via brain functions that are similar to mammalian brain functions.

3.1 Functional domain structure

We found that functional domains in the brain were defined by three *orthodenticle* and *orthopedia* homeobox genes (*DjotxA*, *DjotxB* and *Djotp*) that are exclusively expressed in specific regions of the brain (Umesono et al., 1997; 1999). *DjotxA* is expressed in the optic nerves and medial region of the brain, which form a photosensory domain. *DjotxB* is expressed in the main lobes of the brain, which form a signal processing domain containing a variety of interneurons. *Djotp* is expressed in the lateral branches, which form chemosensory domains. The lateral side of the head region, where *Otx/otp* expression is not detected, contains mechanosensory neurons. In addition, A-P patterning of the brain was shown to be regulated by the expression of *wnt*-family genes (*DjwntA* and *DjfzA*) (Kobayashi et al., 2007). Whereas *DjotxA, DjotxB* and *Djotp* genes were shown to be expressed medio-laterally, *DjwntA* and *DjfzA* genes were expressed antero-posteriorly in the brain. *Wnt* family genes and *Otx/otp* family genes play important roles in domain formation in planarians, as in mammals.

DNA microarray analysis comparing the head region versus the body region of planarians identified many genes that are specifically expressed in the head region (Nakazawa et al., 2003; Mineta et al., 2003). Expression analysis based on whole-mount *in situ* hybridization revealed that many neural genes that are conserved in the vertebrate brain are also expressed in several distinct domains of the planarian CNS (Cebrià et al., 2002a; Mineta et al., 2003). These results indicate that the planarian CNS is functionally regionalized by discrete expression of neural-specific genes.

3.2 Variations of neurotransmitters

Recently, we revealed that planarians have various neural populations defined by neurotransmitters, such as dopamine (DA), serotonin (5-HT), γ-aminobutyric acid (GABA), octopamine (OA; a counterpart of noradrenaline of vertebrates) and acetylcholine (ACh) (Nishimura et al., 2007a, 2007b, 2008a, 2008b, 2008c, 2010; Takeda et al., 2008) (Fig. 2). Immunostaining with specific antibodies against these neurons enables us to visualize their cell morphology and localizations at the single-cell level (Fig. 2). These neurons are distributed in restricted regions in the planarian CNS. In addition, each neuron exclusively uses one neurotransmitter, and forms distinct neural networks in the planarian CNS.

These neurons have also distinct functions, such as locomotion activity and photorecognition. Combined RNAi and pharmacological approaches revealed that dopaminergic neurons positively regulate muscle-mediated behavior. Upregulation of the DA level induced by methamphetamine (DA releaser) caused hyperkinetic conditions such as screw-like hyperkinesia and C-like hyperkinesia, and treatment with DA receptor antagonists (sulpride and reserpine) and reduction of the DA level by RNAi suppressed these hyperkinetic conditions (Nishimura et al., 2007a). Moreover, although an increase of the ACh level by physostigmine (acetylcholinesterase inhibitor) treatment induced sudden muscular contraction, treatment with ACh receptor antagonists (tubocrarine and atropine) or reduction of the ACh level by RNAi extended these behavioral changes (Nishimura et al., 2010). Our histological analysis indicated that cholinergic neurons elongated at neighboring positions of the body-wall musculature (DjMHC-B-positive cells), but dopaminergic neurons did not elongate to the body-wall musculature. These results suggest that although both dopaminergic and cholinergic neurons regulate motor functions, cholinergic neurons act as motor neurons whilst dopaminergic neurons act as interneurons in planarians. These results also indicate that similar gene sets function in both the planarian CNS and the vertebrate CNS.

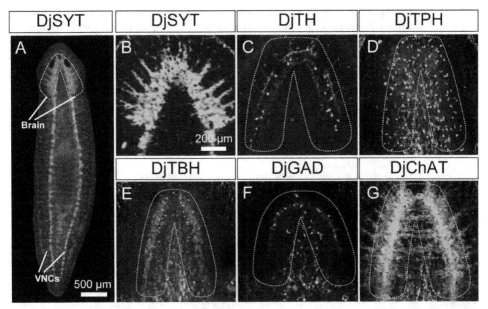

Fig. 2. The neural networks of neurotransmitter-synthesizing neurons. Distribution of pan-neural networks (DjSYT-positive neurons) of the whole body (A) and head (B). Distribution of dopaminergic neurons (DjTH-positive neurons) (C), serotonergic neurons (DjTPH-positive neurons) (D), octopaminergic neurons (DjTBH-positive neurons) (E), GABAergic neurons (DjGAD-positive neurons) (F), and cholinergic neurons (DjChAT-positive neurons) (G) in intact planarian head. White broken line indicates the outline of the brain (B-G).

4. Whole brain regeneration after head amputation

One of most interesting regeneration phenomena in planarians is that they can regenerate a functional brain from any portion of the body within 7-10 days after amputation, utilizing the pluripotent stem cell system. Although non-brain fragments just after decapitation show very little response external stimulation, they can restore normal behaviors such as feeding and negative phototaxis within one week. How can planarians regenerate their CNS not only morphologically but also functionally in one week? This regenerative process can be divided into at least five steps as defined by sequential gene expression alterations, which are similar to those in mammalian brain development (Agata & Umesono et al., 2008). That is, (1) anterior blastema formation, (2) brain rudiment formation, (3) pattern formation, (4) neural network formation, and (5) functional recovery (Fig. 3).

4.1 The stem cell system for brain regeneration

The first step of head regeneration after decapitation involves wound healing and subsequently the formation of the blastema, which is defined by a mass of morphologically undifferentiated cells at the edge of the amputated site. Dorso-ventral attachment induces initiation of the expression of *noggin-like gene A* (*DjnlgA*) at the edge of the amputated site after wound healing, and this expression leads to blastema formation in the first step of planarian regeneration (Ogawa et al., 2002). Mitotic cells are never observed in the blastema, in spite of the increasing mass of the blastema during regeneration (Wenemoser & Reddien, 2010; Tasaki et al, 2001a, 2001b). Recently, it was shown that the blastema cells are supplied from the postblastema region via mitosis from G2 phase-pluripotent stem cells, and that c-Jun-N-terminal kinase (JNK) is involved in this G2/M transition, and that extracellular signal-related kinase (ERK) is required for exit from the proliferative undifferentiated state during blastema formation (Tasaki et al., 2011a, 2011b). It is thought that BMP/noggin signal might be involved in activation of the ERK signal in cooperation with the JNK signal to form the blastema after wound closure.

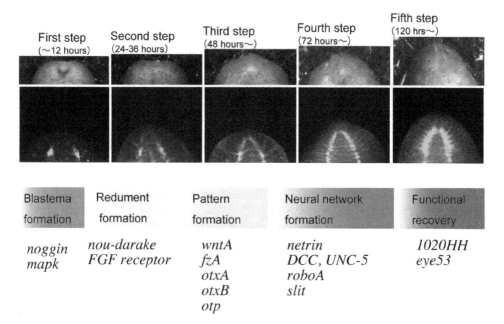

First step (~12 hours)	Second step (24-36 hours)	Third step (48 hours~)	Fourth step (72 hours~)	Fifth step (120 hrs~)
Blastema formation	Redument formation	Pattern formation	Neural network formation	Functional recovery
noggin mapk	nou-darake FGF receptor	wntA fzA otxA otxB otp	netrin DCC, UNC-5 roboA slit	1020HH eye53

Fig. 3. Brain regeneration process after decapitation. This process can be divided into at least five steps according to sequential gene expression alterations. Abbreviations used; mapk, mitogen-activated protein kinase; FGF, fibroblast growth factor; DCC, deleted in colorectal cancer; UNC-5, uncoordinated-5; robo, roundabout.

After the formation of blastemas, the ERK signal is suppressed in the posterior blastema, but enhanced in the anterior blastema. Recently, we found that the hedgehog (Hh) signal has an important role in causing the difference between the anterior and posterior blastemas. In planarians, Hh is produced in the nervous system and Hh-containing vesicles might be transported from anterior to posterior along microtubules inside of the neurites (Yazawa et al., 2009). After amputation of the planarian body, Hh may be secreted from the posterior end of the amputated neurites, and then the Hh signal activates the Wnt signal in the posterior blastema to suppress the ERK signal and activate posterior-specific genes. In contrast, in the anterior blastema, the ERK signal forms a positive feedback loop to activate brain rudiment formation. A fibroblast growth factor receptor (FGFR)-like molecule, *nou-*

darake (*ndk*; meaning "brains everywhere" in Japanese), may have an important role in defining the region forming the positive feedback loop of the ERK signal in the anterior blastema (Cebrià et al., 2002b). The *ndk* gene was identified in *D. japonica* as a gene expressed in the brain rudiment at an early stage of brain regeneration. Interestingly, silencing of the *ndk* gene by RNAi induces the ectopic brain formation in all regions of the body. Thus, *ndk* is essential for defining the region where the brain rudiment is formed.

After formation of the brain rudiment, the Wnt and bone morphogenic protein (BMP) signaling pathways may regulate pattern formation of the brain along the A-P (Kobayashi et al., 2007; Gurley et al., 2008; Petersen & Reddien, 2008) and D-V (Molina et al., 2011; Gavino & Reddien, 2011) polarity, respectively. In conclusion, stem cells may be regulated by various signals in spatial- and temporal manners to form a functional brain.

4.2 Axon guidance and neural network formation during brain regeneration

New brain neurons have to project toward appropriate target sites to reconstruct their neural networks during regeneration. Recently, several axon guidance molecules, including netrin, uncoordinated-5 (UNC-5), deleted in colorectal cancer (DCC), slit, and roundabout (robo) were identified as key molecules regulating axon guidance during eye and brain regeneration in planarians (Cebrià & Newmark 2005, 2007; Cebrià et al., 2007; Yamamoto & Agata, 2011). It is known that netrin is a secreted protein that regulates the direction of axon growth by chemo-attractive and repulsive responses mediated by two types of receptor, UNC-5 and DCC (Hong et al., 1999). Slit is also a secreted protein, and acts as a chemo-repulsive factor for commisure axons by binding to robo in various animals (Brose et al., 1999). RNAi-mediated functional analysis revealed that the silencing of these guidance molecules caused abnormal neural network formation in the CNS and optic nerves during regeneration.

4.3 Functional recovery after completion of whole brain regeneration

In order to analyze the brain function during brain regeneration, we focused on negative phototaxis behavior. We found that there is a time gap between morphological and functional recovery. Although the optic nerves were reconstructed within 4 days after decapitation, negative phototaxis behavior began to recover from 5 days after decapitation (Inoue et al., 2004). Interestingly, two genes, *1020HH* and *eye53* genes, were activated just after completion of the morphological recovery (Cebrià et al., 2002c). Silencing of either *1020HH* or *eye53* caused a defect of the complete recovery of negative phototaxis. These findings suggest that these genes might be involved in the functional recovery, and morphological regeneration and functional regeneration can be distinguished according to their respective gene expression alterations (Inoue et al., 2004).

5. Neurogenesis after selective neuronal lesioning

Recently, we established an experimental model system for selective neuronal elimination to analyze the neurogenesis after selective neuronal lesioning without amputation. For this, we employed 6-hydroxydopamine (6-OHDA)-induced lesioning. 6-OHDA is a cytotoxic substance that induces dopaminergic neuronal cell death, and is widely used for killing dopaminergic neurons and creating parkinsonian animal models (Ungerstedt & Arbuthnott,

1970; Schwarting & Huston, 1996; Nass et al., 2002; Parish et al., 2007). In rodents, the nigro-striatal dopaminergic system is acutely and selectively degenerated by 6-OHDA-microinjection into the substantia nigra, and never recovers the missing neurons (Ungerstedt & Arbuthnott, 1970; Schwarting & Huston, 1996). We succeeded in selective degeneration of dopaminergic neurons in planarians, like that in higher animals. Interestingly, we found that planarians can regenerate only the dopaminergic neurons within 14 days after 6-OHDA-incuded selective dopaminergic neural degeneration (Fig. 4A). Although it has been reported that dopaminergic neurons are also regenerated during the head regeneration process after decapitation (Nishimura et al., 2007a; Takeda et al., 2009), our findings with 6-OHDA are the first showing that planarians are able to regenerate dopaminergic neurons after the selective degeneration of only dopaminergic neurons in the brains of non-amputated animals (Nishimura et al., 2011). According to our observations, dopaminergic neurons were completely degenerated and this degeneration was accompanied by reductions of DA content and locomotion activity within 24 hours after

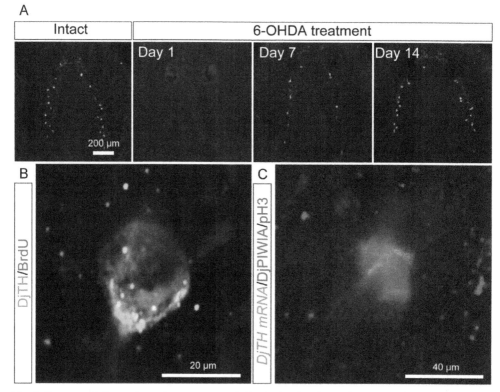

Fig. 4. Process of dopaminergic neurogenesis in the brain after 6-OHDA-induced-lesioning. Immunostaining of brain dopaminergic neurons in intact planarian and 1 day, 7 days, and 14 days after 6-OHDA-administration (A). BrdU-signal can be detected in newly generated dopaminergic neurons 10 days after 6-OHDA-administration (B). Newly generated dopaminergic neurons are produced from stem cells via cell division (C).

6-OHDA-administration. Then, newly generated dopaminergic neurons began to be detected in the brain 4 days after the 6-OHDA-induced lesion. Thereafter, the numbers and axons of dopaminergic neurons gradually recovered over a period of several days. Finally, dopaminergic neurons were completely recovered within 14 days after the 6-OHDA-induced lesion. We confirmed that in this process (1) X-ray-irradiated planarians never regenerate dopaminergic neurons after the 6-OHDA-induced lesion, (2) newly generated dopaminergic neurons are derived from pluripotent stem cells, as demonstrated by long-term trace experiments using BrdU. The dopaminergic neurogenesis after selective degeneration can be divided into three steps: (i) selective dopaminergic neurodegeneration (~24 hr after 6-OHDA-induced lesion), (ii) a transition period (24~72 hr), (iii) dopaminergic neurogenesis and dopaminergic neural network regeneration (96 hr~).

5.1 Recruitment of new dopaminergic neurons from pluripotent stem cells

Long-term chase experiments after BrdU-labeling clearly demonstrated that newly generated dopaminergic neurons are derived from proliferative stem cells. However, a BrdU-pulse chase analysis revealed that BrdU-incorporating cells were detected only in the trunk region but not around the brain region at all. In addition, immunohistochemical analysis using anti-proliferating cell nuclear antigen (PCNA) antibody revealed that PCNA-positive cells were never observed around the brain region (Orii et al., 2005). These results support the notion that essentially no proliferating stem cells that enter S-phase exist around the brain region. Thus, BrdU-positive cells detected in the brain by long term-chase experiments may migrate from the trunk region after proliferation (Newmark & Sánchez Alvarado 1999) (Fig. 4B). Therefore, we carefully investigated when proliferating stem cells are committed to differentiate into dopaminergic neurons during regeneration. Finally, we found that G2 phase stem cells are committed around the brain area to differentiate into dopaminergic neurons after lesioning. The most critical result was obtained by triple staining experiments immunostaining with anti-DjPIWIA antibody and anti-pH3 antibody and *in situ* hybridization using *a planarian tyrosine hydroxylase homologue (DjTH)* riboprobe. We detected *DjTH* mRNA/DjPIWIA protein/pH3-triple positive cells around the brain (Fig. 4C), suggesting that G2 phase stem cells may be accumulated in the head region and that these cells may participate in both regeneration and homeostatic events of the brain. It has already been suggested that the pluripotent stem cells may be committed at G2 phase into appropriate cell types (Hayashi et al., 2010), consistent with dividing stem cells immediately starting to differentiate to dopaminergic neurons. Based on these observations, we speculate that after proliferating in the trunk region, stem cells may migrate into the head region at G2 phase and then some of them might become committed to producing dopaminergic neurons (Nishimura et al., 2011).

5.2 System for recognition of the ablation of dopaminergic neurons

In planarians, it is known that older differentiated cells are constantly eliminated by apoptosis, and are then replaced by new cells by proliferation of stem cells under physiological conditions in planarians (Inoue et al., 2007; Pellettieri & Sánchez Alvarado, 2007). In our observation, a few BrdU-positive dopaminergic neurons were detected in vehicle-control-injected planarians, indicating that dopaminergic neurons could be replaced by stem cell proliferation in physiological conditions via homeostasis. Importantly, 6-

OHDA-induced lesioning accelerated the number and rate of the brain dopaminergic neurogenesis compared to that under physiological conditions in planarians. These results suggest that the number of dopaminergic neurons might be monitored by their surrounding environment. In the case of newts, a lower vertebrate, neurogenic potential for the repair of lost dopaminergic neurons is maintained even in adults (Parish et al., 2007), and this potential may work under conditions of injury-responsive cell-replacement that are induced by dopaminergic signals mediated by the DA receptor, but not under homeostatic conditions (Berg et al., 2010, 2011). In contrast, rodents have neural stem cells in restrict regions. It is known that the activity (proliferation and migration) of endogenous neural stem cells is enhanced in response to acute brain lesions caused by insults such as stroke and neurotoxin-exposure in the adult state (Arvidsson et al., 2002, Höglinger et al., 2004), suggesting that neural stem cells present in the adult brain can be responsive to alterations of the surrounding environment. In the future, it will be possible to identify the cellular and molecular systems that contribute to the recognition of dopaminergic ablation and the recruitment of new dopaminergic neurons, and it will become possible to use RNAi-mediated gene-knockdown and pharmacological drugs to further clarify the regulatory system of dopaminergic neurogenesis/regeneration.

6. Characterization of stem cell participation in brain regeneration

In both types of regeneration processes (*i.e.*, dopaminergic neurogenesis during brain regeneration and after selective degeneration of dopaminergic neurons), we have never observed the neural stem cell-like cells in planarians. Although commitment occurs at G2 phase, one committed stem cell produces only two differentiated cells. Committed stem cells can never enter into S phase after mitosis. Thus, we speculate that planarians have not yet invented a neural stem cell system. Histological analysis during regeneration supported the notion that pluripotent stem cells may directly give rise to fully differentiated neurons. First, we never observed proliferating cells in the brain rudiment during brain regeneration or in the intact brain. Second, the expression of the planarian *musashi* family genes supports the above hypothesis. *Musashi*, an RNA binding protein, is expressed in neural stem cells and/or progenitor cells in various animals (Okano et al., 2002). We isolated three *musashi*-like genes (*DjmlgA*, *DjmlgB* and *DjmlgC*) from planarians (Higuchi et al., 2008). Although they were expressed in the planarian CNS, their expression was not eliminated by X-ray irradiation, indicating that these genes were expressed after cells entered the differentiated state, not in the proliferative stem cells. Based on these observations, we hypothesized that the neural stem cell system probably evolved at a later stage of evolution independently in higher animals such as insects and vertebrates (Agata *et al.* 2006).

In the case of brain regeneration after decapitation, the brain rudiment is formed inside of the anterior blastema. The cells participating into blastema formation have already existed the proliferative state (Tasaki et al., 2011a, 2011b). A part of these cells then start to form the brain rudiment. Thus, commitment of dopaminergic neurons may occur after pattern formation of the brain. And then the neurons forming the primary brain might start to recruit G2 phase stem cells into brain neurons during enlargement of the brain and homeostasis (Takeda et al., 2009). In the case of dopaminergic neurogenesis after 6-OHDA-induced lesioning, G2 phase stem cells located around the brain may be recruited into dopaminergic neurons. The remaining neurons in the brain after 6-OHDA-induced lesioning may have an important role for sensing loss of dopaminergic neurons and recruiting G2 phase stem cells into dopaminergic neurons. Planarians thus have two different ways to regenerate dopaminergic neurons, although pluripotent stem cells become the source of regeneration in both cases. The latter case may provide a unique system for considering how to recruit dopaminergic neuron-committed cells into the lesioned regions (Nishimura et al., 2011). One of the important findings is that commitment occurs at the G2 phase of stem cells. We should consider to what extent committed cells can be incorporated into the lesioned regions, and whether the location of commitment is an important factor for future incorporation of committed stem cells into appropriate positions. As our future work, we will make an attempt to answer several important questions. "How do the remaining cells recognize the loss of dopaminergic neurons?" "How are surrounding stem cells recruited into dopaminergic neurons?" "What kind of signaling pathway(s) are activated in the G2 phase stem cells to differentiate dopaminergic neurons" "How do the committed cells find the pathways to the lesion points?" Answers to the above questions may provide hints about how to realize cell-transplantation therapy in the future.

7. Conclusion

It is difficult to analyze whether dopaminergic neurogenesis/neuroregeneration occurs in the adult mammalian midbrain (Zhao et al., 2003; Frielingsdorf et al., 2004), although it has been demonstrated that neurogenesis occurs in the restricted regions of the adult mammalian brain (Doetsch et al., 1997; Eriksson et al., 1998). However, it is still controversial whether dopaminergic neurogenesis/neuroregeneration potential is "lost" or "quiescent" in the adult mammalian midbrain. In any case, the potential for dopaminergic neurogenesis/neuroregeneration is not sufficient to recover the missing dopaminergic neurons in mammals. Our findings in planarians provide unique opportunities to consider how pluripotent stem cells respond to their surrounding environment, and how new dopaminergic neurons are recruited after the degeneration of dopaminergic neurons.

Cell-transplantation therapy is one possible way to compensate the missing dopaminergic neurons in Parkinson's disease patients. One of the important issues for cell-transplantation therapy is what state of dopaminergic neural precursor cells can be accepted into the host brain environment. For clinical application, non-regulated proliferative ability of donor cells may cause abnormal conditions such as tumor formation after grafting, and therefore, proliferative cells, including undifferentiated cells, should be eliminated as donor cells (Fukuda et al., 2006). Another approach would be to block proliferative ability artificially before grafting. Recently, it was demonstrated that N-[N-(3,5-difluorophenacetyl)-L-alanyl]-S-phenylglycine t-butyl ester (DAPT)-mediated Notch inhibition delays G1/S-phase transition of human ESC-derived neural stem cells, and promotes the onset of neuronal differentiation. However, the outcome of striatal transplantation of DAPT-treated neural stem cells was not different from that of non-DAPT-treated neural stem cells at a late period after grafting (Borghese et al., 2010). Consequently, inhibition of the G1/S-phase transition of donor cells to block proliferation may not enhance the efficiency of transplantation. Our findings from planarian studies suggest that G2-phase stem cells may be in a suitable cell state for harmonization with the host brain environment. Planarians are suitable model animals for analyzing the system that recognizes the ablation of dopaminergic signals and the system for recruitment of new dopaminergic neurons. Thus, our findings give useful suggestions about which state and type(s) of cells would be suitable for cell-replacement therapy with integration into the host brain environment using ESCs and/or iPSC-derived neural precursor cells to treat diseases such as Parkinson's disease.

8. Acknowledgments

We thank Dr. Elizabeth Nakajima (gCOE program A06, Kyoto University) for critical reading of the manuscript. This study was supported in part by a Grant-in-Aid for Global COE Program A06, Scientific Research on Innovative Areas to K. A. (22124001), Creative Scientific Research to K. A. (17GS0318) from the Ministry of Education, Culture, Sports, Science and Technology of Japan, and the Naito Foundation.

9. References

Agata, K.; Soejima, Y.; Kato, K.; Kobayashi, C.; Umesono, Y. & Watanabe K. (1998) Structure of the planarian central nervous system (CNS) revealed by neuronal cell markers. *Zoological Science*, Vol.15, No.3, (Jun 1998), pp. 433-440, ISSN 0289-0003

Agata, K.; Nakajima, E.; Funayama, N; Shibata, N; Saito, Y. & Umesono Y. (2006) Two different evolutionary origins of stem cell systems and their molecular basis. *Seminars in Cell & Developmental Biology*, Vol.17, No.4, (August 2006), pp. 503-509, ISSN 1084-9521

Agata, K. & Umesono, Y. (2008) Brain regeneration from pluripotent stem cells in planarian. *Philosophical Transactions The Royal Society B Biological Sciences*, Vol.363, No.1500, (Jun 2008), pp. 2071-2078, ISSN 1471-2970

Arvidsson, A.; Collin, T.; Kirik, D.; Kokaia, Z. & Lindvall, O. (2002) Neuronal replacement from endogenous precursors in the adult brain after stroke. *Nature Medicine*, Vol.8, No.9, (September 2002), pp. 963-970, ISSN 1078-8956

Borghese, L.; Dolezalova, D.; Opitz, T.; Haupt, S.; Leinhaas, A.; Steinfarz, B.; Koch, P.; Edenhofer, F.; Hampl, A. & Brüstle, O. (2010) Inhibition of notch signaling in human embryonic stem cell-derived neural stem cells delays G1/S phase transition and accelerates neuronal differentiation *in vitro* and *in vivo*. *Stem Cells*, Vol.28, No.5, (May 2010), pp. 955-964, ISSN 1066-5099

Berg, D.A.; Kirkham, M.; Beljajeva, A.; Knapp, D.; Habermann, B.; Ryge, J.; Tanaka, E.M. & Simon, A. (2010) Efficient regeneration by activation of neurogenesis in homeostatically quiescent regions of the adult vertebrate brain. *Development*, Vol.137, No.24, (December 2010), pp. 4127-4134, ISSN 0950-1991

Berg, D.A.; Kirkham, M.; Wang, H.; Frisén, J. & Simon, A. (2011) Dopamine controls neurogenesis in the adult salamander midbrain in homeostasis and during regeneration of dopamine neurons. *Cell Stem Cell*, Vol.8, No.4, (April 2011), pp. 426-433, ISSN 1934-5909

Björklund, L.M.; Sánchez-Pernaute, R.; Chung, S.; Andersson, T.; Chen, I.Y.; McNaught, K.S.; Brownell, A.L.; Jenkins, B.G.; Wahlestedt, C.; Kim, K.S. & Isacson, O. (2002) Embryonic stem cells develop into functional dopaminergic neurons after transplantation in a Parkinson rat model. *National Academy of Sciences of the United States of America*, Vol.99, No.4, (February 2002), pp. 2344-2349. ISSN 0027-8424

Brose, K.; Bland, K.S.; Wang, K.H.; Arnott, D.; Henzel, W.; Goodman, C.S.; Tessier-Lavigne, M. & Kidd, T. (1999) Slit proteins bind Robo receptors and have an evolutionarily conserved role in repulsive axon guidance. *Cell*, Vol.96, No.6, (March 1999), pp. 795-806, ISSN 0092-8674

Chambers, S.M.; Fasano, C.A.; Papapetrou, E.P.; Tomishima, M.; Sadelain, M. & Studer, L. (2009) Highly efficient neural conversion of human ES and iPS cells by dual inhibition of SMAD signaling. *Nature Biotechnology*, Vol.27, No.3, (May 2009), pp. 275-280, ISSN 1087-0156

Cebrià, F.; Kudome, T.; Nakazawa, M.; Mineta, K.; Ikeo, K.; Gojobori, T. & Agata, K. (2002a) The expression of neural-specific genes reveals the structural and molecular complexity of the planarian central nervous system. *Mechanisms of Development*, Vol.116, No.1-2, (August 2002), pp. 199-204, ISSN 0925-4773

Cebrià, F.; Kobayashi, C.; Umesono, Y.; Nakazawa, M.; Mineta, K.; Ikeo, K.; Gojobori, T.; Itoh, M.; Taira, M.; Sánchez Alvarado, A. & Agata, K. (2002b) FGFR-related gene *nou-darake* restricts brain tissues to the head region of planarians. *Nature*, Vol.419, No.6907, (October 2002), pp. 620-624, ISSN 0028-0836

Cebrià, F.; Nakazawa, M.; Mineta, K.; Ikeo, K.; Gojobori, T. & Agata, K. (2002c) Dissecting planarian central nervous system regeneration by the expression of neural-specific genes. *Development Growth & Differentiation*, Vol.44, No.2, (April 2002), pp. 135-146, ISSN 0012-1592

Cebrià, F. & Newmark, P.A. (2005) Planarian homologs of *netrin* and *netrin receptor* are required for proper regeneration of the central nervous system and the maintenance of nervous system architecture. *Development*, Vol.132, No.16, (August 2005), pp. 3691-3703, ISSN 0950-1991

Cebrià, F, Guo, T, Jopek, J. & Newmark, P.A. (2007) Regeneration and maintenance of the planarian midline is regulated by a *slit* orthologue. *Developmental Biology*, Vol.307, No.2, (July 2007), pp. 394-406, ISSN 0012-1606

Cebrià, F. & Newmark, P.A. (2007) Morphogenesis defects are associated with abnormal nervous system regeneration following *roboA* RNAi in planarians. *Development*, Vol.134, No.5, (March 2007), pp. 833-837, ISSN 0950-1991

Cebrià, F. (2008) Organization of the nervous system in the model planarian *Schmidtea mediterranea*: an immunocytochemical study. *Neuroscience Resersch*, Vol.61, No.4, (August 2008), pp. 375-384, ISSN 0168-0102

Couch, J.A.; Chen, J.; Rieff, H.I.; Uri, E.M. & Condron, B.G. (2004) *robo2* and *robo3* interact with eagle to regulate serotonergic neuron differentiation. *Development*, Vol.131, No.5, (March 2004) pp. 997-1006, ISSN 0950-1991

Doetsch, F.; García-Verdugo, J.M. & Alvarez-Buylla, A. (1997) Cellular composition and three-dimensional organization of the subventricular germinal zone in the adult mammalian brain. *The Journal of Neuroscience*, Vol.17, No.13, (July 1997), pp. 5046-5061, ISSN 270-6474

Eisenhoffer, G.T.; Kang, H. & Sánchez Alvarado, A. (2008) Molecular analysis of stem cells and their descendants during cell turnover and regeneration in the planarian *Schmidtea mediterranea*. *Cell Stem Cell*, Vol.3, No.3, (September 2008) pp. 327-339, ISSN 1934-5909

Eriksson, P.S.; Perfilieva, E.; Björk-Eriksson, T.; Alborn, A.M.; Nordborg, C.; Peterson, D.A. & Gage, F.H. (1998) Neurogenesis in the adult human hippocampus. *Nature Medicine*, Vol.4, No.11, (November 1998), pp. 1313-1317, ISSN 1078-8956

Fukuda, H.; Takahashi, J.; Watanabe, K.; Hayashi, H.; Morizane, A.; Koyanagi, M.; Sasai, Y. & Hashimoto, N. (2006) Fluorescence-activated cell sorting-based purification of embryonic stem cell-derived neural precursors averts tumor formation after transplantation. *Stem Cells*, Vol.24, No.3, (March 2006), pp. 763-771, ISSN 1066-5099.

Gaviño, M.A. & Reddien, P.W. (2011) A Bmp/Admp regulatory circuit controls maintenance and regeneration of dorsal-ventral polarity in planarians. *Current Biology*, Vol.21, No.4, (February 2011), pp.294-299, ISSN 0960-9822

Gurley, K.A.; Rink, J.C. & Sánchez Alvarado, A. (2008) *ß-catenin* defines head versus tail identity during planarian regeneration and homeostasis. *Science*, Vol.319, No.5861, (January 2008), pp. 323-327, ISSN 0036-8075

Hayashi, T.; Asami, M.; Higuchi, S.; Shibata, N. & Agata K. (2006) Isolation of planarian X-ray-sensitive stem cells by fluorescence-activated cell sorting. *Development Growth & Differentiation*, Vol.48, No.6, (August 2006), pp. 371-380. ISSN 0012-1592

Hayashi, T.; Shibata, N.; Okumura, R.; Kudome, T.; Nishimura, O.; Tarui, H. & Agata, K. (2010) Single-cell gene profiling of planarian stem cells using fluorescent activated cell sorting and its "index sorting" function for stem cell research. *Development Growth & Differentiation*, Vol.52, No.1, (January 2010), pp. 131-144, ISSN 0012-1592

Hendzel, M.J.; Wei, Y.; Mancini, M.A.; Van Hooser, A.; Ranalli, T.; Brinkley, B.R.; Bazett-Jones, D.P. & Allis, C.D. (1997) Mitosis-specific phosphorylation of histone H3 initiates primarily within pericentromeric heterochromatin during G_2 and spreads in an ordered fashion coincident with mitotic chromosome condensation. *Chromosoma*, Vol.106, No.6, (August 2006), pp. 348-360, ISSN 0009-5915

Heikkila, R.E. & Nicklas, W.J. (1971) Inhibition of biogenic amine uptake by hydrogen peroxide: mechanism for toxic effects of 6-hydroxydopamine. *Science,* Vol.172, No.989, (Jun 1971), pp. 1257-1258, ISSN 0036-8075

Higuchi, S.; Hayashi, T.; Hori, I.; Shibata, N.; Sakamoto, H. & Agata K. (2007) Characterization and categorization of fluorescence activated cell sorted planarian stem cells by ultrastructural analysis. *Development Growth & Differentiation*, Vol.49, No.7, (September 2007), pp. 571-581, ISSN 0012-1592

Higuchi, S.; Hayashi, T.; Tarui, H.; Nishimura, O.; Nishimura, K.; Shibata, N.; Sakamoto, H. & Agata, K. (2008) Expression and functional analysis of *musashi*-like genes in planarian CNS regeneration. *Mechanisms of Development,* Vol.125, No.7, (July 2008), pp. 631-645, ISSN 0925-4773

Höglinger, G.U.; Rizk, P.; Muriel, M.P.; Duyckaerts, C.; Oertel, W.H.; Caille, I. & Hirsch, E.C. (2004) Dopamine depletion impairs precursor cell proliferation in Parkinson disease. *Nature Neuroscience*, Vol.7, No.7, (July 2004), pp. 726-735, ISSN 1097-6256

Hong, K.; Hinck, L.; Nishiyama, M.; Poo, M.M.; Tessier-Lavigne, M. & Stein, E. (1999) A ligand-gated association between cytoplasmic domains of UNC5 and DCC family receptors converts netrin-induced growth cone attraction to repulsion. *Cell*, Vol.97, No.7, (Jun 1999), pp. 927-941, ISSN 0092-8674

Inoue, T.; Kumamoto, H.; Okamoto, K.; Umesono, Y.; Sakai, M., Sánchez Alvarado, A. & Agata, K. (2004) Morphological and functional recovery of the planarian photosensing system during head regeneration. *Zoological Science,* Vol.21, No.3, (March 2004), pp. 275-283, ISSN 0289-0003

Inoue, T.; Hayashi, T.; Takechi, K. & Agata, K. (2007) Clathrin-mediated endocytic signals are required for the regeneration of, as well as homeostasis in, the planarian CNS. *Development*, Vol.134, No.9, (May 2007), pp. 1679-1689, ISSN 0950-1991

Kato, K.; Orii, H.; Watanabe, K. & Agata, K. (1999) The role of dorsoventral interaction in the onset of planarian regeneration. *Development,* Vol.126, No.5, (February 1999), pp. 1031-1040, ISSN 0950-1991

Kawasaki, H.; Mizuseki, K.; Nishikawa, S.; Kaneko, S.; Kuwana, Y.; Nakanishi, S.; Nishikawa, S.I. & Sasai, Y. (2000) Induction of midbrain dopaminergic neurons from ES cells by stromal cell-derived inducing activity. *Neuron*, Vol.28, No.1, (October, 2000), pp. 31-40, ISSN 0896-6273

Kobayashi, C.; Saito, Y.; Ogawa K. & Agata K. (2007) *Wnt* signaling is required for antero-posterior patterning of the planarian brain. *Developmental Biology*, Vol.306, No.2, (Jun 2007), pp. 714-724, ISSN 0012-1606

Mineta, K.; Nakazawa, M.; Cebrià, F.; Ikeo, K.; Agata, K. & Gojobori, T. (2003) Origin and evolutionary process of the CNS elucidated by comparative genomics analysis of planarian ESTs. *National Academy of Sciences of the United States of America*, Vol.100, No.13, (Jun 2003), pp. 7666-7671, ISSN 0027-8424

Molina, M.D.; Neto, A.; Maeso, I.; Gómez-Skarmeta, J.L.; Saló, E. & Cebrià, F. (2011) Noggin and noggin-like genes control dorsoventral axis regeneration in planarians. *Current Biology*, Vol.21, No.4, (February 2011), pp. 300-305, ISSN 0960-9822

Morgan, T.H. (1989) Experimental Studies of the regeneration of *Planaria maculata*. *Arch Entwicklungsmech Org.*, Vol.7, pp. 364-397.

Morizane, A.; Doi, D.; Kikuchi, T.; Nishimura, K. & Takahashi, J. (2011) Small-molecule inhibitors of bone morphogenic protein and activin/nodal signals promote highly efficient neural induction from human pluripotent stem cells. *Journal of Neuroscience Research*, Vol.89, No.2, (February 2011), pp. 117-126, ISSN 0360-4012

Nakazawa, M.; Cebrià, F.; Mineta, K.; Ikeo, K.; Agata, K. & Gojobori T. (2003) Search for the evolutionary origin of a brain: planarian brain characterized by microarray. *Molecular Biology & Evolution*, Vol.20, No.5, (May 2003), pp. 784-791, ISSN 0737-4038

Nass, R.; Hall, D.H.; Miller, D.M. 3rd; & Blakely, R.D. (2002) Neurotoxin-induced degeneration of dopamine neurons in *Caenorhabditis elegans*. *National Academy of Sciences of the United States of America*, Vol.99, No.5, (March 2002), pp. 3264-3269, ISSN 0027-8424

Newmark, P.A. & Sánchez Alvarado, A. (2000) Bromodeoxyuridine specifically labels the regenerative stem cells of planarians. *Developmental Biology*, Vol.220, No.2, (April 2000), pp. 142-153, ISSN 0012-1606

Nishimura, K.; Kitamura, Y.; Inoue, T.; Umesono, Y.; Sano, S.; Yoshimoto, K.; Inden, M.; Takata, K.; Taniguchi, T.; Shimohama, S. & Agata, K. (2007a) Reconstruction of dopaminergic neural network and locomotion function in planarian regenerates. *Developmental Neurobiology*, Vol.67, No.8, (July 2007), pp. 1059-1078, ISSN 1932-8451

Nishimura, K.; Kitamura, Y.; Inoue, T.; Umesono, Y.; Yoshimoto, K.; Takeuchi, K.; Taniguchi, T. & Agata, K. (2007b) Identification and distribution of tryptophan hydroxylase (TPH)-positive neurons in the planarian *Dugesia japonica*. *Neuroscience Research*, Vol.59, No.1, (September 2007), pp. 101-106, ISSN 0168-0102

Nishimura, K.; Kitamura, Y.; Umesono, Y.; Takeuchi, K.; Takata, K.; Taniguchi, T. & Agata, K. (2008a) Identification of glutamic acid decarboxylase gene and distribution of GABAergic nervous system in the planarian, *Dugesia japonica*. *Neuroscience*, Vol.153, No.4, (Jun, 2008), pp. 1103-1114, ISSN 0306-4522

Nishimura, K.; Kitamura, Y.; Inoue, T.; Umesono, Y.; Taniguchi, T. & Agata, K. (2008b) Characterization of tyramine ß-hydroxylase in planarian *Dugesia japonica*: Cloning and expression. *Neurochemistry International*, Vol.53, No.6-8, (December 2008), pp. 184-192, ISSN 0197-0186

Nishimura, K.; Yamamoto, H.; Kitamura, Y.; & Agata, K. (2008c) Brain and Neural Network, In: *Planaria: A Model for Drug Action and Abuse*, (Raffa, R.B. & Rawls, S.M., (Ed.), 4-12 Landes Bioscience, ISBN: 978-1-58706-332-9, Texas, USA

Nishimura, K.; Kitamura, Y.; Taniguchi, T. & Agata, K. (2010) Analysis of motor function modulated by cholinergic neurons in planarian *Dugesia japonica. Neuroscience*, Vol.168, No.1, (Jun 2010), pp. 18-30, ISSN 0306-4522

Nishimura, K.; Inoue, T.; Yoshimoto, K.; Taniguchi, T.; Kitamura, Y. & Agata K. Regeneration of dopaminergic neurons after 6-hydroxydopamine-induced lesion in planarian brain. *Journal of Neurochemistry*, Vol.119, No.6, (December 2011), pp. 1219-1231 ISSN 0022-3042

Ogawa, K.; Ishihara, S.; Saito, Y.; Mineta, K.; Nakazawa, M.; Ikeo, K.; Gojobori, T.; Watanabe, K. & Agata K. (2002) Induction of a *noggin*-like gene by ectopic DV interaction during planarian regeneration. *Developmental Biology, Vol.*250, No.1, (October 2002), pp. 59-70, ISSN 0012-1606

Okamoto, K.; Takeuchi, K. & Agata, K. (2005) Neural projections in planarian brain revealed by fluorescent dye tracing. *Zoological* Science, Vol.22, No.5, (May 2005), pp. 535-546. ISSN 0289-0003

Okano, H.; Imai, T. & Okabe, M. (2002) *Musashi*: a translational regulator of cell fate. *Journal of Cell Science*, 2002 Apr Vol.115, No.Pt 7, (April 2002), pp. 1355-1359, ISSN 0021-9533

Orii, H., Sakurai, T. & Watanabe, K. (2005) Distribution of the stem cells (neoblasts) in the planarian *Dugesia japonica. Development Genes & Evolution,* Vol.215, No.3, (March 2005), pp. 143-157. ISSN 0949-944X

Parish, C.L.; Beljajeva, A.; Arenas, E. and Simon, A. (2007) Midbrain dopaminergic neurogenesis and behavioural recovery in a salamander lesion-induced regeneration model. *Development,* Vol.134, No.15, (August 2007), pp. 2881-2887, ISSN 0950-1991

Pellettieri, J. & Sánchez Alvarado, A. (2007) Cell turnover and adult tissue homeostasis: from humans to planarians. *Annual Review of Genetics*, Vol.41, pp. 83-105, ISSN 0066-4197

Perrier, A.L.; Tabar, V.; Barberi, T.; Rubio, M.E.; Bruses, J.; Topf, N.; Harrison, N.L. & Studer, L. (2004) Derivation of midbrain dopamine neurons from human embryonic stem cells. *National Academy of Sciences of the United States of America,* Vol.101, No.34, (August 2004), pp. 12543-12548, ISSN 0027-8424

Petersen, C.P. & Reddien, P.W. (2008) Smed-*βcatenin-1* is required for anteroposterior blastema polarity in planarian regeneration. *Science*, Vol.319, No.5861, (January 2008), pp. 327-330, ISSN 0036-8075

Petersen, C.P. & Reddien, P.W. (2009) Wnt signaling and the polarity of the primary body axis. *Cell,* Vol.139, No.6, (December 2009), pp. 1056-1068, ISSN 0092-8674

Reddien, P.W. & Sánchez Alvarado, A. (2004) Fundamentals of planarian regeneration. *Annual Review of Cell Developmental Biology,* Vol.20, pp. 725-757, ISSN 1081-0706

Reddien, P.W.; Oviedo, N.J.; Jenning, J.R.; Jenkin, J.C. & Sánchez Alvarado, A. (2005) SMEDWI-2 is a PIWI-like protein that regulates planarian stem cells. *Science,* Vol.310, No.5752, (November 2005), pp. 1327-1330, ISSN 0036-8075

Reddien, P.W. (2011) Constitutive gene expression and the specification of tissue identity in adult planarian biology. *Trends in Genetics,* Vol.27, No.7, (July 2011), pp. 277-285, ISSN 0168-9525

Rink, J.C.; Gurley, K.A.; Elliott, S.A. & Sánchez Alvarado, A. (2009) Planarian Hh signaling regulates regeneration polarity and links Hh pathway evolution to cilia. *Science,* Vol.326, No.5958, (December 2009), pp. 1406-1410, ISSN 0036-8075

Sachs, C. & Jonsson, G. (1975) Mechanisms of action of 6-hydroxydopamine. *Biochemical Pharmacology*, Vo.24, No.1, (January 1975), pp. 1-8, ISSN 0006-2952

Saito, Y.; Koinuma, S.; Watanabe, K. & Agata, K. (2003) Mediolateral intercalation in planarians revealed by grafting experiments. *Developmental Dynamics*, Vol.226, No.2, (February 2003), pp. 334-340, ISSN 1058-8388

Salvetti, A.; Rossi, L.; Deri, P. & Batistoni, R. (2000) An MCM2-related gene is expressed in proliferating cells of intact and regenerating planarians. *Developmental Dynamics*, Vol.218, No.4, (August 2000), pp. 603-614, ISSN 1058-8388

Salvetti, A.; Rossi, L.; Lena, A.; Batistoni, R.; Deri, P.; Rainaldi, G.; Locci.; M.T.; Evangelista, M. & Gremigni, V. (2005) *DjPum*, a homologue of *Drosophila Pumilio*, is essential to planarian stem cell maintenance. *Development*, Vol.132, No.8, (April 2005), pp. 1863-1874, ISSN 0950-1991

Sakai, F.; Agata, K.; Orii, H. & Watanabe, K. (2000) Organization and regeneration ability of spontaneous supernumerary eyes in planarians -eye regeneration field and pathway selection by optic nerves-. *Zoological Science*, Vol.17, No.3, (April 2000), pp. 375-81, ISSN 0289-0003

Sanchez-Pernaute, R.; Lee, H.; Patterson, M.; Reske-Nielsen, C.; Yoshizaki, T.; Sonntag, K.C.; Studer, L. & Isacson, O. (2008) Parthenogenetic dopamine neurons from primate embryonic stem cells restore function in experimental Parkinson's disease. *Brain*, Vol.131, No. Pt.8, (August 2008), pp. 2127-2139, ISSN 0006-8950

Schwarting, R.K. & Huston, J.P. (1996) The unilateral 6-hydroxydopamine lesion model in behavioral brain research. Analysis of functional deficits, recovery and treatments. *Progress in Neurobiolgy*, Vol.50, No.2-3, (October 1996), pp. 275-331, ISSN 0301-0082

Shibata, N.; Umesono, Y.; Orii, H.; Sakurai, T.; Watanabe, K. & Agata, K. (1999) Expression of *vasa(vas)*-related genes in germline cells and totipotent somatic stem cells of planarians. *Developmental Biology*, Vol.206, No.1, (February 1999), pp. 73-87, ISSN 0012-1606

Shibata, N.; Rouhana, L. & Agata K. (2010) Cellular and molecular dissection of pluripotent adult somatic stem cells in planarians. *Development Growth & Differentiation*, Vol.52, No.1, (January 2010), pp. 27-41, ISSN 0012-1592

Tasaki, J.; Shibata, N.; Nishimura, O.; Itomi, K.; Tabata, Y.; Son, F.; Suzuki, N.; Araki, R.; Abe, M.; Agata, K. & Umesono, Y. (2011a) ERK signaling controls blastemacell differentiation during planarian regeneration. *Development*, Vol.138, No. 12, (Jun 2011), pp. 2417-2427, ISSN 0950-1991

Tasaki., J.; Shibata, N.; Sakurai, T.; Agata, K. & Umesono, Y. (2011b) Role of c-JunN-terminal kinase activity in blastema formation during planarian regeneration. *Development Growth & Differentiation*, Vol.53, No.3, (April 2011), 389-400, ISSN 0012-1592

Takagi, Y.; Takahashi, J.; Saiki, H.; Morizane, A.; Hayashi, T.; Kishi, Y.; Fukuda, H.; Okamoto, Y.; Koyanagi, M.; Ideguchi, M.; Hayashi, H.; Imazato, T.; Kawasaki, H.; Suemori, H.; Omachi, S.; Iida, H.; Itoh, N.; Nakatsuji, N.; Sasai, Y. & Hashimoto, N. (2005) Dopaminergic neurons generated from monkey embryonic stem cells function in a Parkinson primate model. *The Journal of Clinical Investigation*, Vol.115, No.1, (January 2005), pp. 102-109. ISSN 0021-9738

Takano, T.; Pulvers, J.N.; Inoue, T.; Tarui, H.; Sakamoto, H.; Agata, K. & Umesono, Y. (2007) Regeneration-dependent conditional gene knockdown (Readyknock) in planarian: demonstration of requirement for Djsnap-25 expression in the brain for negative phototactic behavior. *Development Growth & Differentiation*, Vol.49, No.5, (Jun 2007), pp. 383-394, ISSN 0012-1592

Takeda, H.; Nishimura, K. & Agata K. (Jun 2008) Planaria nervous system, In: *Scholarpedia*, 3, 5558, 2008, Available from http://www.scholarpedia.org/article/Planaria_nervous_system

Takeda, H.; Nishimura, K. & Agata K. (2009) Planarians maintain a constant ratio of different cell types during changes in body size by using the stem cell system. *Zoological Science*, Vol.26, No.12, (December 2009), pp. 805-813, ISSN 0289-0003

Tazaki, A.; Gaudieri, S.; Ikeo, K.; Gojobori, T.; Watanabe, K. & Agata, K. (1999) Neural network in planarian revealed by an antibody against planarian synaptotagmin homologue. *Biochemical and Biophysical Research Communications* Vol.260, No.2, (July 1999), pp. 426-432. ISSN 0006-291X

Umesono, Y.; Watanabe, K. & Agata, K. (1997) A planarian *orthopedia* homolog is specifically expressed in the branch region of both the mature and regenerating brain. *Development Growth & Differentiation*, Vol.39, No.6, (December 1997), pp. 723-727, ISSN 0012-1592

Umesono, Y.; Watanabe, K. & Agata, K. (1999) Distinct structural domains in the planarian brain defined by the expression of evolutionarily conserved homeobox genes. *Development Genes & Evolution*, Vol.209, No.1, (January 1999), pp. 31-39, ISSN 0949-944X

Umesono, Y.; & Agata, K. (2009) Evolution and regeneration of the planarian central nervous system. *Development Growth & Differentiation*, Vol.51, No.3, (April 2009), pp. 185-195, ISSN 0012-1592

Umesono, Y.; Tasaki, J.; Nishimura, K.; Inoue, T. & Agata, K. Regeneration in an evolutionarily primitive brain: the planarian *Dugesia japonica* model. *European Journal of Neuroscience.*,Vol.34, No.6, (September 2011), pp. 863-839. ISSN 0953-816X

Ungerstedt, U. & Arbuthnott, G.W. (1970) Quantitative recording of rotational behavior in rats after 6-hydroxy-dopamine lesions of the nigrostriatal dopamine system. *Brain Research,* Vol.24, No.3, (Decmber 1970), pp. 485-493, ISSN 0006-8993

Yamamoto, H. & Agata, K. (2011) Optic chiasm formation in planarian I: Cooperative *netrin*- and *robo*-mediated signals are required for the early stage of optic chiasm formation. *Development Growth & Differentiation*, Vol.53, No.3, (April 2011), pp. 300-311, ISSN 0012-1592

Yazawa, S.; Umesono, Y.; Hayashi, T.; Tarui, H. & Agata, K. (2009) Planarian Hedgehog/Patched establishes anterior-posterior polarity by regulating Wnt signaling. *National Academy of Sciences of the United States of America*, Vol.106, No.52, (December 2009), pp. 22329-22334, ISSN 0027-8424

Wagner, D.E.; Wang, I.E., & Reddien, P.W. (2011) Clonogenic neoblasts are pluripotent adult stem cells that underlie planarian regeneration. *Science*, Vol.332, No.6031, (May 2011), pp. 811-816, ISSN 0036-8075

Wenemoser, D. & Reddien, P.W. (2010) Planarian regeneration involves distinct stem cell responses to wounds and tissue absence. *Developmental Biology*, Vol.344, No.2, (August 2010), pp. 979-991, ISSN 0012-1606

Wernig, M.; Zhao, J.P.; Pruszak, J.; Hedlund, E.; Fu, D.; Soldner, F.; Broccoli, V.; Constantine-Paton, M.; Isacson, O. & Jaenisch, R. (2008) Neurons derived from reprogrammed fibroblasts functionally integrate into the fetal brain and improve symptoms of rats with Parkinson's disease. *National Academy of Sciences of the United States of America,* Vol.105, No.15, (April 2008), pp. 5856-5861, ISSN 0027-8424

7

Formation of Nervous Systems and Neural Stem Cells in Ascidians

Kiyoshi Terakado
Saitama University
Japan

1. Introduction

Phylum Chordata comprises three subphyla, Cephalochordata, Urochordata and Vertebrata. Urochordates (tunicates) are morphologically very diverse, but recent phylogenetic analyses revealed that urochordates and not chephalochordates are the closest living relatives of vertebrates (Blair and Hedges, 2005; Delsuc et al., 2006, 2008; Putnam et al., 2008).

The central nervous system of the ascidian embryo is formed from the neural plate by its rolling into a hollow tube on the dorsal surface. This feature is unique to and common in chordates (synapomorphy). Cell number of mature tadpole remains nearly constant until metamorphosis begins. From earlier, two histological features are noticed in the tissues of the swimming larva; the first is the cessation of cell division in all the larval tissues and also in rudiments of adult organs, and the second is that functional cells are restricted to the larval organs. These cells differentiate almost synchronously in the larva. Larvae swim first for distribution and then for search the settlement places for metamorphosis without feeding. After onset of metamorphosis, the cells of larval organ disintegrate and/or rearrangement and those of adult rudiments begin to divide and differentiate into functional organs. Body wall muscle begins to contract intermittently, concomitant with the beginning of the feeding. That is, the cells of adult organs inhibited by some factors during swimming stage. The adult ascidian neural complex comprises the cerebral ganglion and the neural gland/its derived organ. The former is formed from the primodium of the cerebral ganglion constructed by rearrangement of the larval central nervous system during metamorphosis, and the latter is formed from a thin tube called the neurohypophyseal duct, respectively. The larval central nervous system contains functional neurons and glial cells, called the ependymal cells. Most of functional neurons and the glial cells in the tail region are lost during metamorphosis. Neurohypophyseal duct cells, located in the anterior left side of the sensory vesicle of swimming larvae, are derived from the anterior embryonic neural plate, which expresses common transcription factors in vertebrates and urochordates. After metamorphosis begins, the duct elongates anteriorly and fuses with the stomodeal ectoderm, where the dorsal tubercle, a large ciliated structure that opens into the upper part of the pharynx, later develops. The rudiment of the cerebral ganglion and the duct elongate posteriorly. The duct also differentiates into the neural gland. The dorsal wall of the neural gland in more developed ascidians has a thick epithelium (placode), the central part of which forms the dorsal strand by repeated invaginations along the visceral nerve. Both gonadotropin-releasing hormone (GnRH) neurons and prolactin-like (non-GnRH) neurons are generated in the dorsal strand and migrate to the cerebral ganglion along the visceral nerve throughout adulthood. Thus, the epithelium of the dorsal strand derived from the neurohypophyseal duct possesses neurogenic potential for such neurons during life (neural stem cells). The GnRH and prolactin-like neurons are mutually in close contact in the dorsal strand and their concurrent seasonal changes also occur in relation to the reproduction. The generation of GnRH and prolactin-like neurons and their migration into the brain suggest that the ascidian dorsal strand is homologous to the craniate olfactory placode, and provide unequivocal support for the clade Olfactores.

2. Formation of central nervous systems

Recently, the notion about the formation of adult central nervous system in ascidians is greatly changed; earlier view is that the neural complex comprising the cerebral ganglion and the neural gland is formed from the neurohypophyseal duct positioned at left side of the cerebral ganglion (Wiley, 1893; Mackie and Burighel, 2005; Manni et al., 2004; Manni et al., 2005). However, Takamura (2002) using neuron-specific antibody and Horie et al. (2011) using light-labeled fluorescent protein clearly revealed that the larval central nervous system contributes to the formation of the adult central nervous system. The contributed cells, called the ependymal cells, remain unchanged in number and state of differentiation until metamorphosis. Based on the formation of the adult central nervous system from the larval ependymal cells, these cells are claimed to act as neural stem cell-like cells (Horie et al., 2011). The anterior-posterior axis of the larval central nervous system is also inherited to form the adult central nervous system, indicating that the anterior-posterior axis of the central nervous system is already determined by developmental regulatory genes (Wada et al., 1998; Horie et al., 2011). Experimental ablation of the cerebral ganglion in C. intestinalis, it regenerates in its entirety within a few weeks (Bollner et al., 1997). This indicates that the regeneration of the adult central nervous system does not require preexisting cells (neurons and glial cells) from the central nervous system; i.e., it accomplishes entirely by cell supply from other tissues and organs than those of the central nervous system. The regenerated central nervous system may also acquire the anterior-posterior axis identical to that of normal development. In the regenerating brain, no mitotic figures were detected, indicating that migration of post-mitotic cells to the site of ganglion regeneration (Bollner et al., 1995, 1997). Initial concentration of GnRH-like cells along the ventral surface of the regenerating brain in C. intestinalis (Bollner et al., 1997) suggests that these cells originate in the dorsal strand and migrate to the surface of regenerating brain as those in normal development. Because the adult brain possesses various types of neurons (cholinergic, GABAergic, glycinergic, and glutamatergic ones), trans-differentiation of the cells from existing tissue must be involved in brain regeneration. The regeneration of the neural gland epithelium and then the neural gland luminal cells after neural complex ablation suggests to be caused by extensive cell divisions of the remaining epithelial cells of the dorsal strand by a heavy BrdU labeling (Bollner et al., 1995).

In the larval central nervous system, non-functional cells are generated in excess as compared with the functional neurons; i.e., larval functional neurons are approximately 100 and non-functional cells, called the ependymal cells, are 245 in *Ciona* central nervous system

(Horie et al., 2011). With regard to the ependymal cells, another explanation may be possible that they are neural progenitor cells that remain quiescent during larval stages and differentiate into adult neurons (and provably also to glial cells) after metamorphosis. They might not be neural stem cells because they occupy large numbers of cells (over 70%) of the larval central nervous system. It has not also been ascertained whether these cells have the ability of self-renew or persistent cell division to yield new neurons and/or glial cells, that the ability is the primary characteristic of neural stem cells.

2.1 Formation of peripheral nervous system

There are two common routs of origin of neurons in vertebrates and urochordates, i.e., the origin in central nervous system (most neurons) and that in peripheral nervous system (very restricted neurons including GnRH neurons). The presence of the olfactory placode in vertebrates and that of its homologous organ in ascidians which both generate the GnRH neurons is a very conspicuous phenomenon in animal kingdom and makes an important morphological characteristic of the clade Olfactores (vertebrates + tunicates).

GnRH is the hypothalamic neurohormone that activates the release of gonadotropin from gonadotropes of the pituitary in vertebrates. These GnRH neurons originate from the olfactory placode and migrate into the brain (GnRH1 or GnRH3 in some teleosts). The other GnRH neurons that originate in the midbrain tegmentum (GnRH2) seem to have a co-transmitter or a neuromodulater function. In ascidians, GnRH that is so called even in invertebrates devoid of the pituitary, because of the composition of the identical number of amino acid residues, conserved sequences, and may involved in reproduction (Powell et al., 1996; Terakado 2001; Adams et al., 2003) or in neuromodulation (Tsutsui et al., 1998). GnRH fibers distribute widely through the body, such as innerside of gonoduct, surface of gonads, branchial basket, surface of muscle bands, ciliated epithelium of pharynx, tentacles, etc.,. Synaptic button was not observed in fiber tips, suggesting that one of the functions of ascidian GnRHs is a neuromodulator or a paracrine secretion. Collectively, there are, at least, four common characteristics between vertebrate and ascidian GnRHs, such as decapeptide, conserved sequence, relation to reproduction, origination in peripheral organ and persistent neurogenesis throughout the adult life.

The evolutionary origin of neurogenic placodes remains controversial because of morphological divergence in chordates. Despite the importance of neurogenic placodes for understanding real functions and phylogenetic relationships among chordates, morphological and developmental data remain scarce. In craniates, peripheral GnRH neurons arise from the olfactory placode, whose cells are derived from the anterior region of the embryonic neural plate (Okubo et al., 2006; Cariboni et al., 2007; Schwarting et al., 2007; Bhattacharyya and Bronner-Fraser, 2008; Chen et al., 2009; Kanaho et al., 2009). Generation of peripheral neurons is a unique phenomenon that does not conform to the central nervous system origin of most neurons. The possible presence of a neurogenic placodal structure in invertebrate chordates has long been debated (Manni et al., 2004, 2005, 2006; Mackie and Burighel, 2005; Mazet et al., 2005, 2006; Schlosser, 2005). Recently, it was directly shown that, using one of the biggest solitary ascidian *Halocynthia roretzi* (Fig.1), GnRH neurons are generated in the dorsal strand and migrate into the cerebral ganglion (Terakado, 2009). It was then hypothesized that the dorsal strand is homologous to the craniate olfactory placode, an idea that are based on the topological relations and generation of peripheral GnRH neurons, which are commonly derived from the anterior region of the embryonic neural plate (Elwyn, 1937; Satoh, 1994; Cole and Meinertzhagen, 2001, 2004). The anterior region of the embryonic neural plate has been suggested to be the territory of the olfactory/adenohypophyseal placodes of vertebrates (Mazet et al., 2005) and expresses certain transcription factors common in craniates. Similarly, prolactin (PRL)-like neurons generated in close contact with GnRH neurons in the dorsal strand, which is formed from the dorsal epithelium of the neural gland by repeated invaginations (Fig. 2A).

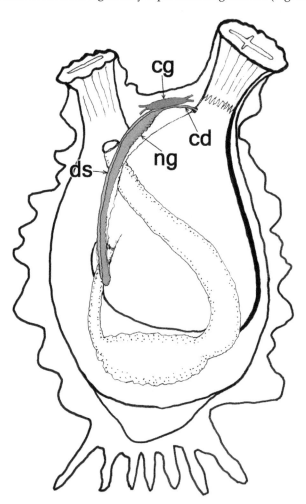

Fig. 1. Schematic drawing of the neural complex in a 3-year-old Halocynthia roretzi. The cerebral ganglion (cg) lies between the atrial and branchial siphons. The neural gland (ng) is located just beneath the ganglion, and its lumen opens anteriorly to upper part of the pharynx through the ciliated duct (cd). The neural gland extends posteriorly with the dorsal strand (ds).

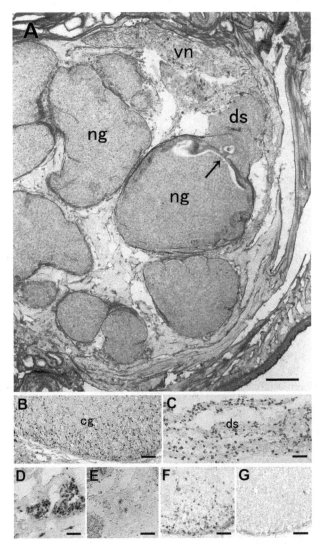

Fig. 2. Formation of the dorsal strand, localization of GnRH and PRL-like neurons and controls.

A. Formation of the dorsal strand (ds) from the placode (arrow) in the dorsal epithelium of the neural gland (ng) by invagination facing the visceral nerve (vn). Aldehyde fuchsin stain. B and C. Occurrence of PRL-like neurons in the cerebral ganglion (cg) and the dorsal strand (ds). PRL-like neurons in the cerebral ganglion are located mostly in the cortical region and possess long neurites, while neurons in the dorsal strand possess very short or lack neurites. Anti–bullfrog PRL stain. D and E. Specificity of GnRH immunoreactivity. Anti-human GnRH reactivity (D) is completely abolished by treatment with antiserum (E) that had been preabsorbed with the same antigen (2 ug/ml). F and G. Specificity of PRL-like immunoreactivity. Anti–bullfrog PRL reactivity (F) is completely abolished by treatment with antiserum (G) that had been preabsorbed with the same antigen (10 ug/ml). Bars: (A) 100 um; (B-G) 50 um.

Urochordates are now thought to be the sister group of vertebrates. Therefore, it is likely that developmental novelties of chordates (neural crest and placode) arose during evolution of the common ancestor of urochordates and vertebrates.

In cephalochordates (amphioxus), the similarity to vertebrates during embryonic development and in the expression of certain common transcription factors in the anterior region suggests the possible presence of a placode(s) that is homologous with those in craniates (Gorbman, 1995; Yasui et al., 2000; Boorman and Shimeld, 2002). However, the proposed placode generates neither neuroendocrine cells that give rise to GnRH neurons nor endocrine cells that give rise to adenohypophyseal endocrine cells. Thus, the first chordate may have lacked placodes (Meulemans and Bronner-Fraser, 2007). These observations provide support the clade Olfactores.

Several neuronal populations are generated from the olfactory placode of vertebrates. Recent results have demonstrated certain morphological, developmental (Burighel et al., 1998; Manni et al., 2004; Terakado, 2009), and molecular (such as *Six*, *Pitx*, *Eya*, *Pax*, *Coe*, *Dach*, *POUIV* gene families) commonalities between urochordates and vertebrates (Bassham and Postlethwait, 2005; Boorman and Shimeld, 2002; Christiaen et al., 2002; Mazet et al., 2005; Mazet and Shimeld, 2005; Schlosser, 2005), but information on the localization of these transcription factors and on the sites of emergence of neuroendocrine/endocrine cells remains controversial.

Because the novel structure, termed the dorsal strand placode, is for the first time histologically observed in invertebrate chordates, definition of the structure is seriously evaluated based the previous criteria (Northcut and Gans, 1983; Schlosser, 2005). The dorsal strand "placode" has the following characteristics; (1) generation from thickened epithelium. (2) invagination at the center of thickened epithelium. (3) generation of many types of cells including neurons. (4) delamination from the invaginated epithelium. (5) migration into the brain and to some other regions. All criteria are fit for the dorsal strand "placode", indicating that generation of placode really occurred in ascidians as an important developmental novelty in a common ancestor of vertebrates and urochordates. Additionally, expression of some transcription factors suggest the establishment of gene network to yield neuroendocrine/endocrine cells, but are often contradict between expression site and real occurrence of cells (see review by Schlosser, 2005) by provably an incomplete establishment of network or by its regression.

The aim of this review is to describe the recent findings on the origin of adult nervous systems, the persistent proliferation of GnRH and PRL-like neurons in the dorsal strand through lifetime, the morphological features of GnRH and PRL-like non-GnRH neurons, and to provide the morphological bases for further cellular, molecular and neural stem cell studies.

2.1.1 Animals

Following species are used in most ascidian studies.

Ciona intestinalis (Enterogona) is a cosmopolitan solitary ascidian that has become the model species of urochordates. Generation time is about 3 months.

Halocynthia roretzi (Pleurogona) is one of the biggest solitary ascidian and produce large eggs. Generation time is about 3-4 years (Fig.1).

Phallusia mammillata is a large solitary ascidian and found in the Atlantic and Mediterranean Sea. Generation time is about 8 months.

Botryllus schlosseri is a cosmopolitan colonial ascidian that has become the model species for the study of blastogenesis (asexual reproduction).

Description of conventional histological and immunohistlogical methods is omitted. Some sections were immunostained with a swine ACTH primary antiserum (Tanaka and Kurosumi, 1986) to illustrate the intimate topological relationships between the neural gland, the dorsal strand, and the visceral nerve.

2.1.2 Immunoelectron microscopy

The neural complexes were cut into small pieces and fixed for 4 hrs at 4°C in 0.2 M sodium phosphate buffer, pH 7.4, containing 4% paraformaldehyde (Merck) and 0.5% glutaraldehyde (TAAB). Tissue was washed overnight at 4°C in phosphate-buffered saline, post-fixed for 1 hr at 4°C with 1% osmium tetroxide in 0.15 M phosphate buffer, dehydrated, and embedded in Epon-Araldite. Ultrathin sections (approximately 8 nm thick) were collected and mounted on nickel grids (Nisshin EM, Tokyo) coated with Formvar (TAAB) which had been stored in a refrigerator at −20°C in order to ensure the adhesion of ultrathin sections, and treated with 1% meta-periodic acid for 10-30 min. As the primany antibody, an antiserum to bullfrog PRL (1:120) or to salmon GnRH (1:200) was used. The sections were then treated with gold-labeled (10 nm) secondary antibody (1:20; British BioCell International, Cardiff, UK) for 1 hr, washed, double-stained lightly with aqueous uranyl acetate and lead citrate, and examined with an electron microscope.

2.1.3 Specificity of immunoreactivity for PRL-like or GnRH neurons

Immunocytochemistry using anti–bullfrog PRL revealed numerous PRL-like neurons in the dorsal strand and the cerebral ganglion (Terakado et al., 1997; Figs. 2B, C). In control sections using preabsorbed antibody, immunoreactivity was undetectable (compare Figs. 2F and G). Using immunoelectron microscopy in control sections with the same preabsorbed antibody, no gold particles were observed in any neurons or endocrine cells. Because GnRH and PRL-like neurons are often localized side by side, the specificity of the GnRH antiserum for the dorsal strand or the cerebral ganglion was also examined. We observed no GnRH immunoreactivity when sections were stained with preabsorbed GnRH antiserum (compare Figs. 2D and E).

2.2 Development of the neurohypophyseal duct

The neurohypophyseal duct (ND) is a thin duct located on the anterior left side of the sensory vesicle of larvae, and remains a duct-like structure until the onset of metamorphosis (Satoh, 1994; Cole and Meinertzhagen, 2001, 2004; Manni et al., 2005). In metamorphosed juveniles, the rudiment of the cerebral ganglion appears as a small mass of cells on the dorsal side of the preexisting neurohypophyseal duct (Figs. 3A, B, C). Brain development proceeds slowly in *H. roretzi*, and thickening of the epidermis (placode formation) and delamination/migration of pioneer cells into the brain is not discernible with light microscopy (Figs. 3A, B, C). The ND elongates anteriorly and fuses with the stomodeal ectoderm (3B), later forming the dorsal tubercle. The cerebral ganglion elongates posteriorly to form a thin, long ganglion in young juveniles (Fig. 3D). Formation and development of the neural gland are more delayed than those of the adult central nervous sytem (Fig. 3D).

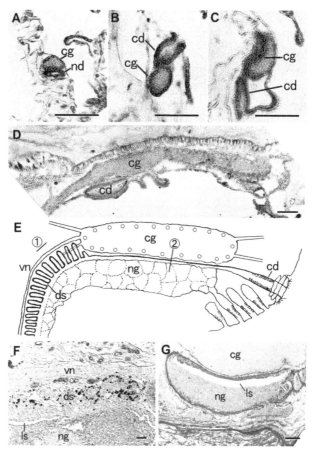

Fig. 3. Development of the neural complex and the topological relationships of the dorsal strand.

A, B, C. Early stages of neural complex formation. The rudiment of the cerebral ganglion (cg) appears on the dorsal side of the neurohypophyseal duct (nd), attaching closely to it (A, anterior is bottom). The neurohypophyseal duct elongates to fuse with the stomodial epithelium (B, anterior is top. cd; ciliated duct). The cerebral ganglion begins to elongate posteriorly (C, anterior is bottom). Hematoxylin/eosin stain. D. The cerebral ganglion in a 5-mm juvenile. The cerebral ganglion (cg) elongates further posteriorly to form a thin, long structure. The nerve fibers run along the long axis. The ciliated duct (cd) is seen in the anterior ventral side (anterior to the left). Hematoxylin stain. E. Schematic representation of the adult neural complex. The epithelium of the dorsal strand (ds) is continuous to the ciliated duct (cd) through the dorsal region of the neural gland (ng, anterior to the right. vn; visceral nerve). F. Longitudinal section along the neural gland (ng)–dorsal strand (ds)–visceral nerve (vn) axis at the position indicated by ① in panel E. The dorsal strand (ds) is closely associated with the visceral nerve (vn). The luminal space of the neural gland lies just under the dorsal epithelium. Dense cells in the dorsal strand are ACTH-positive cells. Anti–swine ACTH stain. G. Transverse section at the position indicated by ② in panel E. The cerebral ganglion (cg) is separated by the dorsal epithelium of the neural gland (ng). The luminal space (ls) lies in the most dorsal region of the neural gland. Aldehyde fuchsin stain. Bars: 50 um.

2.3 Formation of neural complex

The adult neural complex of *H. roretzi* is schematically described, with special reference to the continuation of the epithelium of dorsal strand (ds, Fig. 3E). The most anterior part is the dorsal tubercle, which opens into the upper part of the pharyngeal cavity, where it presents as a screw-like structure in which cilia on the outer surface move towards the pharyngeal cavity. In contrast, cilia on the inner surface move towards the interior of the body. Next to the dorsal tubercle towards the inside is the ciliated duct, in which cells are elongated. The ciliated duct contains both young cells, as judged by their small size and high nucleus/cytoplasm ratio, and degenerating cells, as judged by degenerating cells, as judged by disintegrating organelles. Cilia are embedded in prominent microvilli, and are arranged obliquely to point towards the interior. The region between the ciliated duct and the anterior part of the neural gland body is non-ciliated and has an exocrine function; some large granules (0.3-0.8 um in diameter) lie on the apical side and are often exposed to the lumen (Terakado et al., 1997). In the neural gland region, the epithelial structure is apparent in the dorsal side that faces the cerebral ganglion or the visceral nerve, but is indistinct in other regions. The luminal spaces that are continuous through the ciliated duct, the neural gland, and the dorsal strand terminate at the tips of the tubular structures of the dorsal strand (Figs. 3E, F, G).

Other than the dorsal epithelial cells, the cells of the neural gland are mostly, if not entirely, binucleate and loosely connected, and have no secretory granules. The neural gland elongates posteriorly along the visceral nerve and forms the dorsal strand from the dorsal epithelium by invagination towards the visceral nerve (Fig. 2A). There is an intimate topological relationship between the neural gland, the dorsal strand, and the visceral nerve (Figs. 3E, F). Why is the dorsal strand formed along the visceral nerve? One possibility may be that induction phenomenon might exist between them. Neuroendocrine cells containing GnRH and non-GnRH (PRL-like) neurons are localized in the dorsal strand and the cerebral ganglion. Adenohypophyseal-like cells such as adrenocorticotropic hormone-, growth hormone-, prolactin-, and gonadotropic hormone-immunoreactive cells were also present in the dorsal strand of *H. roretzi* (unpublished observation), which are compatible with the close proximal development of the olfactory and hypophyseal placodes in vertebrates (Mazet et al., 2005), though no such immunoreactivities are obtained in *C. intestinalis* which are compatible with the genome (Holland et al., 2008) and peptidomic (Kawada et al., 2011) analyses. Those differences between two species might be caused by loss of hypophyseal hormone genes in *C. intestinalis*. However, its exact understanding requires further studies.

2.4 Formation of the neural gland and the dorsal strand

The origin of the neural gland is unclear because of the absence of a specific marker (Takamura, 2002; Horie et al., 2011) and least studies on wide range of adult development. Our observations clearly revealed that the epithelium of the ciliated duct is continuous with the dorsal epithelium of the neural gland and further with that of the dorsal strand. Therefore, it is evident that the ciliated funnel (ciliated duct)–neural gland–dorsal strand system is a single entity (Fig. 3E) that is derived from the neurohypophyseal duct. The rudiment of the cerebral ganglion in *H. roretzi* appears immediately on the dorsal side of the neurohypophyseal duct of metamorphosed larvae (Fig. 3A). Delamination/migration of cells from the neurohypophyseal duct to the rudiment of the cerebral ganglion was not ascertained in our studies. The above results suggest that the adult neural complex is formed from dual origins and that its components may develop separately in an early phase (before migration of neurons to the cerebral ganglion) in normal development, although the rudiments of the cerebral ganglion and the neural gland are closely associated. This hypothesis is compatible with the proposition that the larval central nervous system contributes to the formation of the adult central nervous system (Takamura, 2002; Horie et al., 2011), rather than the hypothesis that the entire adult neural complex is generated from the neurohypophyseal duct (Willey, 1893). Peripheral GnRH and PRL-like neurons are generated in the dorsal strand, the epithelium of which is derived from the dorsal wall of the neurohypophyseal duct. In colonial ascidians, neurogenesis may also occur in the dorsal strand (if present), which remains fused with the cerebral ganglion for a long time, supplying neural cells (Manni et al., 1999; Koyama, 2002). The vertebrate olfactory epithelium (derived from the olfactory placode) is capable of prolonged neurogenesis that continues throughout adulthood (Beites et al., 2005; Murdoch and Roskams, 2007). This phenomenon also occurs during regeneration of neurons in the olfactory epithelium (Beites et al., 2005). This observation shows that the neurohypophyseal duct (and its derivatives) is homologous to the olfactory placode of vertebrates and can generate neural cells (neural stem cells) throughout the life of the organism, and that this phenomenon has been maintained throughout evolution from urochordates to mammals. Urochordate species that lack a dorsal strand, such as thaliaceans, appendicularians, and some colonial ascidians, seem not to generate peripheral neurons such as the GnRH and PRL-like neurons. These species may have been regressed the peripheral neurogenesis as an adaptation to asexual reproduction and/or perhaps because of a gross downsizing of body size.

It is well known that in appendicularians, cell division does not occur throughout the body after metamorphosis, and adults of chephalochordate (amphioxus) do not regenerate when injured, suggesting devoid of multipotent stem cells including neural ones.

2.5 Neurogenesis in the neural complex

Although ascidian neural complex contains several organs and distinct regions (cerebral ganglion, neural gland, dorsal strand, ciliated duct, and non-ciliated duct), neurogenesis occurs in the cerebral ganglion and the dorsal strand. The latter is probably the exclusive site of peripheral neurogenesis under normal conditions. Using immunostaining with anti–bullfrog PRL, we observed PRL-like cells along the dorsal strand and in the cerebral ganglion (Terakado et al., 1997). Using electron microscopy, two types of morphologically distinct neurons that occur side by side were discernible (Fig. 4A). In contrast to the generation of GnRH neurons, which occurs both within and adjacent to the epithelium (Terakado, 2009), PRL-like neurons were primarily generated adjacent to the epithelium (Figs. 4A, B, 5A). GnRH neurons contained a single kind of moderately dense secretory granules. On the other hand, PRL-like neurons contained both very dense and moderately dense granules of similar diameter (Figs. 4A, B). Young PRL-like neurons, as judged by a high nucleus/cytoplasm ratio and the presence of a few secretory granules, were frequently found within cell masses lying beside the epithelium (Fig. 5B). Using immunoelectron microscopy, PRL-immunoreactive material was detected in dense granules but not in moderately dense ones (compare Figs. 6A, B).   Granules of one cell were often immunopositive for GnRH, whereas those of a neighboring cell were immunonegative (Fig.

6C). Similarly, granules of one cell were frequently immunopositive for PRL, whereas those of a neighboring cell were immunonegative (Fig. 6D). Most notably, GnRH and PRL immunoreactivities were mutually exclusive, suggesting that these neurons are distinct.

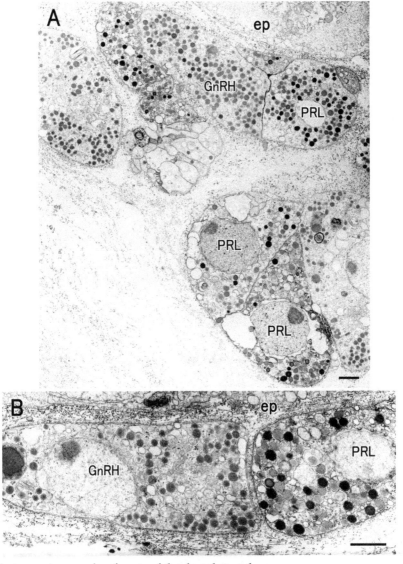

Fig. 4. Electron micrographs of parts of the dorsal strand.

A. Many young and developing GnRH (GnRH) and PRL-like (PRL) neurons are localized beside the epithelium (ep) of the dorsal strand. B. Two types of neurons in the dorsal strand. PRL-like neurons possess dense and moderately dense secretory granules, while GnRH neurons contain similar, moderately dense granules. Uranyl acetate-lead citrate double stain. Bars: 1 um.

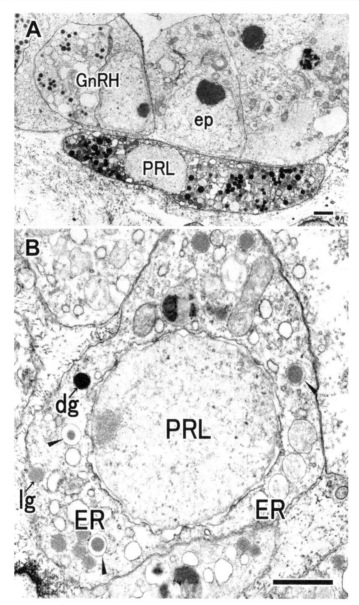

Fig. 5. Localization and ultrastructural features of young PRL-like neurons.

A. PRL-like neurons (PRL) with dense and moderately dense granules are often located beside the epithelium (ep). Growing GnRH neurons (GnRH) are seen in the epithelium of the dorsal strand. B. A young PRL-like neuron is shown possessing a few dense (dg) and moderately dense (lg) granules (arrows) that are membrane-bound. Developing granules (arrowheads), which are centrally condensed, were often observed. Rough endoplasmic reticulum (ER) is distended in several places, which is indicative of extensive protein synthesis. Uranyl acetate-lead citrate double stain. Bars: 1 um.

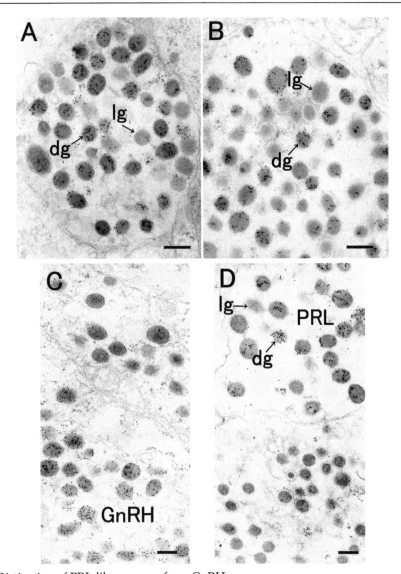

Fig. 6. Distinction of PRL-like neurons from GnRH neurons.

A and B. Immunoelectron micrographs of PRL-like neurons in the cerebral ganglion (A) and the dorsal strand (B). Gold particles are localized on the dense granules (dg) in both neurons. Gold particles are not localized in the moderately dense granules (lg). Anti–bullfrog PRL labeling. C and D. Comparison of anti-GnRH and anti-PRL immunoreactivity between GnRH neuron and probable PRL-like neuron, and between PRL-like neuron and probable GnRH neuron. C. GnRH immunoreactivity in the cerebral ganglion reveals that granules in one cell type are GnRH immunopositive (bottom), whereas those in the other cell type are GnRH immunonegative (top). D. PRL-like immunoreactivity in the cerebral ganglion reveals that granules in the cell on the top are PRL-like immunopositive, whereas those of the cell on the bottom are immunonegative. Bars: (A, B) 250 nm; (C, D) 500 nm.

2.6 Homology of the dorsal strand to the olfactory placode

The dorsal strand of *H. roretzi* is generated by repeated invaginations of the dorsal strand placode, and it produces GnRH and PRL-like neurons, some of which migrate into the cerebral ganglion through the visceral nerve (Terakado, 2009, 2010). Cells derived from the anterior region of the embryonic neural plate and their topological relationships indicate striking similarities between the dorsal strand and the olfactory placode, which suggests that the dorsal strand of urochordate ascidians is homologous to the olfactory placode of vertebrates (Terakado, 2009). Because the ascidian dorsal strand is a single organ, this notion is compatible with the formation of a single olfactory placode in agnathans (Uchida et al., 2003). The dorsal strand also generates many PRL-like (non-GnRH) neurons (Figs. 2C, 4A, B), a finding that has been reported in other species. Anti–salmon PRL also stains some cells of the dorsal strand in *H. roretzi* (unpublished observation). The presence of PRL-like cells has been reported in the cerebral ganglion of *Ciona* (Fritsch et al., 1982) and *Styela* (Pestalino, 1983), and in the brain of vertebrates (Fuxe et al., 1977; Krieger and Liotta, 1979; Toubeau et al., 1979; Hansen and Hansen, 1982). We previously suggested that these PRL-immunoreactive neurons in the vertebrate brain may be homologous to those in the cerebral ganglion of ascidians (Terakado et al., 1997). It is well known that molecular features of prolactin in the adenohypophysis resemble those of vertebrate growth hormones (Kawauchi and Sower, 2006). Immunoreactivity of some neurons of the cerebral ganglion and some cells of the dorsal strand to anti-PRL and anti–growth hormone antisera (unpublished observation) suggests the presence of ancestral molecule(s) of the growth hormone family in ascidians. Even the presence of a single molecule in ascidians raises the possibility that multiple antisera raised against molecules belonging to growth hormone family members react to ascidian prolactin due to the presence of common epitopes. Additional informations are needed to elucidate this problem.

2.7 Significance of neurogenesis in the peripheral organ

Most neurons are generated in the central nervous system in vertebrates and invertebrates. However, the vertebrate olfactory placode (peripheral organ) commonly generates GnRH neurons as well as other non-GnRH neurons (Murakami and Arai, 1994; Hilal et al., 1996; Yamamoto et al., 1996). Prior to or during the breeding season, the number of secretory granules greatly increases in the visceral nerve (Fig. 8). Generation of PRL-like neurons in the peripheral organ of chordates has not been reported other than the present species. The reason(s) why the GnRH neurons originate peripherally in vertebrates and ascidians is unknown; however, it is evident that GnRH neurons generated in peripheral organs are crucial for reproduction. PRL-like neurons in *H. roretzi* also concomitantly originate with the GnRH neurons side by side and migrate into the brain. Quantity of both neurons reveals a year-round change on a large scale which provably accompanies neuron loss after breeding season or winter in mature individuals and recovery thereafter by cell supply to the cerebral ganglion from the dorsal strand.

2.8 Migration of GnRH and PRL-like neurons to the brain

The observation that granulated PRL-like neurons are often found among the fibers of the visceral nerve (Fig. 7) suggests that they migrate towards the cerebral ganglion, similar to the GnRH neurons (Terakado, 2009). The PRL-like neurons in the dorsal strand mostly oval, whereas those in the cerebral ganglion have long neurites (compare Figs. 2B and C). This suggests that PRL-like neurons elongate after entering the brain. Unattached GnRH and PRL-like neurons were numerous and were located also near the visceral nerve (Fig.7 left). The intimate morphological relationship between the dorsal strand and the visceral nerve (Figs. 3E, F) has long been emphasized (see review by Goodbody, 1974; Chiba et al., 2004). In *H. roretzi*, this relationship may now be explained by the possibility that GnRH and PRL-like neurons generated in the dorsal strand invade the bundles of visceral nerve fibers and migrate towards the brain. This close topological relationship may be very important for invasion and migration from the site of generation (the dorsal strand) to the cerebral ganglion. This morphological relationship may partly explain the observation that the brain of *H. roretzi* easily reverts from a thin, cord-like structure (after breeding season, in winter) to the normal brain shape via migration of neurons from the dorsal strand. Similar phenomena are observed during regeneration of other brain structures; for example, after extirpation of the brain in *C. intestinalis*, the regenerating brain contains GnRH neurons, suggesting that GnRH neurons originate in the dorsal strand and subsequently migrate into the regenerating brain (Bollner et al., 1997). Together with the previous demonstration which GnRH neurons are generated in the dorsal strand and migrate into the brain (Terakado, 2009), the current results reveal that PRL-like neurons are generated in the dorsal strand and migrate into the brain during normal development. They both maintain the brain function throughout the life of the organism with other neurons. Even in colonial ascidians, dorsal strand cells divide frequently and become incorporated directly into the cerebral ganglion (Koyama, 2002) and/or enter into the circulation and participate in the formation of blastozooids as neural stem cells.

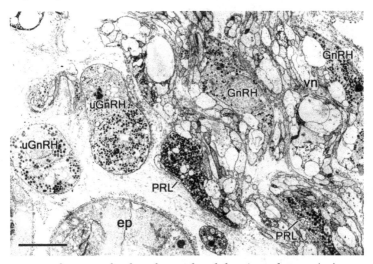

Fig. 7. Contact region between the dorsal strand and the visceral nerve (vn).

GnRH neurons and PRL-like neurons are often attached to the nerve, elongated along the nerve fibers, and distributed continuously towards the cerebral ganglion. Unattached GnRH neurons (uGnRH) are seen in the left. Uranyl acetate-lead citrate double stain. Bar: 5 um.

The neurohypophyseal duct and its derived tissues and cells generate a number of cell types including the ciliated duct cells, epithelial cells of the neural gland, luminal cells of the neural gland, epithelial cells of the dorsal strand, and neuroendocrine/endocrine cells in the dorsal strand. Similarly, the rudiment of the adult central nervous system may generate various kinds of neural cells in the developing brain. Of these cell types, those that are generated in the dorsal strand and migrate into the brain via the visceral nerve may be exclusively GnRH neurons in *Ciona* or GnRH and PRL-like neurons in *Halocynthia*. Abundance of both neurons in the cerebral ganglion and the dorsal strand in *H. roretzi* may correspond to the gigantism seen in this species and the corresponding necessity for a large neural network (provably relating to gametogenesis at expense of the body-wall muscle) to adjust to external/internal changes in the environment.

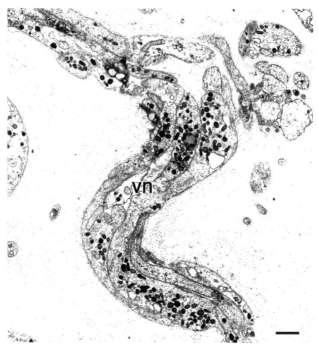

Fig. 8. Electron micrograph of the visceral nerve fibers at breeding season. The secretory granules in the fibers (vn) increase greatly prior to or during the breeding season. Bar: 1 um

2.9 Role of the neurohypophyseal duct

What is the significance of the neurohypophyseal duct in ascidians, in spite of solitary or colonial ones? From the neurohypophyseal duct, the neural gland and then the dorsal strand are formed in all the solitary ascidians and in some colonial ascidians. In the vegetative reproduction (the latter), migratory cells are produced from the dorsal strand (Manni et al, 1999; Koyama, 2002) and may participate in the formation of adult central nervous system of blastozooids as neural stem cells. Above results lead to the hypothesis that the neurohypophyseal duct is a cell reservoir that sets the undifferentiated cells aside for the post-metamorphic formation of the neural gland and the dorsal strand that contains neural stem cells. Peripheral organ origin of the GnRH neurons and their migration into the brain shares in vertebrates and urochordates, and may have evolved in the common ancestor of vertebrates and urochordates. In colonial ascidians that lack or reduced immunological staining to GnRH may be the result of regression due to the exceeding of asexual reproduction.

3. Conclusion

Urochordate ascidians share some morphological and developmental characteristics with those of vertebrates. About one thirds of the larval central nervous system is functional neurons and the rest is glial cells, called the ependymal cells. At metamorphosis, most of functional neurons and glial cells in the tail region disappear. Adult central nervous system is generated from the rearranged ependymal cells (undifferentiated neural cells) of the larval central nervous system after onset of metamorphosis. On the other hand, the peripheral nervous system is later generated from the dorsal strand which is formed by repeated invaginations of the thickened dorsal epithelium of the neural gland. The olfactory placode in vertebrates and the dorsal strand in ascidians are both derived from the anterior region of embryonic neural plate and generate GnRH and some other neurons. In some solitary ascidians, GnRH and PRL-like neurons are continuously generated in the dorsal strand throughout life. Therefore, ascidians are very useful for neural stem cell studies in providing important informations about fundamental processes of neural stem cell formation.

4. Acknowledgment

I am grateful to Emer. Prof. Hideshi Kobayashi of The University of Tokyo for continuous encouragement during studies and to the members of the Department of Regulation Biology, Saitama University for facilitation of the study. The author is also grateful to Emer. Prof. Sakae Kikuyama of Waseda University for gift of the bullfrog prolactin PRL antiserum.

5. References

Adams BA, Tello JA, Erchegyi J, Warby C, Hong DJ, Akinsanya KO, Mackie GO, Vale W, Rivier JE, Sherwood NM (2003) Six novel gonadotropin-releasing hormones are encoded as triplets on each of two genes in the protochordate, Ciona intestinalis. Endocrinology 144: 1907-1919

Bassham S, Postlethwait JH (2005) The evolutionary history of placodes: a molecular genetic investigation of the larvacean urochordate Oikopleura dioica. Development 132: 4259–4272

Beites CL, Kawauchi S, Crocker CE, Calof AL (2005) Identification and molecular regulation of neural stem cells in the olfactory epithelium. Exp Cell Res 306: 309–316

Bhattacharyya S, Bronner-Fraser M (2008) Conpetence, specification and commitment to an olfactory placode fate. Development 135: 4165–4177

Blair JE, Hedges SB (2005) Molecular phylogeny and divergence times of deuterostome animals. Mol Biol Evol 22: 2275–2284

Bollner T, Beesley PW, Thorndyke MC (1997) Investigation of the contribution from peripheral GnRH-like immunoreactive 'neuroblast' to the regenerating central nervous system in the protochordate Ciona intestinalis. Proc Roy Soc Lond B264: 1117–1123

Boorman CJ, Shimeld SM (2002) Pitx homeobox genes in Ciona and amphioxus show left-right asymmetry is a conserved chordate character and defines the ascidian adenohypophysis. Evol Dev 4: 354–365

Burighel P, Lane NJ, Zaniolo G, Manni L (1998) Neurogenic role of the neural gland in the development of the ascidian, Botryllus schlosseri (Tunicata, Urochordata). J Comp Neurol 394: 230-241

Cariboni A, Maggi R, Parnavelas JG (2007) From nose to fertility: the long migratory journey of gonadotropin-releasing hormone neurons. Trends Neurosci 30: 638-644

Chen B, Kim EH, XU PX (2009) Initiation of olfactory placode development and neurogenesis is blocked in mice lacking both Six1and Six4. Bev Biol 326: 75-85

Chiba S, Sasaki A, Nakayama A, Takamura K, Satoh N (2004) Development of *Ciona intestinalis* juveniles (through 2nd ascidian stage). Zool Sci 21: 285-298

Christiaen L, Burighel P, Smith WC, Vernier P, Bourrat F, Joly J-S (2002) *Pitx* genes in Tunicates provide new molecular insight into the evolutionary origin of pituitary. Gene 287: 107-113

Cole AG, Meinertzhagen IA (2001) Tailbud embryogenesis and the development of the neurohypophysis in the ascidian *Ciona intestinalis*. In "Biology of ascidians" Ed by H Sawada, H Yokosawa, CC Lambert, Tokyo, Springer-Verlag pp 137-141

Cole AG, Meinertzhagen IA (2004) The central nervous system of the ascidian larva: mitotic history of cells forming the neural tube in late embryonic *Ciona intestinalis*. Dev Biol 271: 239-262

Delsuc F, Brinkmann H, Chourrout D, Philippe H (2006) Tunicate and not cephalochordates are the closest living relatives of vertebrates. Nature 439: 965-968

Delsuc F, Tsagkogeorga G, Lartillot N, Phillippe H (2008) Additional Molecular support for the new chordate phylogeny. Genesis 46: 592-604

Elwyn A (1937) Some stages in the development of the neural complex in Ecteinascida turbinate. Bull Neurol Inst NY6: 163-177

Fritsch HA, Van Noorden S, Pearse AG (1982) Gastro-intestinal and neurohormonal peptides in the alimentary tract and cerebral complex of *Ciona intestinalis* (Ascidiaceae). Cell Tissue Res 223: 369-402

Fuxe K, Haekfelt T, Eneroth P, Gustafsson JA, Skett P (1977) Prolactin-like immunoreactivity: localization in nerve terminals of rat hypothalamus. Science 196: 899-900

Goodbody I (1974) The physiology of ascidians. Adv Mar Biol 12: 1-140

Gorbman A (1995) Olfactory origins and evolution of the brain-pituitary endocrine system: facts and speculation. Gen Comp Endocrinol 97: 171-178

Hansen BL, Hansen GN (1982) Immunocytochemical demonstration of somatotropin-like and prolactin-like activity in the brain of *Calamoichtes calabaricus* (Actinopterygii). Cell Tissue Res 222: 615-6627

Hilal EM, Chen JH, Silverman AJ (1996) Joint migration of gonadotropin-releasing hormone (GnRH) and neuropeptide Y (NPY) neurons from olfactory placode to central nervous system. J Neurobiol 31: 487-502

Holland LZ, Albalat R, Azumi K, Benito-Gutierrez E, Blow MJ, Bronner-Fraser M, Brunet F, Butts T, Candiani S, Dishaw LJ, Ferrir DEK, Garcia-Fernandez J, Gibson-Brown JJ, Gissi C, Godzik A, Hallbook F, Hirose D, Hosomichi K, Ikuta T, Inoko H, Kasahara M, Kasamatsu L, Kawashima T, Kimura A, Kobayashi M, Kozmik Z, Kubokawa K, Laudet V, Litman GW, McHardy AC, Meulemans D, Nonaka M, Olinski RP, Pancer Z, Pennacchio LA, Pestarino M, Rast JP, Rigoutsos I, Robinson-Rechavi M, Roch G, Saiga H, Sasakura Y, Satake M, Satou Y, Schubert M, Sherwood N, Shiina T, Takatori N, Tello J, Vopalensky P, Wada S, Xu A, Ye Y, Yoshida K, Yoshizaki F, Yu Jr-K, Zhang Q, Zmasek CM, Putnam NH, Rokhsar DS, Satoh N, Holland PWH (2008) Genome Res 18: 1100-1111

Horie T, Shinki R, Ogura Y, Kusakabe TG, Satoh N, Sasakura Y (2011) Ependymal cells of chordate larvae are stem-like cells that form the adult nervous system. Nature 469: 525-528

Kanaho Y, Enomoto M, Endo D, Maehiro S, Park MK, Murakami S (2009) Neurotrophic effect of gonadotropin-releasing hormone of neurite extension and neuronal migration of embryonic gonadotropin-releasing hormone neurons in chick olfactory nerve bundle culture. J Neurosci Res 87: 2237-2244

Kawada K, Ogasawara M, Sekiguchi T, Aoyama M, Hotta K, Oka K, Satake H (2011) Peptidomic analysis of the central nervous system of the protochordate, *Ciona intestinalis*: Homologs and prototypes of vertebrate peptides and novel peptides. Endocrinology 152: 2416-2427

Kawauchi H, Sower SA (2006) The down and evolution of hormones in the adenohypophysis. Gen Comp Endocrinol 148: 3-14

Koyama H (2002) The dorsal strand of *Polyandrocarpa misakiensis* (Protochordata: Ascidiacea): a light and electron microscope study. Acta Zool (Stockh), 83: 231-243

Krieger DT, Liotta AS (1979) Pituitary hormones in brain: where, how, and why? Science 205: 366-372

Mackie GO, Burighel P (2005) The nervous system in adult tunicates: current research directions. Can J Zool. 83: 151-220

Manni L, Lane NJ, Sorrentino M, Zaniolo G, Burighel P (1999) Mechanism of neurogenesis during the embryonic development of a tunicate. J Comp Neurol 412: 527-541

Manni L, Lane NJ, Joly JS, Gasparini F, Tiozzo S, Caicci F, Zaniolo G, Burighel P (2004) Neurogenic and non-neurogenic placodes in ascidians. J Exp Zool (Mol Dev Evol) 302: 483-504

Manni L, Agnelletto A, Zaniolo G., Burighel P (2005) Stomodial and neurohypophysial placodes in *Ciona intestinalis*: Insights into the origin of the pituitary gland. J Exp Zool (Mol Dev Evol) 300B: 324-339

Manni L, Mackie GO, Caicci F, Zaniolo G, Burighel P (2006) Coronal organ of ascidians and the evolutionary significance of secondary sensory cells in chordates. J Comp Neurol 495: 363-37

Mazet F (2006) The evolution of sensory placodes. Sci World J 6: 1841-1850

Mazet F, Hutt JAA, Milloz J, Millard J, Graham A, Shimeld SM (2005) Molecular evidence from Ciona intestinalis for the evolutionary origin of vertebrate sensoiry placodes. Dev Biol 282: 494-508

Mazet F, Shimeld SM (2005) Molecular evidence from ascidians for the evolutionary origin of vertebrate cranial sensory placodes. J Exp Zool (Mol Dev Evol) 304B:340-346

Meulemans D, Bronner-Fraser M (2007) The amphioxus Sox family: implications for the evolution of vertebrate placodes. Int J Biol Sci 3: 356-364

Murakami S, Arai Y (1994) Transient expression of somatostatin immunoreactivity in the olfactory-forebrain region in the chick embryo. Brain Res Dev Brain Res 82: 277-285

Murdoch B, Roskams AJ (2007) Olfactory epithelium progenitors: Insights from transgenic mice and in vitro biology. J Mol Histol 38: 581-899

Northcutt RG, Gans C (1983) The genesis of neural crest and epidermal placode: a reinterpretation of vertebrate origins. Q Rev Biol 58: 1-28

Okubo K, Sakai F, Lau EL, Yoshizaki G, Takeuchi Y, Naruse K, Aida K, Nagahama Y (2006) Forebrain gonadotropin-releasing hormone neuronal development: insights from transgenic medaka and the relevance to X-linked Kallman syndrome. Endocrinology 147: 1076-1084

Pestalino M (1983) Prolactinergic neurons in a protochordate. Cell Tissue Res 233: 471-474

Powell JF, Reska-Skinner SM, Prakash MO, Fischer WH, Park M, Rivier JE, Craig AG, Mackie GO, Sherwood NM (1996) Two new forms gonadotropin-releasing hormone in a protochordate and the evolutionary implications. Proc Natl Acad Sci USA 93: 10461-10464

Putnam NH, Butts T, Ferrier DEK, Furlong RF, Hellsten U, Kawashima T, Robinson-Rechavi
    M, Shoguchi E, Terry A, Yu J-K, Benito-Gutierrez E, Dubchak I, Garcia-Fernandez J,
    Gibson-Brown JJ, Grigoriev IV, Horton AC, de Jong PJ, Jurka J, Kapitonov VV,
    Kohara Y, Kuroki Y, Lindquist E, Lucas S, Osoegawa K, Pennacchio LA, Salamov AA,
    Satou Y, Sauka-Spengler T, Schmutz J, Shin-I T, Toyoda A, Bronner-Fraser M,
    Fujiyama A, Holland LZ, Holland PWH, Satoh N, Rokhsar DS (2008) The amphioxus
    genome and the evolution of the chordate karyotype. Nature 453: 1064-1071
Satoh N (1994) Developmental biology of ascidians. Cambridge University Press,
    Cambridge, UK
Schlosser G (2005) Evolutionary origins of vertebrate placodes: insights from
    developmental studies and from comparisons with other deuterostomes. J Exp
    Zool (Mol Dev Evol) 304B: 347-399
Schwarting GA, Wierman ME, Tobet SA (2007) Gonadotropin-releasing hormone neuronal
    migration. Semin Reprod Med 25: 305-312
Takamura K (2002) Changes in the nervous systems from larva to juvenile in *Ciona
    intestinalis*. Rep Res Inst Mar Biores Fukuyama Univ 12: 27-35
Tanaka S, Kurosumi K (1986) Differential subcellular localization of ACTH and α-MSH in
    corticotropes of the rat anterior pituitary. Cell Tissue Res 243: 229-238
Terakado K (2010) Generation of prolactin-like neurons in the dorsal strand of ascidians.
    Zool Sci 27: 581-588
Terakado K (2009) Placode formation and generation of gonadotropin-releasing hormone
    (GnRH) neurons in ascidians. Zool Sci 26: 389-405
Terakado K (2001) Induction of gamete release by gonadotropin-releasing hormone in a
    protochordate, *Ciona intestinalis*. Gen Comp Endocrinol 124:277-284
Terakado K, Ogawa M, Inoue K, Yamamoto K, Kikuyama S (1997) Prolactin-like
    immunoreactivity in the granules of neural complex cells in the ascidian
    Halocynthia roretzi. Cell Tissue Res 289: 63-71
Toubeau G, Desclin J, Parmentier M, Pasteels JL (1979) Compared localization of prolactin-
    like and adrenocorticotropin immunoreactivity within the brain of the rat.
    Neuroendocrinology 29: 374-384
Tsutsui H, Yamamoto N, Ito H, Oka Y (1998) GnRH-immunoeactive neuronal system in the
    presumptive ancestral chordate, Ciona intestinalis (Ascidian). Gen Comp
    Endocrinol 112: 426-432
Uchida K, Murakami Y, Kuraku S, Hirano S, Kuratani S (2003) Development of the
    adenohypophysis in the lamprey: evolution of epigenetic patterning programs in
    organogenesis. J Exp Zool (Mol Dev Evol) 300B: 32-47
Wada H, Saiga H, Satoh N, Holland PW (1998) Tripartite organization of the ancestral
    chordate brain and the antiquity of placodes: insight from ascidian *Pax-2/5/8, Hox*
    and *Otx* genes. Development 125: 1113-1122
Willey A (1893) Studies on the Protochordata. II The development of neuro-hypophyseal
    system in *Ciona intestinalis* and *Clavelina lepadiformis*, with an account of the origin
    of sense organs in Ascidia mentula. Q J Microsc Sci 35: 295-334
Yamamoto N, Uchiyama H, Ohki-Hamazaki H, Tanaka H, Ito H (1996) Migration of GnRH-
    immunoreactive neurons from the olfactory placode to the brain: a study using
    avian embryonic chimeras. Brain Res Dev Brain Res 95: 234-244
Yasui K, Zhang S, Uemura M, Saiga H (2000) Left-right asymmetric expression of BbPtx-
    related gene, in a lancelet species and the developmental left-sidedness in
    deuterostomes. Development (Camb.) 127: 187-195

Part 3

Regulation of Neural Stem Cell Development

8

Musashi Proteins in Neural Stem/Progenitor Cells

Kenichi Horisawa and Hiroshi Yanagawa
Department of Bioscience and Informatics, Keio University
Japan

1. Introduction

Many RNA-binding proteins are encoded in the genomes of various organisms and play a critical role in several life systems. The human genome contains thousands of RNA-binding proteins (Glisovic *et al.*, 2008). The most important biological role for these proteins involves the post-transcriptional events in gene expression, *e.g.*, splicing, export, stabilization, localization, and translation. Recent studies have shown that these post-transcriptional events are of similar importance to transcriptional and post-translational events and are highly orchestrated (Keene *et al.*, 2007).

Musashi is an RNA-binding protein that contains typical RNA-recognition motifs (RRMs). The gene encoding the Musashi protein was originally identified in *Drosophila* and is responsible for the asymmetrical division of sensory organ precursor cells (Nakamura *et al.*, 1994). Later studies determined that Musashi proteins are RNA-binding proteins that bind to a sequence in the 3′untranslated region (UTR) of *tramtrack69* (*ttk69*) mRNA (Lai & Li, 1999). The binding of these proteins prevents the translation of *ttk69* mRNA, resulting in asymmetric cell division (Hirota *et al.*, 1999; Okabe *et al.*, 2001).

Subsequently, two highly conserved mammalian homolog proteins, Musashi1 (Msi1) and Musashi2 (Msi2), were discovered in mice (Sakakibara *et al.*, 1996, 2001). Over 90 Musashi and Musashi-like proteins have been discovered in various multicellular animals; however, these proteins have not been found in prokaryotes, plants, or monocellular organisms. The expression pattern and structure of these proteins are highly similar among various organisms (Good *et al.*, 1998; Yoda *et al.*, 2000; Kawashima *et al.*, 2000; Cuadrado *et al.*, 2002; Lowe *et al.*, 2003; Asai *et al.*, 2005; Higuchi *et al.*, 2008).

Musashi proteins are highly expressed in the vertebrate nervous system. (Kaneko *et al.*, 2000). In the mammalian central nervous system, Msi1 appears specifically in undifferentiated neural stem/precursor cells during both the embryonic and adult stages (Sakakibara *et al.*, 1996; Kaneko *et al.*, 2000; Sakakibara & Okano, 1997). Interestingly, Msi1 expression was also observed in many kinds of somatic stem cells in adult tissues, such as the eye (Raji *et al.*, 2007), intestine (Potten *et al.*, 2003), stomach (Akasaka *et al.*, 2005), mammary gland (Clarke *et al.*, 2005), and hair follicles (Sugiyama-Nakagiri *et al.*, 2006).

Later studies revealed that Msi1 maintains the stemness of the neural stem/precursor cells through the translational suppression of m-Numb, a regulator protein of the Notch signal pathway (Imai *et al.*, 2001; Kawahara *et al.*, 2008). Although other target mRNAs of Msi1 have been recently reported, the full function of Msi1 in maintaining stem/precursor cells remains to be elucidated (Battelli *et al.*, 2006; de Sousa Abreu *et al.*, 2009; Horisawa *et al.*, 2009).

Furthermore, the relationship between Musashi proteins and several disease states have recently been reported. Msi1 is reported to play a role in a variety of cancers (Toda *et al.*, 2001; Shu *et al.*, 2002; Sakatni *et al.*, 2005) and neural disorders (Lovell & Markesbery, 2005; Ziabreva *et al.*, 2006; O'Sullivan *et al.*, 2011; Oki *et al.*, 2010; Nakayama *et al.*, 2010; Crespel *et al.*, 2005).

In this chapter, we present an overview of Musashi proteins, especially mammalian Msi1, and consider possible directions for further research.

2. The discovery of Musashi proteins and their function

Musashi was originally identified in a *Drosophila* mutant with abnormal external sensory organs (Fig.1A&B). In the early '90s, Nakamura and co-workers showed that the *musashi* gene is responsible for the asymmetrical division of sensory organ precursor (SOP) cells in *Drosophila*, which are precursors for the ectodermal system common to both neural and non-neural cell lineages in loss-of-function experiments (Nakamura *et al.*, 1994). In wild-type animals, the SOP cell divides into a non-neural precursor cell (green in Fig.1C) and a neural precursor cell (white in Fig.1C), whereas in *musashi* mutants, two non-neural precursor cells (white in Fig.1D) are produced instead. The symmetrically divided non-neural precursor cells differentiate to hair-forming cells (Sf and So in Fig.1A&B), leading to a double-bristle phenotype instead of the single-hair wild-type phenotype (Fig.1 A&B). Based on this double-hair shape, the gene was named "Musashi" after a famous Japanese swordsman who fought with two swords, Musashi Miyamoto (A.D. 1584-1645).

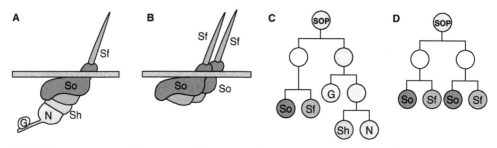

Fig. 1. Structures and cell lineages of the external sensory organs in *Drosophila*
(A & B) Structures of the adult external sensory organs (mechanosensory bristles) in wild-type (A) and musahi mutant (B) animals. The cell lineages contain neuron (N; green) and non-neuronal support cells (magenta), a shaft cell (Sf), a socket cell (So), a sheath cell (Sh) and glia (G); (C & D) Cell lineages of the mechanosensory bristle in wild-type (C) and *musashi* mutant (D) animals. Cells with neuronal potential are green, and non-neuronal cells are magenta and white.

Subsequent studies revealed that the Musashi protein, which has RNA-binding activity, introduces neural differentiation potential for one daughter cell of the SOP cell via selective translational repression of the mRNA of a neural differentiation inhibitory factor (a transcription repressor possessing a BTB domain and zinc-finger domain) called *ttk69*

(Okabe *et al.*, 2001). The ttk69 protein is located downstream in the Notch signaling pathway and acts as a determinant of non-neural identity.

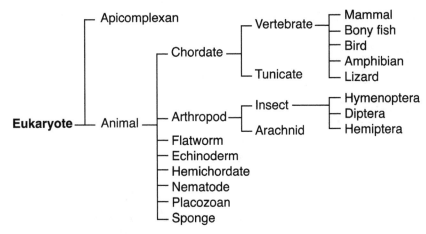

All listed organisms are multi-cellular eukaryotes.

Fig. 2. A dendrogram of the organisms bearing the *musashi* or *musashi*-related genes.

The Systematic Evolution of Ligands by EXponential enrichment (SELEX) assay (Tuerk & Gold, 1990), an *in vitro* selection method for RNA, was employed to identify the specific target RNA motifs of Musashi proteins from a synthesized random-sequence RNA library. Uridine-rich sequences containing two or three (GUU...UAG) or (GUU...UG) repeats were identified as Musashi binding targets (Okabe *et al.*, 2001). Indeed, *ttk69* mRNA contains 15 of these motif sequences in the 3'UTR, and it has been demonstrated that the Musashi protein binds to the 3'UTR of *ttk69* mRNA and inhibits the translation of a reporter gene linked to the 3'UTR *in vitro* (Okabe *et al.*, 2001).

Musashi and Musashi-like proteins have since been discovered in several multicellular organisms, but these genes have not been found in prokaryotes, plants, or monocellular organisms (Fig.2). This implies that the Musashi protein is specifically required for the development and evolution of multicellular animals.

3. The homologs of Musashi protein in mammals

Further studies in *Drosophila* have revealed that the Musashi protein is also expressed in the compound eye primordium (Hirota *et al.*, 1999), CNS (Nakamura *et al.*, 1994), and neural stem/precursor cells in the larval brain (Nakamura *et al.*, 1994), which have many characteristics in common with mammalian neural stem cells (NSCs) (Ito & Hotta, 1992). Thus, to elucidate the functions of the Musashi gene family in mammals, a homolog search and immunohistochemical studies were performed in mice.

Two highly conserved homolog genes, *musashi1* (*msi1*) (Sakakibara *et al.*, 1996) and *musashi2* (*msi2*) (Sakakibara *et al.*, 2001), were discovered in mice. While the length of these proteins are considerably shorter than that of *Drosophila* Musashi, the RNA-recognition motifs (RRMs) were highly conserved (~95% identical) between mammalian and insect systems (Fig.3).

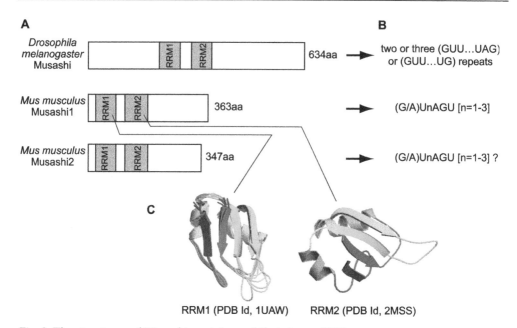

Fig. 3. The structures of Musashi proteins and their target RNA sequences
(A) Primary structures of Musashi proteins in Drosohila melanogaster and Mus musculus.
(B) Musashi binding motifs in target mRNAs. (C) Partial 3D structures of RRMs of Msi1 protein.

A high level of expression of Msi1 in NSCs of the periventricular area and undifferentiated neural precursor cells (Sakakibara *et al.*, 1996; Kaneko *et al.*, 2000; Sakakibara & Okano, 1997) was observed. Therefore, Msi1 is now widely used as a marker of NSCs and progenitor cells in the CNS of a variety of vertebrates. These cells, which can form neurospheres, were identified in the adult human brain using this approach (Pincus *et al.*, 1998). Precise immunohistochemical analyses revealed that Msi1 is strongly expressed in the ventricular zone of the neural tube in embryos and in neurogenic sites within the postnatal brain, including the subventricular zone (SVZ), olfactory bulb, and rostral migratory stream (RMS) (Sakakibara & Okano, 1997). The Msi1 protein is expressed in neural stem/progenitor cells within these tissues and is rapidly down-regulated in post-mitotic neurons (Sakakibara *et al.*, 1996).

The Msi2 protein in mice is a paralog of Msi1, displaying more than 90% homology with the Msi1 protein in the RRMs (Sakakibara *et al.*, 2001) (Fig.3). Although the expression pattern in the CNS is very similar between the members of this family, Msi2 is also continuously expressed in a subset of neuronal lineage cells, such as parvalbumin-containing GABA neurons in the neocortex and neurons in several nuclei of the basal ganglia (Sakakibara *et al.*, 2001). Other reports have also shown a differential expression pattern of these genes in uroepithelial cells (Nikpour *et al.*, 2010). Although the functional properties (*e.g.*, RNA-binding specificity) of the two proteins are similar, these differences in expression might explain the functional assignation of these proteins.

Although the partial 3D structures of RRMs of Msi1 protein have been solved by NMR, the full-length 3D structures of Msi1 and Msi2 remain to be elucidated (Nagata *et al*, 1999; Miyanoiri *et al*, 2003).

The human genome also contains both *msi1* and *msi2* genes (Good *et al.*, 1998; Sakakibara *et al.*, 2001). The structure and expression pattern of these proteins in the CNS highly resemble those in mice. As described below, Musashi proteins are related to several diseases. Functional studies in mice will thus contribute to therapeutic developments for Musashi-related conditions.

Additionally, a small Msi2-like gene, LOC100504473, has been found near the Msi2 locus on the mouse genome, but its expression and function are yet to be defined.

4. Molecular and physiological functions of Musashi proteins in stem/progenitor cells

To identify the target RNAs of Msi1 in mammals, a SELEX analysis from a random-sequence RNA library was performed, similar to those done in *Drosophila*. The selected consensus sequence revealed that the mouse Msi1 protein binds specifically to RNAs that possess a (G/A)UnAGU [n=1-3] sequence (Imai *et al.*, 2001) (Fig.3).

A survey for the motif was performed in mRNAs expressed in the embryonic CNS. The 3'UTR region of *m-numb* mRNA (Zhong *et al.*, 1996) was highlighted as a candidate target. Subsequent experiments found that *m-munb* mRNA is a specific binding target of the Msi1 protein *in vitro* and *in vivo*. Its translation is repressed by the Msi1 protein (Imai *et al.*, 2001; Kawahara *et al.*, 2008).

The m-Numb protein binds to the intracellular domain of the Notch protein, which has nuclear translocation and transactivation activities, and inhibits the Notch signaling pathway (Berdnik *et al.*, 2002), which positively regulates neural stem cell self-renewal (Nakamura *et al.*, 2000; Hitoshi *et al.*, 2002; Tokunaga *et al.*, 2004) (Fig.4). In agreement with this hypothesis, oscillation in the expression of the *hes1* gene, a downstream target of Notch, controls the differentiation of embryonic stem cells to neural cells (Kobayashi *et al.*, 2009). Indeed, the Msi1 protein induces the expression of the *hes1* gene (Imai *et al.*, 2001; Yokota *et al.*, 2004).

Musashi proteins in both mammalian species and *Drosophila* contribute to maintaining the stem/progenitor cell status via translational repression of target mRNA. However, the target mRNAs are, interestingly, not orthologous. This result implies a highly conserved function of Musashi proteins in maintaining the stemness of progenitor/stem cells and the probable presence of other unknown target RNAs of the Musashi proteins.

Recently, mammalian Msi1 protein expression was identified not only in CNS, but also in other tissues and organs in embryonic or adult stages, including the eye (*e.g.*, corneal epithelium, corneal endothelium, stromal keratocyte, progenitor cell of the limbus, equatorial lens stem cell, differentiated lens fiber, and retinal pigment epithelium cells) (Raji *et al.*, 2007; Susaki *et al.*, 2009), intestine (small intestinal crypt, colon crypt, columnar cell, and epithelial cell) (Kayahara *et al.*, 2003; Nishimura *et al.*, 2003; Potten *et al.*, 2003; Asai *et al.*,

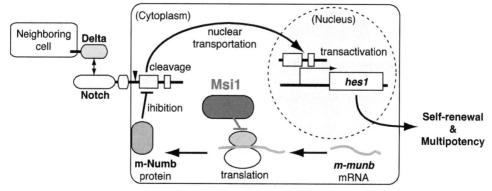

Fig. 4. A model for Msi1 function in the regulation of Notch signaling
Msi1 translationally regulates *m-numb* gene expression. Because m-Numb blocks the activation of the Notch signal induced by Delta on neighboring cells, translational repression of m-Numb by Msi1 stimulates Notch signaling and HES1 pathways.

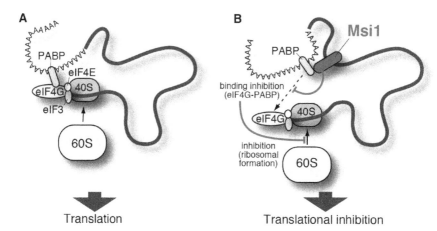

Fig. 5. Schematic representation of the molecular function of Msi1
(A) Translation of a non-target mRNA of Msi1; (B) Translational inhibition of a target mRNA of Msi1. The Msi1 protein interacts with the 3'UTR of its target mRNA and PABP and subsequently inhibits translation initiation by competing with eIF4G for PABP. These sequential events inhibit the formation of the 80S ribosome complex.

2005; Samuel *et al.*, 2008; Murata *et al.*, 2008), stomach (luminal compartment of the mucosa, isthmus/neck region, and fetal pyloric gland) (Nagata *et al.*, 2006; Akasaka *et al.*, 2005; Asai *et al.*, 2005; Murata *et al.*, 2008), breast (mammary gland epithelial cell) (Clarke *et al.*, 2005), and hair follicles (kerationocyte) (Sugiyama-Nakagiri *et al.*, 2006). These studies suggest that the Msi1 protein may be an effective marker for stem/progenitor cells in various tissues and acts as a regulator of the stem cell status of cells.

On the other hand, the function of the Msi2 protein in neural stem/progenitor cells is still unclear, though it is known that Msi1 and Msi2 have similar RNA-binding specificity

(Sakakibara *et al.*, 2001). The results of an Msi1 and Msi2 double knockout experiment suggested that these proteins have mutually complementary functions (Sakakibara *et al.*, 2002).

Recently, the molecular mechanism of translational repression by Msi1 has been uncovered. Kawahara *et al.* identified the poly(A)-binding protein (PABP) as an Msi1-binding protein and found that Msi1 competes with elF4G for PABP binding on its target mRNAs (Fig.5) (Kawahara *et al.*, 2008).

However, the molecular machinery of other functions of Musashi protein (described below) remains to be elucidated. A survey for the co-factors of Musashi proteins is an important future task in order to fully understand the functions of these proteins.

5. Musashi-related diseases - Cancers and neural disorders

Msi1 has been shown to play a role in a variety of cancers and neural disorders.

Several studies have reported high Msi1 protein expression in many types of tumors, including glioma (Toda *et al.*, 2001), hepatoma (Shu *et al.*, 2002), colorectal adenoma (Sakatani *et al.*, 2005; Schulenburg *et al.*, 2007), teratoid/rhabdoid tumors in eye (Fujita *et al.*, 2005), non-small cell lung cancer (Kanai *et al.*, 2006), retinoblastoma (Seigel *et al.*, 2007), medulloblastoma (Nakano *et al.*, 2007; Sanchez-Diaz *et al.*, 2008), ependymoma (Nakano *et al.*, 2007), endometrial carcinoma (Götte *et al.*, 2008), neurocytoma (Yano *et al.*, 2009), glioblastoma (Liu *et al.*, 2006), and cervical carcinoma (Ye *et al.*, 2008). This might because that many carcinoma cells are of epithelial stem cell lineage (Miller *et al.*, 2005) which express the Msi1 protein.

Although the exact function of Msi1 in these cancer cells remains unclear, the knockdown of Msi1 via siRNA resulted in arrested tumor growth in colon adenocarcinoma xenografts transplanted in athymic nude mice, reduced cancer cell proliferation, and increased apoptosis (Sureban *et al.*, 2008). These results suggest an important potential role for Msi1 in tumorigenesis and tumor proliferation.

It has also been shown that some tumors express the Msi2 protein in addition to Msi1 (Seigel *et al.*, 2007). This may indicate a complementary role of the two proteins in tumors.

Msi1 is also hypothesized to be a key player in neuronal disorders. Several reports indicate that Msi1 is relevant to neurodegenerative disorders, such as Alzheimer's disease (AD). Ectopic expression of Msi1 was observed in the hippocampus of AD patients (Lovell & Markesbery, 2005), while a significant decrease in Msi1-expressing cells was observed in the SVZ (Ziabreva *et al.*, 2006). Although it is difficult to explain these phenomena at present, the function of Msi1 in maintaining the stemness of NSCs might play a role in the pathogenesis of the disease.

Msi1 may also play a role in Parkinson's disease (PD), an another type of neurodegenerative disorder. A clinical experiment found that chronic treatment with an anti-PD drug increased Msi1-positive cells in the SVZ of PD patients. The authors suggested that impaired neurogenesis may contribute to the decline in this neurodegenerative disease (O'Sullivan *et al.*, 2011).

Oki *et al.* (2010) reported an up-regulation in Msi1 expression in collapsed nervous system tissue arising from a blood circulation defect. In the ischemic striatum induced by middle cerebral artery occlusion (MCAO), an increase in Msi1-immunoreactivity was observed in reactive astrocytes beginning at 2 days after MCAO and persisting until 14 days after MCAO. The proliferation of Msi1-positive cells was observed beginning at 4 days after MCAO and reached a peak at 7 days after MCAO (Oki *et al.*, 2010)

Nakayama *et al.* (2010) also observed an induction of Msi1-positive cells at the site of ischemic lesions beginning on day 1 after stroke in humans. This result indicates the presence of a regional regenerative response in the human cerebral cortex and the importance of Msi1 in this phenomenon (Nakayama *et al.*, 2010).

Interestingly, Msi1 protein-expressing cells are increased in the hippocampus of mesial temporal lobe epilepsy (MTLE) patients (Crespel *et al.*, 2005). Large numbers of Msi1-positive cells were also observed in the SVZ in these patients (Crespel *et al.*, 2005). Increased neurogenesis has been reported in animal models of MTLE (Crespel *et al.*, 2005). The abnormal proliferation of such Msi1-expressing neural progenitors in the hippocampus might cause epilepsy.

Unlike Msi1, the relevance of Msi2 to various diseases has not yet been elucidated. However, it was recently demonstrated that Msi2 triggers the acute transformation of chronic myelogenous leukaemia (CML) through translational control of the Numb protein in humans (Ito *et al.*, 2010; Kharas et al., 2010; Nishimoto & Okano, 2010). Byers et al. (2011) reported that Msi2 protein expression can be a clinical prognostic biomarker of human myeloid leukaemia (Byers *et al.*, 2011)

6. Novel finding for the functions of Musashi proteins

Although Musashi proteins are thought to act as translational suppressors, MacNicol and co-workers found a novel function of Musashi in *Xenopus* oocytes. In this system, it activates the translation of *mos* mRNA (Charlesworth *et al.*, 2006), a gene that is related to the meiotic cell cycle progression (Sagata *et al.*, 1988). This is an opposite result from previous findings on the translational effect of Msi1. Interestingly, in human oocytes, a parallel physiological phenomenon is controlled by factors other than the Musashi homolog proteins (Prasad *et al.*, 2008).

A similar translation-activating effect of Msi1 was also observed in mammals. Kuwako *et al.* (2010) found that the Msi1 protein up-regulates the translation of the Robo3 protein and controls midline crossing in precerebellar neurons. While previous studies reported that the Msi1-binding sites are in the 3'UTR of mRNAs, the Msi1-binding region in Robo3 mRNA is in the protein-coding region and does not bear the Msi1-binding consensus sequence (Kuwako *et al.*, 2010). This result implies that the discovery of novel Msi1 co-factors will be an important task for understanding the molecular mechanism of the Msi1 proteins in translational control.

Until recently, only a small number of Msi1-targeted mRNAs (Imai *et al.*, 2001; Battelli *et al.*, 2006) had been reported. De Sousa Abreu *et al.* (2009) performed an RNA immnoprecipitation (RIP)-Chip assay in HEK293T cells, a cell line derived from human embryonic kidney, to comprehensively identify the target mRNAs (de Sousa Abreu, 2009). They identified a group of 64 mRNAs whose genes belong to two main functional categories pertinent to tumorigenesis and protein modification. A subsequent proteomics study also revealed that

Msi1 can have not only negative but also positive effects on gene expression for some of the targets (de Sousa Abreu *et al.*, 2009). This result is consistent with other recent findings.

Our group also performed *in vitro* screening analysis to detect specific binding targets of Msi1 controlling the stem cell status of NSCs. We succeeded in identifying a novel target mRNA of Msi1, *doublecortin* (*dcx*), from an mRNA library of embryonic mouse brain tissue (Horisawa *et al.*, 2009).

The *dcx* is a gene related to the migration of newborn neurons and neural development. Mutations in this gene cause an X-linked dominant disorder characterized by classic lissencephaly with severe mental retardation and epilepsy in hemizygous males and subcortical laminar heterotopia, also known as double cortex syndrome, associated with milder mental retardation and epilepsy in heterozygous females (Gleeson *et al.*, 1998; des Portes *et al.*, 1998; Sossey-Alaoui *et al.*, 1998).

The Msi1 protein specifically bound to the 3'UTR region of the mRNA *in vitro*, which contains an Msi1 binding motif, and repressed translation of a reporter gene linked to the mRNA fragment (Horisawa *et al.*, 2009).

We hypothesize that the Msi1 protein prevents inappropriate migration of NSCs through translational inhibition of the *dcx* gene. Several findings support our hypothesis. First, the Dcx protein is expressed only in neuronal precursors just differentiated from NSCs (Couillard-Despres *et al.*, 2005). Secondly, mutually exclusive protein expression of Msi1 and Dcx in human brains was observed (Crespel *et al.*, 2005). Finally, a knock-out of the Musashi family genes reduced the number of neurospheres isolated from embryonic mouse brains, while the knock-down of *dcx* prevented migration of the cells from neurospheres, leaving their structure intact (Ocbina *et al.*, 2006).

Gene symbols	Functions of the encoded proteins	Spices	Effects	References
ttk69	Notch signaling	*Drosophila melanogaster*	Translational suppression	Okabe *et al*, 2001
m-numb	Notch signaling	*Mus musculus* (Msi1)	Translational suppression	Imai *et al*, 2001
*p21*WAF1	Cell cycle control	*Mus musculus* (Msi1)	Translational suppression	Battelli *et al*, 2006
mos	Meiotic cell cycle progression	*Xenopus laevis* (Msi1)	Translational activation	Charlesworth *et al*, 2006
dcx	Neural migration	*Mus musculus* (Msi1)	Translational suppression?	Horisawa *et al*, 2009
robo3	Axonal guidance	*Mus musculus* (Msi1)	Translational activation	Kuwako *et al*, 2010
let-7	Non coding RNA	*Mus musculus* (Msi1)	Nuclear translocation of Lin28	Kawahara *et al*, 2010
numb	Notch signaling	*Homo sapiens* (Msi2)	Translational suppression	Ito *et al*, 2010

Table 1. Known target RNAs of Musashi proteins

In addition, we also identified another candidate Msi1-binding mRNA that is related to neuronal migration and axon outgrowth (unpublished data). Thus, Msi1 might repress the maturation of neural stem/progenitor cells to neurons through direct translational inhibition of the genes that influence neuronal maturation and migration.

All of the known target RNAs of Musashi proteins, which have been validated in previous studies, are listed in Table 1.

The precise mechanism through which the function of Msi1 is controlled remains unclear. Although Wang et al. (2008) proposed that the Msi1 protein is involved in both Notch and Wnt signaling pathways as a novel autocrine process (Nagata et al., 2006; Glazer et al., 2008), details of the mechanism remain unclear, and direct regulators of Msi1 have not been identified.

On the other hand, Ratti et al. (2006) reported post-transcriptional regulation of Msi1 mRNA by embryonic lethal abnormal vision (ELAV), an RNA-binding protein of *Drosophila* (Ratti et al., 2006). This is an interesting result because it may imply that some kind of cascade of post-transcriptional regulation contributes to neurogenesis, in addition to other machinery, *i.e.*, signal transduction, transcriptional regulation, and post-translational modification.

Upstream mechanisms regulating Msi1 transcription have also been studied. Kawase et al. (2011) found that the sixth intron of the *msi1* gene has a regulatory element for *msi1* transcription in neural stem/progenitor cells. The identification of transcription factors for the *msi1* gene will help elucidate the role of the Msi1 protein in stem cells (Kawase et al., 2011).

More recently, Kawahara et al. (2011) discovered a novel function of the Msi1 protein. They showed that Msi1 works in concert with Lin28 to regulate post-transcriptional microRNA (miRNA) biogenesis in the cropping step, which occurs in the nucleus. This indicates that Msi1 can influence stem cell maintenance and differentiation by controlling the subcellular localization of proteins involved in miRNA synthesis, as well as by regulating the translation of its target mRNA (Kawahara et al., 2011).

7. Conclusion

Somatic stem/precursor cells, including neural stem cells, are promising targets for regenerative medicine. Because these cells are derived from the patients themselves, they are not subject to the ethical questions and possible immunological rejection that are common problems in regenerative therapies using embryonic stem (ES) cell.

The Musashi family proteins are key factors for the understanding and application of somatic stem cells. Musashi proteins control the stem cell state through the translational regulation of target mRNAs, and the Musashi family is a highly conserved RNA-binding protein group expressed in undifferentiated stem/precursor cells at both embryonic and adult stages.

Although several studies have revealed that a Notch signal inhibitor, *m-numb*, and a cell cycle regulator, *p21WAF1*, are direct targets of Msi1, a mouse homolog of Musashi and that the machinery involved is located in the context of both the Notch and Wnt signaling pathways (Glazer et al., 2008), the full picture of Msi1 function in neural stem/precursor cells remains to be uncovered. Recently, de Sousa Abreu et al. employed an RNA immunoprecipitation (RIP)-chip technique to comprehensively detect Msi1 targeted mRNAs, and they identified a group of 64 mRNAs from HEK293T cells, whose genes belong to two main functional categories pertinent to tumorigenesis: 1) cell cycle, proliferation, differentiation, and apoptosis and 2) protein modification (de Sousa Abreu *et al.*, 2009). However, a more specific survey is necessary to identify the key factors that regulate stemness. We speculate that Msi1 might have specific targets in each cell type or site, such as *dcx*, in addition to the previously discovered targets, which are related to the cell cycle, proliferation, and self-renewal.

While Musashi proteins were originally thought to act as translational suppressors, recent findings indicate that these proteins can activate the translation of specific targets (Charlesworth *et al.*, 2006; de Sousa Abreu *et al.*, 2009; Kuwako *et al.*, 2010). This result indicates that currently unknown molecular machinery may exist that differs from the translational suppression machinery (Kawahara *et al.*, 2008). Components of this machinery, *e.g.*, binding proteins of Msi1, need to be comprehensively clarified using high-throughput techniques (Rigaut *et al.*, 1999; Horisawa *et al.*, 2004, 2008).

Many researches indicate that Musashi proteins have strong associations with some diseases, such as cancers and neuronal disorders. A more complete understanding of the Musashi proteins will also contribute to the development of therapies for these diseases.

8. Acknowledgment

We thank Dr. Takao Imai and Prof. Hideyuki Okano (Department of Physiology, Keio University School of Medicine) for valuable advice and discussion.

9. References

Akasaka, Y.; Saikawa, Y.; Fujita, K.; Kubota, T.; Ishikawa, Y.; Fujimoto, A.; Ishii, T.; Okano, H. & Kitajima, M. (2005) Expression of a candidate marker for progenitor cells, Musashi-1, in the proliferative regions of human antrum and its decreased expression in intestinal metaplasia. *Histopathology*, Vol.47, No.4, (October 2005), pp.348-356, ISSN 1365-2559

Asai, R.; Okano, H. & Yasugi, S. (2005) Correlation between Musashi-1 and c-hairy-1 expression and cell proliferation activity in the developing intestine and stomach of both chicken and mouse. *Dev Growth Differ.*, Vol.47, No.8, (October 2005) pp.501-510, ISSN 0012-1592

Battelli, C.; Nikopoulos, G.N.; Mitchell, J.G. & Verdi, J.M. (2006) The RNA-binding protein Musashi-1 regulates neural development through the translational repression of p21WAF-1. *Mol Cell Neurosci.*, Vol.31, No.1, (January 2006), pp.85-96, ISSN 1044-7431

Berdnik, D.; Török, T.; González-Gaitán, M. & Knoblich, J.A. (2002) The endocytic protein alpha-Adaptin is required for numb-mediated asymmetric cell division in *Drosophila. Dev Cell.* Vol.3, No.2, (August 2002), pp.221-231, ISSN 1534-5807

Byers, R.J.; Currie, T.; Tholouli, E.; Rodig, S.J. & Kutok, J.L. MSI2 protein expression predicts unfavorable outcome in acute myeloid leukemia. (2011) *Blood*, in press, (July 2011), ISSN 0006-4971

Charlesworth, A.; Wilczynska, A.; Thampi, P., Cox, L.L. & MacNicol, A.M. (2006) Musashi regulates the temporal order of mRNA translation during Xenopus oocyte maturation. *EMBO J.*, Vol.25, No.12, (June 2006), pp.2792-2801, ISSN 0261-4189

Clarke, R.B.; Spence, K.; Anderson, E.; Howell, A.; Okano, H. & Potten, C.S. (2005) A putative human breast stem cell population is enriched for steroid receptor-positive cells. *Dev Biol.*, Vol.277, No.2, (January 2005), pp.443-456, ISSN 0012-1606

Couillard-Despres, S.; Winner, B.; Schaubeck, S.; Aigner, R.; Vroemen, M.; Weidner, N.; Bogdahn, U.; Winkler, J.; Kuhn, H.G. & Aigner, L. (2005) Doublecortin expression levels in adult brain reflect neurogenesis. *Eur J Neurosci.*, Vol.21, No.1, (January 2005), pp.1-14, ISSN 1460-9568

Crespel, A.; Rigau, V.; Coubes, P.; Rousset, M.C.; de Bock, F.; Okano, H.; Baldy-Moulinier, M.; Bockaert, J. & Lerner-Natoli, M. (2005) Increased number of neural progenitors in human temporal lobe epilepsy. *Neurobiol Dis.*, Vol.19, No.3, (August 2005), pp.436-450, ISSN 0969-9961

Cuadrado, A.; García-Feríndez, L.F.; Imai, T.; Okano, H. & Muñoz, A. (2002) Regulation of tau RNA maturation by thyroid hormone is mediated by the neural RNA-binding protein musashi-1. *Mol Cell Neurosci.*, Vol.20, No.2, (June 2002), pp.198-210, ISSN 1044-7431

de Sousa Abreu, R.; Sanchez-Diaz, P.C.; Vogel, C.; Burns, S.C.; Ko, D.; Burton, T.L.; Vo, D.T.; Chennasamudaram, S.; Le, S.Y.; Shapiro, B.A. & Penalva, L.O. (2009) Genomic analyses of musashi1 downstream targets show a strong association with cancer-related processes. *J Biol Chem.*, Vol.284, No.18, (May 2009), pp.12125-12135, ISSN 0021-9258

des Portes, V.; Pinard, J.M.; Billuart, P.; Vinet, M.C.; Koulakoff, A.; Carrié A.; Gelot, A.; Dupuis, E.; Motte, J.; Berwald-Netter, Y.; Catala, M.; Kahn, A.; Beldjord, C. & Chelly, J. (1998) A novel CNS gene required for neuronal migration and involved in X-linked subcortical laminar heterotopia and lissencephaly syndrome. *Cell*, Vol.92, No.1, (January 1998), pp.51-61, ISSN 0092-8674

Fujita, M.; Sato, M.; Nakamura, M.; Kudo, K.; Nagasaka, T.; Mizuno, M.; Amano, E.; Okamoto, Y.; Hotta, Y.; Hatano, H.; Nakahara, N.; Wakabayashi, T. & Yoshida J. (2005) Multicentric atypical teratoid/rhabdoid tumors occurring in the eye and fourth ventricle of an infant: case report. *J Neurosurg.*, Vol.102, No.3, (April 2005), pp.299-302, ISSN 0022-3085

Glazer, R.I.; Wang, X.Y.; Yuan, H. & Yin, Y. (2008) Musashi1: a stem cell marker no longer in search of a function. *Cell Cycle*, Vol.7, No.17, (September 2008) pp.2635-2639, ISSN 1538-4101

Gleeson, J.G.; Allen, K.M.; Fox, J.W.; Lamperti, E.D.; Berkovic, S.; Scheffer, I.; Cooper, E.C.; Dobyns, W.B.; Minnerath, S.R.; Ross, M.E. & Walsh, C.A. (1998) Doublecortin, a brain-specific gene mutated in human X-linked lissencephaly and double cortex syndrome, encodes a putative signaling protein. *Cell*, Vol.92, No.1, (January 1998), pp.63-72, ISSN 0092-8674

Glisovic, T.; Bachorik, J.L.; Yong, J. & Dreyfuss, G. RNA-binding proteins and post-transcriptional gene regulation. (2008) *FEBS Lett.*, Vol.582, No.14, (January 2008), pp.1977-1986, ISSN 0014-5793

Good, P.; Yoda, A.; Sakakibara, S.; Yamamoto, A.; Imai, T.; Sawa, H.; Ikeuchi, T.; Tsuji, S.; Satoh, H. & Okano, H. (1998) The human Musashi homolog 1 (MSI1) gene encoding the homologue of Musashi/Nrp-1, a neural RNA-binding protein putatively expressed in CNS stem cells and neural progenitor cells. *Genomics*, Vol.52, No.3, (September 1998), pp.382-384, ISSN 0888-7543

Götte, M.; Wolf, M.; Staebler, A.; Buchweitz, O.; Kelsch, R.; Schüring, A.N. Kiesel, L. (2008) Increased expression of the adult stem cell marker Musashi-1 in endometriosis and endometrial carcinoma. *J Pathol.*, Vol.215, No.3, (July 2008), pp.317-329, ISSN 1096-9896

Higuchi, S.; Hayashi, T.; Tarui, H.; Nishimura, O.; Nishimura, K.; Shibata, N.; Sakamoto, H. & Agata, K. (2008) Expression and functional analysis of musashi-like genes in planarian CNS regeneration. *Mech Dev.*, Vol.125, No.7, (July 2008), pp.631-645, ISSN 0047-6374

Hirota, Y.; Okabe, M.; Imai, T.; Kurusu, M.; Yamamoto, A.; Miyao, S.; Nakamura, M.; Sawamoto, K. & Okano, H. (1999) Musashi and seven in absentia downregulate Tramtrack through distinct mechanisms in *Drosophila* eye development. *Mech Dev.*, Vol.87, No.1-2, (September 1999), pp.93-101, ISSN 0047-6374

Hitoshi, S.; Alexson, T.; Tropepe, V.; Donoviel, D.; Elia, A.J.; Nye, J.S.; Conlon, R.A.; Mak, T.W.; Bernstein, A. & van der Kooy, D. (2002) Notch pathway molecules are essential for the maintenance, but not the generation, of mammalian neural stem cells. *Genes Dev.*, Vol.16, No.7, (April 2002), pp.846-858, ISSN 0890-9369

Horisawa, K.; Tateyama, S.; Ishizaka, M.; Matsumura, N.; Takashima, H.; Miyamoto-Sato, E.; Doi, N. & Yanagawa, H. (2004) *In vitro* selection of Jun-associated proteins using mRNA display. *Nucleic Acids Res.*, Vol.32, No.21, (December 2004), e169, ISSN 0305-1048

Horisawa, K.; Doi, N. & Yanagawa, H. (2008) Use of cDNA tiling arrays for identifying protein interactions selected by in vitro display technologies. *PLoS One*, Vol.3, No.2, (February 2008), e1646, ISSN 1932-6203

Horisawa, K.; Imai, T.; Okano, H. & Yanagawa, H. (2009) 3'-Untranslated region of doublecortin mRNA is a binding target of the Musashi1 RNA-binding protein. *FEBS Lett.*, Vol.583, No.14, (July 2009), pp.2429-2434, ISSN 0014-5793

Imai, T.; Tokunaga, A.; Yoshida, T.; Hashimoto, M.; Mikoshiba, K.; Weinmaster, G.; Nakafuku, M. & Okano, H. (2001) The neural RNA-binding protein Musashi1 translationally regulates mammalian numb gene expression by interacting with its mRNA. *Mol Cell Biol.*, Vol.21, No.12, (June 2001), pp.3888-3900, ISSN 0270-7306

Ito, K. & Hotta, Y. (1992) Proliferation pattern of postembryonic neuroblasts in the brain of *Drosophila melanogaster*. *Dev Biol.*, Vol.149, No.1 (January 1992), pp.134-148, ISSN 0012-1606

Ito, T.; Kwon, H.Y.; Zimdahl, B.; Congdon, K.L.; Blum, J.; Lento, W.E.; Zhao, C.; Lagoo, A.; Gerrard, G.; Foroni, L.; Goldman, J.; Goh, H.; Kim, S.H.; Kim, D.W.; Chuah, C.; Oehler, V.G.; Radich, J.P.; Jordan, C.T. & Reya, T. (2010) Regulation of myeloid leukaemia by the cell-fate determinant Musashi. *Nature*, Vol.466, No,7307, (August 2010), pp.765-768, ISSN 0028-0836

Kanai, R.; Eguchi, K.; Takahashi, M.; Goldman, S.; Okano, H.; Kawase, T. & Yazaki, T. (2006) Enhanced therapeutic efficacy of oncolytic herpes vector G207 against human non-small cell lung cancer--expression of an RNA-binding protein, Musashi1, as a marker for the tailored gene therapy. *J Gene Med.*, Vol.8, No.11, (November 2006), pp.1329-1340, ISSN 1099-498X

Kaneko, Y.; Sakakibara, S.; Imai, T.; Suzuki, A.; Nakamura, Y.; Sawamoto, K.; Ogawa, Y.; Toyama, Y.; Miyata, T. & Okano, H. (2000) Musashi1: an evolutionarily conserved marker for CNS progenitor cells including neural stem cells. *Dev Neurosci.*, Vol.22, No.1-2, pp.139-153, ISSN 0378-5866

Kawahara, H.; Imai, T.; Imataka, H.; Tsujimoto, M.; Matsumoto, K. & Okano, H. (2008) Neural RNA-binding protein Musashi1 inhibits translation initiation by competing with eIF4G for PABP. *J Cell Biol.*, Vol.181, No.4, (May 2008), pp.639-653, ISSN 0021-9525

Kawahara, H.; Okada, Y.; Imai, T.; Iwanami, A.; Mischel, P.S. & Okano, H. (2011) Musashi1 cooperates in abnormal cell lineage protein 28 (Lin28)-mediated let-7 family microRNA biogenesis in early neural differentiation. *J Biol Chem.*, Vol.286, No.18, (May 2011), pp.16121-16130, ISSN 0021-9258

Kawase, S.; Imai, T.; Miyauchi-Hara, C.; Yaguchi, K.; Nishimoto, Y.; Fukami, S.; Matsuzaki, Y.; Miyawaki, A.; Itohara, S. & Okano H. (2011) Identification of a novel intronic enhancer responsible for the transcriptional regulation of musashi1 in neural stem/progenitor cells. *Mol Brain*, Vol.4, (April 2011), 14, ISSN 1756-6606

Kawashima, T.; Murakami, A.R.; Ogasawara, M.; Tanaka, K.; Isoda, R.; Sasakura, Y.; Nishikata, T.; Okano, H. & Makabe, K.W. (2000) Expression patterns of musashi homologs of the ascidians, *Halocynthia roretzi* and *Ciona intestinalis*. *Dev Genes Evol.*, Vol.210, No.3, (March 2000), pp.162-165, ISSN 0949-944X

Kayahara, T.; Sawada, M.; Takaishi, S.; Fukui, H.; Seno, H.; Fukuzawa, H.; Suzuki, K.; Hiai, H.; Kageyama, R.; Okano, H. & Chiba, T. (2003) Candidate markers for stem and early progenitor cells, Musashi-1 and Hes1, are expressed in crypt base columnar cells of mouse small intestine. *FEBS Lett.*, Vol.535, No.1-3, (January 2003), pp.131-135, ISSN 0014-5793

Keene, J.D. (2007) RNA regulons: coordination of post-transcriptional events. *Nat Rev Genet.*, Vol.8, No.7, (July 2007), pp.533-543, ISSN 1471-0056

Kharas, M.G.; Lengner, C.J.; Al-Shahrour, F.; Bullinger, L.; Ball, B.; Zaidi, S.; Morgan, K.; Tam, W.; Paktinat, M.; Okabe, R.; Gozo, M.; Einhorn, W.; Lane, S.W.; Scholl, C.; Fröhling, S.; Fleming, M.; Ebert, B.L.; Gilliland, D.G.; Jaenisch, R. & Daley, G.Q. Musashi-2 regulates normal hematopoiesis and promotes aggressive myeloid leukemia. (2010) *Nat. Med.*, Vol. 16, No.8, (August 2010), pp.903-908, ISSN 1078-8956

Kobayashi, T.; Mizuno. H.; Imayoshi, I.; Furusawa, C.; Shirahige, K. & Kageyama, R. (2009) The cyclic gene Hes1 contributes to diverse differentiation responses of embryonic stem cells. *Genes Dev.*, Vol.23, No.16, (August 2009), pp.1870-1875, ISSN 0890-9369

Lai, Z.C. & Li, Y. (1999) Tramtrack69 is positively and autonomously required for *Drosophila* photoreceptor development. *Genetics*, Vol.152, No.1, (May 1999), pp.299-305, ISSN 0016-6731

Liu, G.; Yuan, X.; Zeng, Z.; Tunici, P.; Ng, H.; Abdulkadir, I.R.; Lu, L.; Irvin, D.; Black, K.L. & Yu J.S. (2006) Analysis of gene expression and chemoresistance of CD133+ cancer stem cells in glioblastoma. *Mol Cancer*, Vol.5, (December 2006), 67, ISSN 1476-4598

Lovell, M.A. & Markesbery, W.R. (2005) Ectopic expression of Musashi-1 in Alzheimer disease and Pick disease. *J Neuropathol Exp Neurol.*, Vol.64, No.8, (August 2005), pp.675-680, ISSN 0022-3069

Lowe, C.J.; Wu, M.; Salic, A.; Evans, L.; Lander, E.; Stange-Thomann, N.; Gruber, C.E.; Gerhart, J. & Kirschner, M. (2003) Anteroposterior patterning in hemichordates and the origins of the chordate nervous system. *Cell*, Vol.113, No.7, (June 2003), pp.853-865, ISSN 0092-8674

Miller, S.J.; Lavker, R.M. & Sun, T.T. (2005) Interpreting epithelial cancer biology in the context of stem cells: tumor properties and therapeutic implications. *Biochim Biophys Acta.*, Vol.1756, No.1, (September 2005), pp.25-52, ISSN 0006-3002

Miyanoiri, Y.; Kobayashi, H.; Imai, T.; Watanabe, M.; Nagata, T.; Uesugi, S.; Okano, H. and Katahira, M. (2003) Origin of higher affinity to RNA of the N-terminal RNA-binding domain than that of the C-terminal one of a mouse neural protein, musashi1, as revealed by comparison of their structures, modes of interaction, surface electrostatic potentials, and backbone dynamics. *J Biol Chem.*, Vol.278 No. 42, (October 2003), pp.41309-41315, ISSN 0021-9258

Murata, H.; Tsuji, S.; Tsujii, M.; Nakamura, T.; Fu, H.Y.; Eguchi, H.; Asahi, K.; Okano, H.; Kawano, S. & Hayashi, N. (2008) *Helicobacter pylori* infection induces candidate stem cell marker Musashi-1 in the human gastric epithelium. *Dig Dis Sci.*, Vol.53, No,2, (February 2008), pp.363-369, ISSN 0163-2116

Murayama, M.; Okamoto, R.; Tsuchiya, K.; Akiyama, J.; Nakamura, T.; Sakamoto, N.; Kanai, T. & Watanabe, M. (2009) Musashi-1 suppresses expression of Paneth cell-specific genes in human intestinal epithelial cells. *J Gastroenterol.*, Vol.44, No.3, (February 2009), pp.173-182, ISSN 0002-9270

Nagata, H.; Akiba, Y.; Suzuki, H.; Okano, H. and Hibi, T. (2006) Expression of Musashi-1 in the rat stomach and changes during mucosal injury and restitution. *FEBS Lett.*, Vol.580, No.1, (January 2006), pp.27-33, ISSN 0014-5793

Nagata, T.; Kanno, R.; Kurihara, Y.; Uesugi, S.; Imai, T.; Sakakibara, S.; Okano, H. and Katahira, M. (1999) Structure, backbone dynamics and interactions with RNA of the C-terminal RNA-binding domain of a mouse neural RNA-binding protein, Musashi1. *J Mol Biol.*, Vol.287, No.2, (March 1999), pp.315-330, ISSN 0022-2836

Nakamura, M.; Okano, H.; Blendy, J.A. and Montell, C. (1994) Musashi, a neural RNA-binding protein required for *Drosophila* adult external sensory organ development. *Neuron,*Vol.13, No.1, (July 1994), pp.67-81, ISSN 0896-6273

Nakamura, Y.; Sakakibara, S.; Miyata, T.; Ogawa, M.; Shimazaki, T.; Weiss, S.; Kageyama, R. & Okano, H. (2000) The bHLH gene hes1 as a repressor of the neuronal commitment of CNS stem cells. *J Neurosci.*, Vol.20, No.1, (January 2000), pp.283-293, ISSN 0270-6474

Nakano, A.; Kanemura, Y.; Mori, K.; Kodama, E.; Yamamoto, A.; Sakamoto, H.; Nakamura, Y.; Okano, H.; Yamasaki, M. and Arita, N. (2007) Expression of the neural RNA-binding protein Musashi1 in pediatric brain tumors. *Pediatr Neurosurg.*, Vol.43, No.4, pp.279-284, ISSN 8755-6863

Nakayama, D.; Matsuyama, T.; Ishibashi-Ueda, H.; Nakagomi, T.; Kasahara, Y.; Hirose, H; Kikuchi-Taura, A.; Stern, D.M.; Mori, H. & Taguchi, A. Injury-induced neural stem/progenitor cells in post-stroke human cerebral cortex. (2010) *Eur J Neurosci.*, Vol.31, No.1, (January 2010), pp.90-98, ISSN 0953-816X

Nikpour, P.; Baygi, M.E.; Steinhoff, C.; Hader, C.; Luca, A.C.; Mowla, S.J. & Schulz, W.A. (2011) The RNA binding protein Musashi1 regulates apoptosis, gene expression and stress granule formation in urothelial carcinoma cells. *J Cell Mol Med.*, Vol.15, No.5, (May 2011), pp.1210-1224, ISSN 1582-1838

Nishimoto, Y. and Okano, H. New insight into cancer therapeutics: induction of differentiation by regulating the Musashi/Numb/Notch pathway. (2010) *Cell Res.*, Vol.20, No.10, (October 2010), pp.1083-1085, ISSN 1001-0602

Nishimura, S.; Wakabayashi, N.; Toyoda, K.; Kashima, K. & Mitsufuji, S. (2003) Expression of Musashi-1 in human normal colon crypt cells: a possible stem cell marker of human colon epithelium. *Dig Dis Sci.*, Vol.48, No.8, (August 2003), pp.1523-1529, ISSN 0163-2116

Ocbina, P.J.; Dizon, M.L.; Shin, L. & Szele, F.G. (2006) Doublecortin is necessary for the migration of adult subventricular zone cells from neurospheres. *Mol. Cell Neurosci.*, Vol.33, No.2, (October 2006), pp.126-135, ISSN 1044-7431

Okabe, M.; Imai, T.; Kurusu, M.; Hiromi, Y. & Okano, H. (2001) Translational repression determines a neuronal potential in *Drosophila* asymmetric cell division. *Nature*, Vol.411, No.6833, (May 2001), pp.94-98, ISSN 0028-0836

Okano, H.; Imai, T. & Okabe, M. (2002) Musashi: a translational regulator of cell fate. *J Cell Sci.*, Vol.115, Pt7, (April 2002), pp.1355-1359, ISSN 0021-9533

Okano, H.; Kawahara, H.; Toriya, M.; Nakao, K.; Shibata, S. & Imai, T. (2005) Function of RNA-binding protein Musashi-1 in stem cells. *Exp Cell Res.*, Vol.306, No.2, (June 2005), pp.349-356, ISSN 0014-4827

Oki, K.; Kaneko, N.; Kanki, H.; Imai, T.; Suzuki, N.; Sawamoto, K. & Okano, H. (2010) Musashi1 as a marker of reactive astrocytes after transient focal brain ischemia. *Neurosci Res.*, Vol.66, No.4, (April 2010), pp.390-395, ISSN 0168-0102

O'Sullivan, S.S.; Johnson, M.; Williams, D.R.; Revesz, T.; Holton, J.L.; Lees, A.J. & Perry, E.K. (2011) The effect of drug treatment on neurogenesis in Parkinson's disease. *Mov Disord.*, Vol.26, No.1, (January 2011), pp.45-50, ISSN 0885-3185

Pincus, D.W.; Keyoung, H.M.; Harrison-Restelli, C.; Goodman, R.R.; Fraser, R.A.; Edgar, M.; Sakakibara, S.; Okano, H.; Nedergaard, M. & Goldman, S.A. (1998) Fibroblast growth factor-2/brain-derived neurotrophic factor-associated maturation of new neurons generated from adult human subependymal cells. *Ann Neurol.*, Vol.43, No.5, (May 1998), pp.576-585, ISSN 0364-5134

Potten, C.S.; Booth, C.; Tudor, G.L.; Booth, D.; Brady, G.; Hurley, P.; Ashton, G.; Clarke, R.; Sakakibara, S. & Okano, H. (2003) Identification of a putative intestinal stem cell and early lineage marker; musashi-1. *Differentiation*, Vol.71, No.1, (January 2003), pp.28-41, ISSN 0301-4681

Prasad, C.K.; Mahadevan, M.; MacNicol, M.C. & MacNicol, A.M. (2008) Mos 3' UTR regulatory differences underlie species-specific temporal patterns of Mos mRNA cytoplasmic polyadenylation and translational recruitment during oocyte maturation. *Mol Reprod Dev.*, Vol.75, No.8, (August 2008), pp.1258-1268, ISSN 1040-452X

Raji, B.; Dansault, A.; Leemput, J.; de la Houssaye, G.; Vieira, V.; Kobetz, A.; Arbogast, L.; Masson, C.; Menasche, M. & Abitbol, M. (2007) The RNA-binding protein Musashi-1 is produced in the developing and adult mouse eye. *Mol Vis.*, Vol.13, (August 2007), pp.1412-1427, ISSN 1090-0535

Ratti, A.; Fallini, C.; Cova, L.; Fantozzi, R.; Calzarossa, C.; Zennaro, E.; Pascale, A.; Quattrone, A. and Silani, V. (2006) A role for the ELAV RNA-binding proteins in neural stem cells: stabilization of Msi1 mRNA. *J Cell Sci.*, Vol.119, Pt7, (April 2006), pp.1442-1452, ISSN 0021-9533

Rigaut, G.; Shevchenko, A.; Rutz, B.; Wilm, M.; Mann, M. & Séraphin, B. (1999) A generic protein purification method for protein complex characterization and proteome exploration. *Nat Biotechnol.*, Vol.17, No.10, (October 1999), pp.1030-1032, ISSN 1087-0156

Sagata, N.; Oskarsson, M.; Copeland, T.; Brumbaugh, J. and Vande Woude, G.F. (1988) Function of c-mos proto-oncogene product in meiotic maturation in Xenopus oocytes. *Nature*, Vol.335, No.6190, (October 1988), pp.519-525, ISSN 0028-0836

Sakakibara, S.; Imai, T.; Hamaguchi, K.; Okabe, M.; Aruga, J.; Nakajima, K.; Yasutomi, D.; Nagata, T.; Kurihara, Y.; Uesugi, S.; Miyata, T.; Ogawa, M.; Mikoshiba, K. & Okano, H. (1996) Mouse-Musashi-1, a neural RNA-binding protein highly enriched in the mammalian CNS stem cell. *Dev Biol.*, Vol.176, No.2, (June 1996), pp.230-242, ISSN 0012-1606

Sakakibara, S. & Okano, H. (1997) Expression of neural RNA-binding proteins in the postnatal CNS: implications of their roles in neuronal and glial cell development. *J Neurosci.*, Vol.17, No.21, (November 1997), pp.8300-8312, ISSN 0270-6474

Sakakibara, S.; Nakamura, Y.; Satoh, H. & Okano, H. (2001) RNA-binding protein Musashi2: developmentally regulated expression in neural precursor cells and subpopulations of neurons in mammalian CNS. *J Neurosci.*, Vol.21, No.20, (October 2001), pp.8091-8107, ISSN 0270-6474

Sakakibara, S.; Nakamura, Y.; Yoshida, T.; Shibata, S.; Koike, M.; Takano, H.; Ueda, S.; Uchiyama, Y.; Noda, T. & Okano, H. (2002) RNA-binding protein Musashi family: roles for CNS stem cells and a subpopulation of ependymal cells revealed by targeted disruption and antisense ablation. *Proc Natl Acad Sci USA*, Vol.99, No.23, (November 2002), pp.15194-15199, ISSN 0027-8424

Sakatani, T.; Kaneda, A.; Iacobuzio-Donahue, C.A.; Carter, M.G.; de Boom Witzel, S.; Okano, H.; Ko, M.S.; Ohlsson, R.; Longo, D.L. & Feinberg, A.P. (2005) Loss of imprinting of Igf2 alters intestinal maturation and tumorigenesis in mice. *Science*, Vol.307, No.5717, (March 2005), pp.1976-1978, ISSN 0036-8075

Samuel, S.; Walsh, R.; Webb, J.; Robins, A.; Potten, C. & Mahida, Y.R. (2009) Characterization of putative stem cells in isolated human colonic crypt epithelial cells and their interactions with myofibroblasts. *Am J Physiol Cell Physiol.*, Vol.296, No.2, (February 2009), pp.C296-305, ISSN 0363-6143

Sanchez-Diaz, P.C.; Burton, T.L.; Burns, S.C.; Hung, J.Y. & Penalva, L.O. (2008) Musashi1 modulates cell proliferation genes in the medulloblastoma cell line Daoy. *BMC Cancer*, Vol.8, (September 2008), 280, ISSN 1471-2407

Schulenburg, A.; Cech, P.; Herbacek, I.; Marian, B.; Wrba, F.; Valent, P. Ulrich-Pur, H. (2007) CD44-positive colorectal adenoma cells express the potential stem cell markers musashi antigen (msi1) and ephrin B2 receptor (EphB2). *J Pathol.*, Vol.213, No.2, (October 2007), pp.152-160, ISSN 1096-9896

Seigel, G.M.; Hackam, A.S.; Ganguly, A.; Mandell, L.M. & Gonzalez-Fernandez, F. (2007) Human embryonic and neuronal stem cell markers in retinoblastoma. *Mol Vis.* Vol.13, (June 2007), pp.823-832, ISSN 1090-0535

Shu, H.J.; Saito, T.; Watanabe, H.; Ito, J.I.; Takeda, H.; Okano, H. & Kawata, S. (2002) Expression of the Musashi1 gene encoding the RNA-binding protein in human hepatoma cell lines. *Biochem Biophys Res Commun.*, Vol.293, No.1, (April 2002), pp.150-154, ISSN 0006-291X

Sossey-Alaoui, K.; Hartung, A.J.; Guerrini, R.; Manchester, D.K.; Posar, A.; Puche-Mira, A.; Andermann, E.; Dobyns, W.B. & Srivastava, A.K. (1998) Human doublecortin (DCX) and the homologous gene in mouse encode a putative Ca2+-dependent signaling protein which is mutated in human X-linked neuronal migration defects. *Hum Mol Genet.*, Vol.7, No.8, (August 1998), pp.1327-1332, ISSN 0964-6906

Sugiyama-Nakagiri, Y.; Akiyama, M.; Shibata, S.; Okano, H. & Shimizu, H. (2006) Expression of RNA-binding protein Musashi in hair follicle development and hair cycle progression. *Am J Pathol.*, Vol.168, No.1, (January 2006), pp.80-92, ISSN 0887-8005

Sureban, S.M.; May, R.; George, R.J.; Dieckgraefe, B.K.; McLeod, H.L.; Ramalingam, S.; Bishnupuri, K.S.; Natarajan, G.; Anant, S. & Houchen, C.W. (2008) Knockdown of RNA binding protein musashi-1 leads to tumor regression *in vivo. Gastroenterology,* Vol.134, No.5, (May 2008), pp.1448-1458, ISSN 0016-5085

Susaki, K.; Kaneko, J.; Yamano, Y.; Nakamura, K.; Inami, W.; Yoshikawa, T.; Ozawa, Y.; Shibata, S.; Matsuzaki, O.; Okano, H. & Chiba, C. (2009) Musashi-1, an RNA-binding protein, is indispensable for survival of photoreceptors. *Exp Eye Res.,* Vol.88, No.3, (March 2009), pp.347-355, ISSN 0014-4835

Toda, M.; Iizuka, Y.; Yu, W.; Imai, T.; Ikeda, E.; Yoshida, K.; Kawase, T.; Kawakami, Y.; Okano, H. & Uyemura, K. (2001) Expression of the neural RNA-binding protein Musashi1 in human gliomas. *Glia,* Vol.34, No.1, (April 2001), pp.1-7, ISSN 1098-1136

Tokunaga, A.; Kohyama, J.; Yoshida, T.; Nakao, K.; Sawamoto, K. & Okano, H. (2004) Mapping spatio-temporal activation of Notch signaling during neurogenesis and gliogenesis in the developing mouse brain. *J Neurochem.,* Vol.90, No.1, (July 2004), pp.142-154, ISSN 0022-3042

Tuerk, C. & Gold, L. (1990) Systematic evolution of ligands by exponential enrichment: RNA ligands to bacteriophage T4 DNA polymerase. *Science,* Vol.249, No.4968, (August 1990), pp.505-510, ISSN 0036-8075

Wang, X.Y.; Yin, Y.; Yuan, H.; Sakamaki, T.; Okano, H. & Glazer, R.I. (2008) Musashi1 modulates mammary progenitor cell expansion through proliferin-mediated activation of the Wnt and Notch pathways. *Mol Cell Biol.,* Vol.28, No.11, (June 2008), pp.3589-3599, ISSN 0270-7306

Yano, H.; Ohe, N.; Shinoda, J.; Yoshimura, S. & Iwama, T. (2009) Immunohistochemical study concerning the origin of neurocytoma--a case report. *Pathol Oncol Res.,* Vol.15, No.2, (June 2009), pp.301-305, ISSN 1219-4956

Ye, F.; Zhou, C.; Cheng, Q.; Shen, J. and Chen, H. (2008) Stem-cell-abundant proteins Nanog, Nucleostemin and Musashi1 are highly expressed in malignant cervical epithelial cells. *BMC Cancer,* Vol.8, (April 2008), 108, ISSN 1471-2407

Yoda, A.; Sawa, H. & Okano, H. (2000) MSI-1, a neural RNA-binding protein, is involved in male mating behaviour in Caenorhabditis elegans. *Genes Cells.* Vol.5, No.11, (November 2000), pp.885-895, ISSN 1356-9597

Yokota, N.; Mainprize, T.G.; Taylor, M.D.; Kohata, T.; Loreto, M.; Ueda, S.; Dura, W.; Grajkowska, W.; Kuo, J.S. & Rutka, J.T. (2004) Identification of differentially expressed and developmentally regulated genes in medulloblastoma using suppression subtraction hybridization. *Oncogene,* Vol.23, No.19, (April 2004), pp.3444-3453, ISSN 0950-9232

Zhong, W.; Feder, J.N.; Jiang, M.M.; Jan, L.Y. & Jan, Y.N. (1996) Asymmetric localization of a mammalian numb homolog during mouse cortical neurogenesis. *Neuron,* Vol.17, No.1, (July 1996), pp.43-53, ISSN 0896-6273

Ziabreva, I.; Perry, E.; Perry, R.; Minger, S.L.; Ekonomou, A.; Przyborski, S. & Ballard, C. (2006) Altered neurogenesis in Alzheimer's disease. *J Psychosom Res.,* Vol.61, No.3, (September 2006), pp.311-316, ISSN 0022-3999

γ-Secretase-Regulated Signaling Mechanisms: Notch and Amyloid Precursor Protein

Kohzo Nakayama[1], Hisashi Nagase[2],
Chang-Sung Koh[3] and Takeshi Ohkawara[1]
[1]Department of Anatomy,
[2]Department of Immunology and Infectious Diseases,
Shinshu University, School of Medicine,
[3]Department of Biomedical Sciences,
Shinshu University, School of Health Sciences, Matsumoto
Japan

1. Introduction

In *Drosophila*, Notch mutations lost a lateral signaling ability and produced a neurogenic phenotype, where cells destined to become epidermis switch fate and give rise to neural tissue (Artavanis-Tsakonas *et al.* 1995; Lewis 1998). Therefore, when Notch signaling was disrupted, too many neurons were generated. Notch attracted further interest because sel-12, which appears to facilitate the reception of signaling mediated by lin-12 (*C. elegans* Notch), was identified by screening for a suppressor of lin-12 gain-of-function mutation (Levitan and Greenwald 1995). Since sel-12 is thought to be a counterpart of human presenilin (PS), which is a catalytic component of γ-secretase and has been implicated in Alzheimer's disease (AD), it was thought that the Notch signaling pathway might have a close relation with AD. Thus, many scientists have investigated the relationship between Notch signaling and AD. As we focused below, it has become clear that the Notch signaling pathway is controlled by γ-secretase-mediated proteolysis.

Both Notch receptors and their ligands are evolutionarily conserved single transmembrane-spanning proteins (type 1 transmembrane protein; amino terminus is extracellular and carboxyl terminus is cytoplasmic.) that control the fates of numerous cells in both invertebrates and vertebrates (Artavanis-Tsakonas *et al.* 1995; Artavanis-Tsakonas *et al.* 1999; Justice and Jan 2002). For example, Delta, a major Notch ligand, expressing cells inhibit the neural determination of neighboring Notch-expressing neural stem cells (NSCs) during neurogenesis (Nakayama *et al.* 2008a). In addition, it is well known that isoforms of Notch mediate somitogenesis, differentiation of lymphoid cells as well as differentiation of NSCs, and that dysregulation of Notch signaling causes developmental defects or cancer in mammals (Bolos *et al.* 2007).

The molecular mechanism of Notch signaling is quite unique in that it is controlled by proteolytic cleavage reactions (Artavanis-Tsakonas *et al.* 1999; Justice and Jan 2002). In the canonical Notch signaling pathway, ligands bind to the extracellular domain of Notch on neighboring cells, and trigger sequential proteolytic cleavage. Finally, the intracellular domain (ICD) of Notch (NICD) is released from the cell membrane by γ-secretase and translocates to the nucleus to modulate gene expression through binding to transcription factors. Therefore, γ-secretase plays a central regulatory role in Notch signaling. First, we give a detailed interpretation of Notch itself and Notch signaling as well as its role in differentiation of NSCs.

The Notch signaling pathway has long been believed to be mono-directional because ligands for Notch were generally considered unable to transmit signals into the cells expressing them (Fitzgerald and Greenwald 1995; Henderson et al. 1997). However, several groups have shown that Delta is cleaved sequentially by proteases, probably including ADAM and γ-secretase (Ikeuchi and Sisodia 2003; LaVoie and Selkoe 2003; Six et al. 2003), and ICD of Delta is released from the cell membrane and translocates to the nucleus (LaVoie and Selkoe 2003; Six et al. 2003). We have also shown that ICD of mouse Delta binds to Smads, which are transcription factors for TGF-β/Activin signaling pathway, and enhances transcription of specific genes required for neuronal differentiation (Hiratochi et al. 2007). These results suggest that Delta also has a signaling mechanism similar to Notch signaling. Thus, we also review this issue that the Notch-Delta signaling pathway is bi-directional and similar mechanisms regulated by γ-secretase are involved in both directions of the Notch-Delta signaling pathway in developing NSCs.

γ-Secretase was first identified as a protease that cleaves amyloid precursor protein (APP) within the transmembrane (TM) domain and produces Aβ peptides (Haass and Selkoe 1993), which are thought to be pathogenic in AD (Hardy 1997; Selkoe 2001). However, the physiological functions of γ-secretase have not been clarified (Kopan and Ilagan 2004; Selkoe and Wolfe 2007). Recently, it was demonstrated that more than 50 type 1 transmembrane proteins, including APP, Notch and Delta, are substrates for γ-secretase (McCarthy et al. 2009) and their ICDs are also released from the cell membrane, similar to Notch. These observations that the common enzyme, γ-secretase, modulates proteolysis and the turnover of putative signaling molecules have led to the attractive hypothesis that mechanisms similar to the Notch signaling pathway may contribute widely to γ-secretase-regulated signaling pathways (Koo and Kopan 2004; Nakayama et al. 2008a; Nakayama et al. 2011).

Interestingly, it has also been reported that ICD of APP (AICD), which is released from the cell membrane by γ-secretase, translocates to the nucleus (Cupers et al. 2001; Gao and Pimplikar 2001; Kimberly et al. 2001) and may function as a transcriptional regulator (Cao and Sudhof 2001; Guenette 2002). As the apoptotic potential of AICD has been demonstrated, it is likely that APP signaling induces cell death, which leads to AD.

To explore APP signaling, we established embryonic carcinoma P19 cell lines overexpressing AICD (Nakayama et al. 2008b). Although neurons were differentiated from these cell lines with all-*trans*-retinoic acid (RA) treatment, AICD expression induced neuron-specific apoptosis. The effects of AICD were restricted to neurons, with no effects observed on non-neural cells. Furthermore, we evaluated changes in gene expression induced by AICD during this process of neuron-specific cell death using DNA microarrays (Ohkawara et al. 2011). The results of microarray analysis indicated that AICD induces dynamic changes in the gene expression profile. Therefore, it is likely that APP also has a signaling mechanism and that AICD may play a role in APP signaling, which leads to AD.

Here, we focus on molecular mechanisms of the Notch-Delta signaling pathway in a bi-directional manner and discuss the possibility that γ-secretase-regulated mechanisms similar to the Notch-Delta signaling pathway may play a potential role in signaling events involving type 1 transmembrane proteins. In addition, we introduce the current topics of γ-secretase. We also discuss the possibility that APP signaling induces dynamic changes in gene expression, which may be closely correlated with AICD-induced neuron-specific apoptosis, leading to AD.

2. Notch

2.1 Notch and its ligands

The typical Notch gene encodes a 300-kD type 1 transmembrane protein with the large extracellular domain which contains about 36 tandem epidermal growth factor (EGF)-like repeats (Wharton et al. 1985). The 11th and 12th EGF-like repeats are necessary and sufficient for binding to its ligands in Drosophila (Rebay et al. 1991). NICD is also large and has six tandem ankyrin-like (CDC10) repeats (Wharton et al. 1985). The fundamental structures are well conserved throughout evolution, although the numbers of EGF-like repeats vary from 10 in C. elegans (Glp-1) (Yochem and Greenwald 1989) to 36 in Drosophila and some vertebrate Notch .

While Drosophila has only one Notch gene, four Notch isoforms (Notch1 to 4) have been found in mammals. TAN1 (Notch1), which is a first identified mammalian homolog of Notch, was cloned as a gene responsible for human T cell acute lymphoblastic leukemia (T-ALL) (Ellisen et al. 1991). Notch2 was also cloned as an oncogene of cat thymic lymphoma (Rohn et al. 1996). A mutation of the Notch3 gene causes cerebral autosomal dominant arteriopathy with subcortical infarcts and leukoencephalopathy (CADASIL) (Joutel et al. 1996), in which the main symptom is cerebral vascular disorder. Interestingly, Notch4 is a cellular counterpart of the oncogene of mouse mammary tumor virus (int3) and expresses in vascular endothelial cells (Sarkar et al. 1994).

While Drosophila has two different ligands Delta (Kopczynski et al. 1988) and Serrate (Fleming et al. 1990), two families of ligands, Delta family (Delta-like protein: Dll1, 3 and 4) (Bettenhausen et al. 1995; Dunwoodie et al. 1997; Shutter et al. 2000) and Jagged family (Jagged1 and 2) (Lindsell et al. 1995; Shawber et al. 1996), have been identified in mammals to date. C. elegans has two ligands, Lag-2 (Tax et al. 1994) and Apx-1 (Mello et al. 1994). The extracellular domains of all these ligands also contain variable numbers of EGF-like repeats; for example Drosophila Delta has nine, most vertebrate Deltas have eight, and C. elegans Lag-2 has two repeats. All of these ligands also share a single copy of a second cysteine-rich conservative motif called the DSL (Delta: Serrate: Lag-2) domain (Tax et al. 1994), which is essential for binding to Notch (Henderson et al. 1997). In addition, spondylocostal dysostosis (SCD), which is characterized by abnormal vertebral segmentation, is caused by mutations of Dll3 gene (Sparrow et al. 2002). Alagille syndrome, which is a multi-system disorder characterized by paucity of bile ducts and congenital heart disease, is associated with a Jagged1 mutation (Oda et al. 1997) as well as a Notch2 mutation (McCright et al. 2002).

ICDs of all ligands are relatively short compared to those of Notch and it was thought that none of ICDs of Notch ligands display any significant sequence similarity throughout evolution (Henderson *et al.* 1994). As described below, structural evidence supports the idea that ICDs of these ligands are non-functional. However, we have revealed that Delta homologues display significant sequence similarity, which is restricted to vertebrates, in their ICDs (Hiratochi *et al.* 2007). There is no homology between these vertebrate Deltas and *Drosophila* Delta. In addition, Dll3, a divergent type of Delta, does not show any homology to other Delta in ICD.

2.2 The molecular mechanism of the Notch signaling pathway

Fig. 1 shows a diagram of the Notch signaling pathway. In the canonical Notch signaling pathway, ligands bind to the extracellular domain of Notch on neighboring cells. Both Notch (Gupta-Rossi *et al.* 2004) and its ligands (Itoh *et al.* 2003) undergo ubiquitin-regulated internalization. Mind bomb (Mib) is essential for efficient activation of Notch signaling in this step. Mib is a RING-type E3 ubiquitin ligase that ubiquitylates ICDs of Notch ligands and promotes internalization of these ligands in a ubiquitination-dependent manner (Itoh *et al.* 2003). As a result of these reactions, conformations of Notch and its ligands may be changed by pulling each other to trigger sequential proteolytic cleavages called the regulated intramembrane proteolysis (RIP) mechanism (Brown *et al.* 2000). The RIP mechanism requires sequential cleavage steps to occur within the juxtamembrane (JM) and TM domains, and these steps are carried out by metalloproteases and γ-secretase, respectively (Selkoe and Kopan 2003). Since precise steps of Notch processing are recently made clear and those steps are very similar to that of APP, we mentioned about details of these processes in "3.2 Processing mechanisms of several γ-secretase substrates, such as APP, are very similar to that of Notch."

Finally, γ-secretase serves to release NICD from the cell membrane to the cytoplasm and released NICD translocates to the nucleus. Thus, γ-secretase plays a central role in the regulation of Notch signaling. Although NICD has a nuclear localization signal and is accumulated in the nucleus as an activated form of Notch, mechanisms of the transport of NICD from cytoplasm to nucleus have not yet been clarified.

In the nucleus, NICD binds to transcription factors and controls expressions of certain genes. Members of the CSL family (CBF1/RBP-jκ in mammals, Su(H) in *Drosophila* and Lag-1 in *C. elegans*) are major downstream transcription factors of Notch signaling (Artavanis-Tsakonas *et al.* 1995; Kimble and Simpson 1997; Artavanis-Tsakonas *et al.* 1999). NICD binds to CSL transcription factors; six tandem ankyrin-like repeats lying in NICD are essential for binding to CSL transcriptional factors (Roehl *et al.* 1996). As NICD also binds to Mastermind-like proteins (MAML family in mammals) (Wu *et al.* 2000), the CSL-NICD-MAML complex is formed. As a result of forming these complexes, co-repressors are dispersed from CSL and co-activators such as P/CAF and P300 are recruited by these complexes (Wallberg *et al.* 2002). Therefore, the function of CSL complexes is converted from a transcriptional repressor to an activator. Finally, activated CSL complexes bind to the *cis*-acting DNA sequences of target genes and enhance the transcriptional activity of these genes.

The most established target genes for Notch signaling are Hes (Hairy/Enhancer of split in *Drosophila*) genes, which code for the basic helix-loop-helix (bHLH) transcriptional repressor for tissue-specific genes (Kageyama *et al.* 2007). Seven mammalian Hes, designated Hes1 to Hes7, have been identified to date, although the mouse does not have Hes4. Hes1 and Hes5 bind to their target DNA sequences called N box (CACNAG) by forming homodimers or heterodimers with Hey (Hes-related with YRPW motif) 1 or Hey2, and to recruit histone deacetylase (HDAC) activity by associating with Groucho, resulting in transcriptional repression (Akazawa *et al.* 1992; Leimeister *et al.* 1999; Iso *et al.* 2001). Moreover, they associate with E proteins which are ubiquitously expressed bHLH factors and prevent proneural bHLH factors, such as Neurogenin, from forming functional complexes with E protein (Kageyama *et al.* 2007). In this manner, Notch represses the differentiation of cells to specific lineages. In addition, Delta expression is induced by proneural genes that code for bHLH transcriptional factor, although multiple POU-binding factors are also important for Delta expression in mammalian NSCs (Nakayama *et al.* 2004). Thus, Notch signaling strongly inhibits Delta expression.

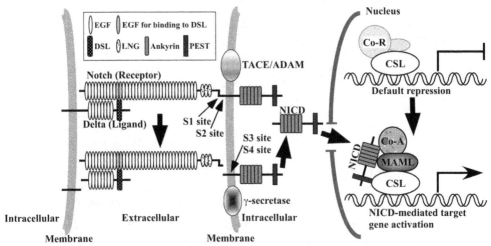

Notch proteins are expressed on the cell surface as heterodimers after cleavage at the S1 site by furin. The binding of Notch to the ligand triggers sequential proteolytic cleavage of RIP. When Notch binds to the ligand, Notch is cleaved at the S2 site in the juxtamembrane region by TACE or ADAM protease. Next, the remaining protein stub is further cleaved by γ-secretase at the S3 and S4 sites within the transmembrane domain and NICD is released from the membrane. Then, NICD translocates into the nucleus and binds to the CSL together with MAML. The resultant CSL–NICD–MAML complex removes co-repressors from CSL transcription factor and recruits a co-activator, resulting in conversion from repressor to activator. Finally, the complexes of CSL-NICD-MAML-co-activators promote transcription of the target genes

Fig. 1. Notch signaling pathway.

2.3 Notch signaling in the differentiation of NSCs

The definition of NSCs is that cells can self-renew and are capable of differentiating into main phenotypes of the nervous system, such as neurons, astrocytes and oligodendrocytes. In mammals, such cells have been isolated from the developing neural tube and more recently from the adult brain. Although there are some data showing that Notch signaling plays a role in the adult NSCs, a large majority of evidence for Notch signaling in controlling NSCs differentiation comes from analysis of embryonic neurogenesis.

In the developing mammalian central nervous system, NSCs repeat self-renewal by symmetric cell division to increase the total number of NSCs as a first step (NSCs/progenitor cells expansion phase). In this phase, Notch signaling is thought to maintain those NSCs in the proliferating and undifferentiating state (Fortini 2009; Kopan and Ilagan 2009; Pierfelice et al. 2011). Recently, it has been shown that expression of Hes1, the target genes for Notch signaling, oscillates with a period of about 2 hours in this phase (Kageyama et al. 2007). Hes1 expression may induce the oscillatory expression of Dll1 gene and the proneural Neurogenin2 (Ngn2) gene by periodic repression. Thus, concentrations of Dll1 mRNA and both Ngn2 mRNA and protein also oscillate with an inverse correlation with Hes1 (Kageyama et al. 2008; Shimojo et al. 2011). It is thought that Ngn2 cannot induce differentiation of neuron when Ngn2 expression oscillated and Dll1 leads to the activation of Notch signaling to maintain NSCs in proliferating state.

In next phase (neurogenic phase), NSCs undergo asymmetric cell division, where each NSC divides into two distinct types, NSC and neuron. In this phase, oscillatory expressions of Hes1 disappear (Kageyama et al. 2008; Shimojo et al. 2011). Since Hes1 expression is repressed, Dll1 and Ngn2 are constitutively expressed in a sustained manner and Ngn2 induces neuronal differentiation. Although the role of Notch signaling is not well understood, numb, which is an antagonist of Notch signaling (Frise et al. 1996; Guo et al. 1996; Spana and Doe 1996), is thought to be a critical component of NSCs asymmetrical division. During NSC divisions in this phase, numb appeared to be asymmetrically distributed to the neuronal daughter cells and was absent in undifferentiated NSCs (Zhong et al. 1996; Zhong et al. 1997; Chenn 2005). Thus, these observations suggest that numb inhibits Notch signaling and promotes differentiation to neuron in the neuronal daughter cells. After the generation of neurons, NSCs differentiate into oligodendrocytes and ependymal cells, followed by differentiation into astrocytes (gliogenic phase).

Recently, it has been shown that Notch signaling may also play an essential role in maintenance and differentiation of adult NSCs (Imayoshi and Kageyama 2011). Usually, adult NSCs are in the dormant state (quiescent state) and Notch signaling may maintain this state of adult NSCs. It is thought that NSCs turn from dormant state into dividing state, when the activity of Notch signaling falls down. Thus, Notch signaling controls the balance between dormant state and differentiation state of adult NSCs.

2.4 Delta signaling may be involved in neuronal differentiation

The Notch signaling pathway has long been thought to be mono-directional because ligands for Notch were generally considered unable to transmit signals into cells expressing these ligands (Henderson et al. 1994; Fitzgerald and Greenwald 1995). Indeed, it was thought that none of ICDs of putative Notch ligands display any significant sequence similarity throughout evolution (Henderson et al. 1994). Moreover, replacement of most of ICD of LAG-2, a C. elegans lin-12 (Notch) ligand, with a β-galactosidase fusion protein has no discernible effect on LAG-2 function (Henderson et al. 1994). In contrast, however, it has been reported that the extracellular domain of Notch expressed in the mesoderm provided a positive signal to the overlaying ectoderm in Drosophila as mentioned below (Baker and Schubiger 1996). Since these observations suggest that signaling in the opposite direction also exists, the important and critical question is whether signaling events occur not only from ligand-expressing cells to Notch-expressing cells but also vice versa, i.e., in a bi-directional manner.

Recently, evidence has been accumulating in support of a functional role of ICD of Notch ligands, which implies the existence of bi-directional signaling mechanisms. For example, Delta has been shown to release ICD from the cell membrane when cleaved by ADAM protease and γ-secretase (Qi et al. 1999; Ikeuchi and Sisodia 2003; LaVoie and Selkoe 2003; Six et al. 2003). Several groups have reported evidences supporting the nuclear localization of Delta ICD (Bland et al. 2003; LaVoie and Selkoe 2003; Six et al. 2003). These observations suggest that Delta ICD is released from the cell membrane by RIP. Indeed, we have shown that Delta homologues display significant sequence similarity, which is restricted to vertebrates, in their ICDs (Hiratochi et al. 2007). It is likely that conservation of these amino acid sequences reflect the functional importance of Delta ICD.

To clarify the question of whether the Notch-Delta signaling pathway is bi-directional, we investigated the effect of Notch on differentiation of NSCs isolated from mouse embryos (Hiratochi et al. 2007). When NSCs were co-cultured on a monolayer of mouse Dll1-expressing COS7 cells, the rate at which neurons emerged was lower than that in controls. As mentioned above, Notch signaling maintains the proliferating and undifferentiating state of NSCs and inhibits the differentiation into neurons (Fortini 2009; Kopan and Ilagan 2009; Pierfelice et al. 2011). Therefore, these observations indicate that Dll1 on COS7 cells generates signals to neighboring NSCs that express Notch and thus activates Notch signaling. Conversely, when NSCs were co-cultured on a monolayer of mouse Notch1-expressing COS7 cells, the rate of neurons developing from NSCs was significantly higher than that in control cultures. These results suggest that Notch1 on COS7 cells may also generate signals to neighboring NSCs and these ligands, probably Delta, may then transmit signals into cells expressing them to promote neuronal differentiation. Thus, signaling events may occur not only from Delta-expressing cells to Notch-expressing cells but also vice versa, that is, in a bi-directional manner, during differentiation of NSCs. Indeed, Baker and Schubiger published results from a mosaic experiment in Drosophila, which showed that expression of Notch in the mesoderm of Notch mutant suppressed the ectodermal defects of this mutant (Baker and Schubiger 1996). This effect was inferred to be due to the extracellular domain of the protein and not its signaling function, since activated Notch failed to produce non-autonomous suppression (Baker and Schubiger 1996). These results indicate that the extracellular domain of Notch expressed in the mesoderm sent a positive signal to the overlying ectoderm. Thus, these observations further support the hypothesis that Notch-expressing cells also send a signal to Delta-expressing cells.

2.5 Delta ICD may modify expression of certain genes

The nuclear localization of Delta ICD suggests that this domain may have effects on the transcription of a specific target gene similar to NICD. To examine this possibility, we searched for transcriptional factors capable of binding to ICD of Dll1 (Dll1IC) using a new method and identified Smads as a Dll1IC binding transcription factor through the differentiation process of mouse NSCs (Hiratochi et al. 2007).

Smads are transcription factors and have been shown to act as mediators of signaling by the TGF-β superfamily. Eight Smads, designated Smad1 to Smad8, have been identified to date in mammal (Miyazawa et al. 2002; Derynck and Zhang 2003). Smad2 and Smad3 are activated by TGF-β and activin (Eppert et al. 1996; Zhang et al. 1996; Nakao et al. 1997), while

Smad1 and Smad5 are major components that are activated by bone morphogenic proteins (BMPs) (Hoodless *et al.* 1996; Kretzschmar *et al.* 1997; Suzuki *et al.* 1997). Although Smad1 and Smad5 did not bind to Dll1IC, Smad2 and Smad3 showed strong binding (Hiratochi *et al.* 2007). These observations indicate that Dll1IC can modify TGF-β/Activin signaling through binding to Smad2 and/or Smad3. However, BMP signaling, which is known to inhibit neurogenesis and to enhance the appearance of astrocytes, may not be affected by Dll1IC, because Dll1IC did not bind to Smad1 or Smad5.

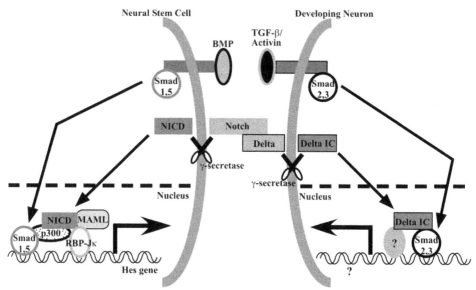

Notch receptor also generates signals to Delta expressed on the surface of neighboring NSCs. Delta is cleaved sequentially by proteases, probably including ADAM and γ-secretase, and finally the intracellular domain of Delta (DeltaIC) is released from the cell membrane and translocates to the nucleus, where it mediates TGF-β/Activin signaling through binding to Smad2/3 and enhances transcription of specific genes leading to neuronal differentiation. It is well known that NICD is also released from the cell membrane by proteases similar to the ones involved in the cleaving of Delta, then translocates to the nucleus to modulate gene expression through binding to the transcription factor, that is, Suppressor of Hairless (Su(H), RBP-jκ in mammals) together with MAML. This means that similar mechanisms are involved in both directions of the bi-directional Notch-Delta signaling pathway. BMPs, another group belonging to the TGF-β superfamily, have recently been shown to inhibit neurogenesis and to enhance the generation of astrocytes from NSCs. It has also been demonstrated that NICD and activated Smad1/5 form a complex with p300 in the specific promoter sequence, which contains both the RBP-jκ and Smad binding sequences. It is therefore possible that the TGF-β superfamily mediates both neurogenesis and gliogenesis from NSCs coupled with the bi-directional Notch-Delta signaling pathway.

Fig. 2. Schematic of the bi-directional model of Notch-Delta signaling pathway in the process of NSC differentiation.

Although we have yet to determine the actual target genes for the Dll1IC-Smad complex, we showed that binding of Dll1IC to Smad enhanced its transcriptional activity using the 9XCAGA-Luc promoter-reporter system that responds specifically to Smad3 (Dennler *et al.* 1998; Jonk *et al.* 1998), as a model system. These results strongly suggest that Dll1IC mediates transcription of certain genes, which are targets of TGF-β/Activin signaling, through binding to Smad2 and/or Smad3.

As mentioned above, it is likely that Delta transmits signals into NSCs expressing them to promote neuronal differentiation. To test this possibility, we established embryonic carcinoma P19 cells stably overexpressing Dll1IC (Hiratochi et al. 2007). Although control P19 cells have been shown to be induced to differentiate into neurons, RA stimulation is essential for the induction of neurons from these P19 cells. However, neurons could be induced from P19 cells stably overexpressing Dll1IC without RA stimulation and this induction was strongly inhibited by SB431542, a specific inhibitor of TGF-β type1 receptor (Laping et al. 2002) that activates Smad2 and Smad3. These results suggest that overexpression of Dll1IC in P19 cells induced neurons through binding to Smad2 and/or Smad3. Therefore, it is highly possible that Delta signaling also plays an important role in neuronal differentiation. Recently, it has been reported that TGF-β inhibits proliferation and accelerates differentiation of the hippocampal granule neuron (Lu et al. 2005). This observation also supports our hypothesis.

A schematic model of Notch-Delta signaling pathway in the process of NSC differentiation is shown in Fig. 2.

3. γ-Secretase

3.1 Overview of γ-secretase

γ-Secretase was first identified as a protease that cleaves APP within the TM domain and produces Aβ peptides (Haass and Selkoe 1993), which are thought to have pathogenic roles in AD. However, the physiological functions of this enzyme have not been clarified (Kopan and Ilagan 2004; Selkoe and Wolfe 2007). The γ-secretase is a complex composed of PS, nicastrin (NCT), anterior pharynx defective-1 (Aph-1), and PS enhancer-2 protein (Pen-2) (Iwatsubo 2004; Kopan and Ilagan 2004; Selkoe and Wolfe 2007). PS is a catalytic component of the γ-secretase complex, and the two PS genes, PS1 gene (PSEN1) (Sherrington et al. 1995) located on chromosome 14 and PS2 gene (PSEN2) (Levy-Lahad et al. 1995; Rogaev et al. 1995) located on chromosome 1, were identified by genetic linkage analyses as the genes responsible for several forms of early-onset familial AD (FAD). PSEN1 and PSEN2 encode polytopic transmembrane proteins of 467 and 448 amino acids, respectively, which show about 65% sequence identity between the two proteins. While PS1 expression level is higher than that of PS2, both proteins are expressed ubiquitously in the brain and peripheral tissues of adult mammals (Lee et al. 1996). The model for PS with eight or nine transmembrane domains is generally accepted and PS has a hydrophilic loop domain between the putative 6th and 7th transmembrane domains facing the cytoplasm (Doan et al. 1996) and is cleaved by an unidentified protease within this loop resulting into two fragments, N- and C-terminal fragment (NTF and CTF), that remain associated as a heterodimer (Thinakaran et al. 1996). This proteolytic cleavage is thought to occur when nascent PS assembles with NCT, Aph-1, and Pen-2 as a γ-secretase complex and activates PS as the catalytic component of aspartyl protease (Iwatsubo 2004; Kopan and Ilagan 2004; Selkoe and Wolfe 2007).

The single-pass membrane protein NCT may recognize the substrate proteins of γ-secretase (Yu et al. 2000; Shah et al. 2005). The extracellular domain of NCT resembles an aminopeptidase, but lacks catalytic residues, and can interact with the N-terminal stubs of γ-secretase substrates after ectodomain shedding (Shah *et al.* 2005). Thus, shedding of membrane proteins may be essential for the production of free N-termini of these proteins retained in the membrane, which can then be recognized by NCT. Aph-1 is thought to act as a scaffold during the process of γ-secretase complex assembly, and Pen-2 was suggested to act as a trigger for the proteolytic cleavage of PS to regulate PS activity (Kopan and Ilagan 2004; Selkoe and Wolfe 2007).

3.2 Processing mechanisms of several γ-secretase substrates, such as APP, are very similar to that of Notch

Precise steps of Notch processing are recently made clear (Fig.3). After translation, Notch is cleaved by furin-like covertase at the S1 site in the *trans*-Golgi network, and the two resulting fragments remain associated to form a functional heterodimer that is expressed on the cell surface (Logeat *et al.* 1998).

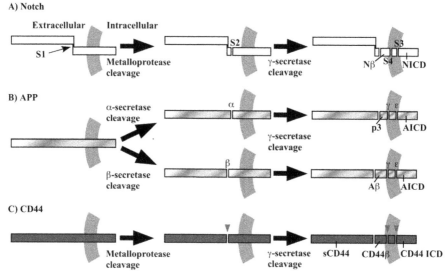

(A) In response to ligand binding, Notch undergoes shedding due to metalloprotease cleavage at the S2 site within the JM domain. After shedding the extracellular domain, the remaining Notch stub is further cleaved by γ-secretase at S3 and S4 sites within the TM domain. This sequential proteolysis produces NICD and Nβ fragment. (B) Cleavage of APP by α-secretase or β-secretase at the α-site or β-site, respectively, within the JM domain results in shedding of almost the entire extracellular domain and generates membrane-tethered α- or β-carboxy terminal fragments (CTFs). Several zinc metalloproteinases and BACE2 can cleave APP at the α-site, while BACE1 cleaves APP at the β-site. After shedding the extracellular domain, the remaining stub is further cleaved at least twice within the TM domain at γ- and ε-sites by γ-secretase, producing either p3 peptide (in combination with α-secretase) or Aβ (in combination with BACE1), respectively, and AICD. (C) Several stimuli, such as PKC activation and Ca²⁺ influx, trigger ectodomain cleavage of CD44 by a metalloprotease at the site within the JM domain, resulting in the secretion of soluble CD44 (sCD44). After shedding the extracellular domain, the remaining CD44 stub is further cleaved by γ-secretase at two sites within the TM domain. This sequential proteolysis produces the CD44 ICD and CD44β, an Aβ-like peptide.

Fig. 3. Similarities in the proteolytic processes among Notch, APP, and CD44.

As mentioned above, the sequential proteolytic cleavage called RIP mechanism is initiated by ligand binding and shedding at the S2 site by TACE or ADAM protease making the truncated Notch (Pan and Rubin 1997; Brou *et al.* 2000). Truncated Notch is further cleaved by γ-secretase in at least two sites within the TM domain, *i.e.*, at the S3 site to release NICD and at the S4 site to release the remaining small peptide (Nβ) (Kopan *et al.* 1996; Schroeter *et al.* 1998; Okochi *et al.* 2002), which resembles Aβ.

The proteolytic process of APP resembles that of Notch and also follows the RIP mechanism (Fig.3). Cleavage of APP by α-secretase (Esch *et al.* 1990) or β-secretase (Vassar *et al.* 1999) at the α-site or β-site, respectively, within the JM region results in shedding of almost the entire extracellular domain and generates membrane-tethered α- or β- CTFs. Several zinc metalloproteinases (Buxbaum *et al.* 1998; Lammich *et al.* 1999) and the aspartyl protease BACE2 can cleave APP at the α-site (Farzan *et al.* 2000), while BACE1 (β-site APP cleaving enzyme) cleaves APP at the β-site (Vassar *et al.* 1999). After shedding, the remaining stub is further cleaved at least twice by γ-secretase within the TM domain at γ- and ε-sites resulting in production of either non-amyloidogenic p3 peptide (in combination with α-secretase) or amyloidogenic Aβ (in combination with BACE1), respectively, and AICD (Kopan and Ilagan 2004; Selkoe and Wolfe 2007). In addition, AICD was shown to be a substrate of caspase and to be cleaved at the group III caspase consensus sequence 16 amino acids from the membrane border within the AICD.

It has been reported that several γ-secretase substrates also follow the RIP mechanism with release of their ICDs from the cell membrane. As shown in Fig. 3, the process of sequential proteolytic cleavage of CD44, which is important for immune system function, is very similar to those of Notch and APP and follows the RIP mechanism (Nagase *et al.* 2011). In addition, the ICD of this protein (CD44ICD) is also translocated to the nucleus, suggesting that CD44ICD may also mediate the gene expression.

3.3 Does γ-secretase mediate signaling events of type 1 transmembrane proteins?

γ-Secretase seems to cleave a diverse set of type1 transmembrane proteins, which have been shed their extracellular domains, in a sequence-independent manner (Struhl and Adachi 2000). As reflected by the flexible sequence specificity of γ-secretase activity, more than 50 type 1 transmembrane proteins have been reported as substrates of γ-secretase (McCarthy *et al.* 2009). As shown in Table 1, these substrates also have a wide range of functions, including roles in cell differentiation (Notch, Delta, and Jagged), cell adhesion (N-cadherin, E-cadherin, and CD44), synaptic adhesion (Nectin-1α), ion conductance regulation (voltage-gated sodium channel β2 subunit), axon guidance and tumor suppression (DCC), neurotrophin receptor (P75NTR), and its homolog (NRADD), lipoprotein receptor (ApoER2), and growth factor-dependent receptor tyrosine kinase (ERBB4).

As mentioned above, proteolytic cleavages of several γ-secretase substrates, such as APP and CD44, follow the RIP mechanism. The ICDs of these substrates are released from the cell membrane to cytoplasm by γ-secretase, and finally these ICDs translocate to the nucleus. These processes are very similar to those involved in Notch signaling. Thus, the observations that the common enzyme, γ-secretase, modulates proteolysis and the turnover of possible signaling molecules led to the signaling hypothesis suggesting that mechanisms similar to those occurring in the Notch signaling pathway may contribute widely to γ-secretase-regulated signaling pathways (Koo and Kopan 2004; Nakayama *et al.* 2008a; Nakayama *et al.* 2011).

Indeed, as mentioned above, Dll1 is cleaved sequentially by proteases, probably including ADAM and γ-secretase, and Dll1IC is released from the cell membrane and undergoes translocation to the nucleus (Hiratochi *et al.* 2007). In the nucleus, Dll1IC enhances transcription of specific genes through binding to Smads. These observations suggest that Dll1 may also have a signaling mechanism similar to Notch signaling.

Substrate	Function	PS or ICD function
ApoER2	Lipoprotein receptor, neuronal migration	Activate nuclear reporter
APP	Precursor to Aβ, adhesion, trophic properties, axonal transport?	Aβ generation, release of ICD, complex with Fe65/Tip60, Cell death?
APLP1/2	Cell adhesion?	Form complex with Fe65 and Tip60
E-cadherin	Cell adhesion	Promote disassembly of adhesion complex
N-cadherin	Cell adhesion	Promote CBP degradation
β-catenin	Transduce Wnt signals stabilize adherens junctions	Facilitate phosphorylation
CD43	Signal transduction	Signaling molecule?
CD44	Cell adhesion	Activate TRE-mediated nuclear transcription
CSF1-R	Protein tyrosine kinase	Unknown
CXCL16 & CX3CL1	Membrane chemokine ligands	Unknown
DCC	Axon guidance, tumor suppressor	Activate nuclear reporter
Delta	Notch ligand	Transcription regulation
ERBB4	Receptor tyrosine kinase	Regulate heregulin-induced growth inhibition
HLA-A2	MHC class I molecule	Unknown
IGIF-R	Receptor tyrosine kinase	Unknown
IFN-αR2	Subunit of type I IFN-α receptor	Transcriptional regulation
IL-1RI	Cytokine receptor	Unknown
IL-1RII	Cytokine receptor	Unknown
Jagged	Notch ligand	Modulate AP-1 mediated transcription
LDLR	Lipoprotein receptor	Unkown
LRP	Scavenger and signaling receptor	Activate nuclear reporter
Na channel β-subunit	Cell adhesion, an auxiliary subunit of voltage-gated Na channel	Alter cell adhesion and migration
Nectin-1α	Adherens junction, synapse receptor	Remodeling of cell junctions?

Substrate	Function	PS or ICD function
Notch1-4	Signaling receptor	Transcription regulation
NRADD	Apoptosis in neuronal cells	Modulate glycosylation/matutaion of NRADD
P75NTR	Neurotrophin co-receptor, dependence receptor	Modulate p75-TrkA complex? Nuclear singaling?
γ-protocadherin	Cell adhesion, neuronal differentiation	Regulation of gene transcription?
Syndecan-3	Cell surface proteoglycan co-receptor	Regulation of membrane-targeting of CASK
Telencephalin	Cell adhesion	Turnover of telencephalin
Tyrosinase, Tyrosinase-related protein 1/2	Pigment synthesis	Intracellular transport of Post-Golgi Tyr-containing vesicles

PS, presenilin; ICD, intracellular domain; APLP, APP like protein; CBP, CREB (cAMP-responsive element binding protein)-binding protein; TRE, TPA (12-o-tetradecanoylphorbol 13-acetate)-responsive element; AP-1, activator protein-1; CASK, calmodulin-dependent serine kinase; Tyr, Tyrosinase.

Table 1. Substrates for γ-secretase

3.4 Is γ-secretase a proteasome of the membrane?

As mentioned above, more than 50 type 1 membrane proteins have been reported as substrates of γ-secretase. This observation raises the simple question of why so many membrane proteins can transmit signals to the nucleus. In contrast to the signaling hypothesis, Kopan and Ilagan proposed another possibility that γ-secretase may act as a proteasome for membrane proteins (Kopan and Ilagan 2004). They pointed out that generally the ICDs of these substrates including AICD, which are released by γ-secretase, are rapidly degraded. Moreover, ectodomain shedding seems to be constitutive for some substrates, and ligand binding has been reported to enhance only intramembrane cleavage of Notch (Schroeter et al. 1998), Delta (Hiratochi et al. 2007), Syndecan-3 (Schulz et al. 2003), and ERBB4 (Ni et al. 2001). In addition, they also pointed out that the most evidence supporting the signaling hypothesis was obtained in overexpression experiments that differ somewhat from physiological conditions. Based on these observations, they proposed the proteasome hypothesis that the primary function of γ-secretase is to facilitate the selective disposal of type 1 membrane proteins (Kopan and Ilagan 2004).

While the proteasome hypothesis of γ-secretase is reasonable, there is no doubt that γ-secretase regulates signaling pathways of some substrates, such as Notch (Artavanis-Tsakonas et al. 1999; Selkoe and Kopan 2003; Koo and Kopan 2004). Although further studies are required to elucidate this issue, it is likely that γ-secretases are not uniform complexes but that different γ-secretase complexes may exist in different combinations with components such as Aph-1, Pen2, and/or PS isoforms, with different cellular functions, such as roles in signaling or degradation (Kopan and Ilagan 2004). Since γ-secretase substrates such as APP are generally more abundant than transcription factors, which are usually rare molecules, it is uncertain whether the majority of the ICDs of these substrates released by γ-secretase are required for the signaling mechanisms (Nakayama et al. 2008a; Nakayama et al.

2011). Although a large proportion of ICDs of these substrates are rapidly degraded, it is likely that a small amount of the remaining ICDs may be suitable for their functions with a small quantity of transcription factors. Thus, the greater part of ICDs of these substrates may be degraded and only a small proportion may play a role in signaling.

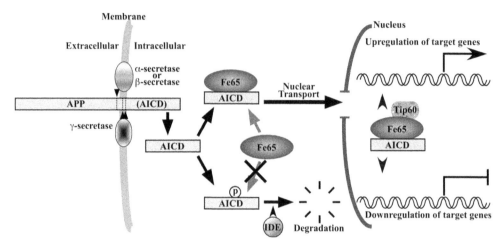

After cleavege of JM domain by α- or β-secretase, AICD is released from the membrane by γ-secretase. Non-phosphorylated AICD binds to the nuclear adaptor protein Fe65, which is thought to be essential for translocation of AICD to the nucleus, and forms complexes, alone or with the histone acetyltransferase Tip60. These complexes can immediately translocate to the nucleus, where they meidate up- and downregulation of certain target genes in association with Tip60. On the other hand, pholphorylated AICD cannot translocate to the nucleus due to the inhibition of binding to Fe65, leading to rapid degradation by the proteasome and/or insulin-degrading enzyme (IDE).

Fig. 4. Putative APP signaling pathway.

In relation to this issue, an attractive model has been proposed (Fig.4) (Buoso *et al.* 2011). Binding to nuclear adaptor protein Fe65 is thought to be essential for translocation of AICD to the nucleus. In this model, since non-phosphorylated AICD binds to Fe65 and forms complexes, these complexes can immediately translocate to the nucleus, where they control the expression of certain genes in association with the histone acetyltransferase Tip60. On the other hand, as other stimuli induce phosphorylation of AICD, which strongly inhibits binding to Fe65, AICD without Fe65 cannot translocate to the nucleus. Phosphorylated AICD left in the cytosol is rapidly degraded, most likely by the proteasome and/or insulin-degrading enzyme (IDE) (Edbauer *et al.* 2002). Indeed, it has been reported that when phosphorylated at Thr[668] in the APP-695 isoform, AICD cannot bind to Fe65 (Kimberly *et al.* 2005).

4. APP signaling?

4.1 Overview of APP

APP was first identified as a cDNA cloned using a partial amino acid sequence of Aβ fragment from the amyloid plaque of AD brains (Kang *et al.* 1987). APP is a type 1 membrane protein expressed in many tissues, especially concentrated in the synapses of neurons. In humans, the APP gene contains at least 18 exons in a total length of 240 kb (Yoshikai *et al.* 1990), and several alternative splicing isoforms of APP have been observed, differing mainly in the absence (APP-695 which is predominately expressed in neurons) or presence (APP-751 and APP-770) of a Kunitz protease inhibitor (KPI) domain located toward the N-terminus of the protein (Sisodia *et al.* 1993). As mentioned above, APP undergoes sequential proteolytic cleavage reactions to yield the extracellular fragment, intracellular fragment (AICD), and Aβ fragment located in the membrane-spanning domain, which is thought to be the main cause of the onset of AD.

While APP has central roles in AD (Hardy 1997; Selkoe 2001), the physiological functions of this protein also remain to be clarified (Zheng and Koo 2006). It has been reported that APP acts as a cell adhesion molecule for cell-cell interaction (Soba *et al.* 2005), and as a neurotrophic and/or synaptogenic factor (Hung *et al.* 1992; Bibel *et al.* 2004; Leyssen *et al.* 2005). In addition, the possibility that APP is a cell-surface receptor is interesting from the signaling perspective. Several evidences support this idea; *e.g.*, Aβ can bind to APP and thus may be a candidate ligand for APP (Lorenzo *et al.* 2000). It has also been reported that F-spondin (Ho and Sudhof 2004) and Nogo-66 receptor (Park *et al.* 2006) could bind to the extracellular domain of APP and regulate Aβ production. Furthermore, the extracellular domain of APP may potentially interact in *trans* suggesting that APP molecules can bind to each other (Wang and Ha 2004).

APP homologs show significant evolutionary sequence conservation in ICD (Nakayama *et al.* 2008b), which may reflect the functional importance of AICD. However, the Aβ region of this protein is not well conserved across species. As mentioned, AICD is thought to form complexes with Fe65 and these complexes translocate to the nucleus. In the nucleus, these complexes may associate with Tip60 and may bind to the *cis*-acting DNA sequence of the tetraspanin protein KAI1 gene to control transcriptional activity (Baek *et al.* 2002).

4.2 AICD induces neuron-specific apoptosis

There is accumulating evidence in support of the idea that APP signaling exists and contributes to the onset of AD. For example, transgenic mice overexpressing both AICD and Fe65 showed abnormal high activity of glycogen synthase kinase 3 beta (*Gsk3b* protein) (Ryan and Pimplikar 2005), leading to hyperphosphorylation and aggregation of TAU, resulting in microtubule destabilization, and reduction of nuclear β-catenin levels causing a loss of cell-cell contact mechanisms that may give rise to neurodegeneration in AD brain. In addition, it was also shown that c-Abl modulates AICD-dependent transcriptional induction, as well as apoptotic responses (Vazquez *et al.* 2009). Interestingly, elevated AICD levels have also been observed in AD brains (Ghosal *et al.* 2009). Therefore, it is highly possible that APP signaling changes expression patterns of certain genes and induces cell death, which may lead to AD pathology.

To explore APP signaling, we established several AICD-overexpressing embryonic carcinoma P19 cell lines (Nakayama *et al.* 2008b). Although neurons were differentiated from these cell lines after aggregation culture with RA treatment, AICD expression induced neuron-specific cell death. Indeed, while neurons from control cells which carried vector alone were healthy, almost all neurons from AICD-overexpressing P19 cells showed severe degeneration four days after induction of differentiation (Fig. 5). Moreover, DNA fragmentation was detected, and all of terminal deoxynucleotidyl transferase (TdT)-mediated deoxyuridine triphosphate (dUTP)-biotin nick end-labeling (TUNEL)-positive cells were also Tuj1-positive neurons. Based on these observations, we concluded that AICD can induce neuron-specific apoptosis (Nakayama *et al.* 2008b). The effects of AICD were restricted to neurons, with no effects observed on non-neural cells. Thus, although further studies are required, these results strongly suggest that AICD plays a role in APP signaling, which leads to the onset of AD.

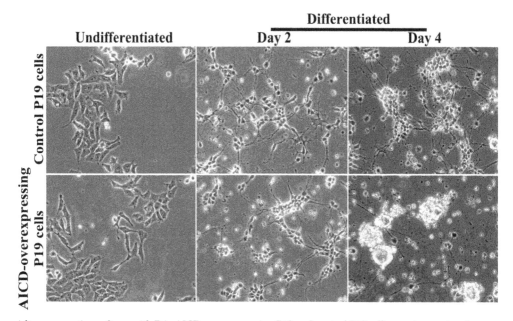

After aggregation culture with RA, AICD-overexpressing P19 and control P19 cells carrying vector alone were replated and cultured for the indicated periods on dishes and allowed to differentiate. Undifferentiated AICD-overexpressing P19 cells retained epithelial cell-like morphology similar to control cells, while the differentiated cells became round and showed a bipolar morphology with neurite extension. Two days after replating (Day 2), all cell lines grew well and neurons with long neurites appeared. Four days after replating (Day 4), control cells still grew well as clusters and many neurons had differentiated from these cells. However, many AICD-overexpressing P19 cells showed severe degeneration, becoming spherical with numerous vacuoles and detached from the culture dishes.

Fig. 5. Overexpression of AICD in P19 cells induces neuronal cell death.

4.3 AICD induces dynamic changes in the gene expression profile

If APP signaling exists, AICD should change expression of certain genes. To test this hypothesis and identify the genes involved in this process of neuron-specific apoptosis, we employed both AICD-overexpressing P19 cells and control P19 cells again and monitored AICD-induced changes in expressions of more than 20,000 independent genes by DNA microarray analysis at 3 time points during culture: the undifferentiated state, after 4 days of aggregation with RA (aggregated state), and 2 days after replating (differentiated state) (Ohkawara *et al.* 2011). Surprisingly, AICD can change expressions of a great many genes:

the expression levels of 277 genes were upregulated by more than 10-fold in the presence of AICD, while 341 genes showed downregulation of expression to less than 10% of the original level (Fig.6).

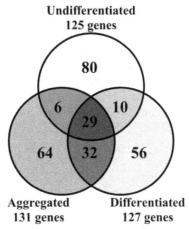

(A) 277 upregulated genes
Undifferentiated
125 genes

80

6   10

29

64   32   56

Aggregated   **Differentiated**
131 genes   **127 genes**

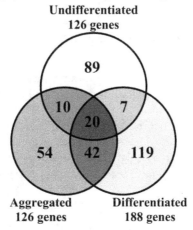

(B) 341 downregulated genes
Undifferentiated
126 genes

89

10   7

20

54   42   119

Aggregated   **Differentiated**
126 genes   **188 genes**

Venn diagrams showing the total numbers of genes upregulated by more than 10-fold in the presence of AICD (A) and genes downregulated to less than 10% of their original level (B) at three states of neural differentiation in P19 cells: undifferentiated, aggregated, and differentiated.

Fig. 6. Upregulated and downregulated genes by AICD.

AICD strongly induced expressions of several genes. For example, AICD-overexpressing P19 cells showed strong expression of protein tyrosine phosphatase receptor T (*Ptprt*) gene at all sampling points: 906-fold, 204-fold, and 116-fold upregulation, in undifferentiated, aggregated, and differentiated states, respectively, estimated from the intensity of hybridization signals. In contrast to these upregulated genes, AICD also strongly inhibited the expression of several genes (Ohkawara *et al.* 2011). For example, *Hes5* was markedly increased through the process of neural differentiation: an increase of almost 300-fold in control P19 cells. However, this extreme induction in control P19 cells could not be detected in AICD-overexpressing P19 cells, indicating that AICD inhibits this induction. These results show that AICD induces both upregulation and downregulation of many genes, suggesting that AICD plays an important role in APP signaling.

We performed Gene Ontology (GO) analysis and classified these upregulated and downregulated genes according to GO terms (Ohkawara *et al.* 2011). While a few genes were classified into GO terms related to cell death, many genes were classified into GO terms unrelated to cell death. Furthermore, we evaluated AICD-induced changes in expression of genes thought to be involved in cell death in AD; however, we found no significant changes in expression of these genes. Therefore, it is likely that AICD does not directly induce the expression of genes involved in cell death, but the extreme dynamic changes in gene expression disrupt the homeostasis of certain neurons and thus give rise to neuron-specific cell death.

4.4 Amyloid hypothesis

Genetic studies indicate that both APP itself and its proteolytic processing are responsible for the onset of AD (Nakayama *et al.* 2011). The amyloid hypothesis is generally accepted as the mechanism of the onset of AD. The traditional amyloid hypothesis is that overproduced Aβ forms insoluble amyloid plaques, which are commonly observed in the AD brain and are believed to be the toxic form of APP responsible for neurodegeneration (Hardy and Selkoe 2002).

However, several issues have been raised regarding these hypotheses. One of the most significant arguments against the amyloid hypothesis is the presence of high levels of Aβ deposition in many non-demented elderly people (Terry RD 1999). This observation implies that Aβ amyloid plaques are not toxic. Based on these observations, the interesting possibility has been proposed that AD may be caused by an APP-derived protein, other than Aβ (Schnabel 2009). As both extracellular fragment and AICD are generated at the same time as Aβ, acceleration of proteolytic processing leads to overproduction of not only Aβ but also of both extracellular fragment and AICD. Therefore, it is likely that neuron-specific apoptosis induced by AICD may also be involved in the onset of AD.

5. Conclusion

Although γ-secretase plays central roles in AD, the physiological functions of this enzyme have yet to be fully elucidated. As reviewed here, Notch signaling is controlled by γ-secretase: intramembrane cleavage of Notch by γ-secretase serves to release ICD that has activity in the nucleus through binding to transcription factors. Recently, it was reported that many type 1 transmembrane proteins are substrates for γ-secretase, and ICDs of these substrates are released from the cell membrane by γ-secretase. These observations that the common enzyme, γ-secretase, modulates proteolysis and the turnover of possible signaling molecules have led to the attractive hypothesis that mechanisms similar to the Notch signaling pathway may widely contribute to γ-secretase-regulated signaling pathways. Indeed, APP signaling induces dynamic changes in gene expression, which may be closely correlated with AICD-induced neuron-specific apoptosis and the onset of AD. Thus, it is likely that γ-secretase controls Notch signaling in NSCs and APP signaling in neurons that may lead to the onset of AD.

6. Abbreviations

AD	Alzheimer's disease
APP	amyloid precursor protein
AICD	the intracellular domain of APP
Aph-1	anterior pharynx defective-1
bHLH	basic helix-loop-helix
BMP	bone morphogenic protein
CTF	C-terminal fragment
Dll	Delta-like protein
Dll1IC	the intracellular domain of Dll1
EGF	epidermal growth factor
FAD	familial AD
GO	gene ontology
Hes	Hairy/Enhancer of split
ICD	intracellular domain
IDE	insulin-degrading enzyme
JM	juxtamembrane
Mib	Mind bomb
NCT	nicastrin
Ngn2	Neurogenin2
NICD	the intracellular domain of Notch
NSC	neural stem cell
NTF	N-terminal fragment
Pen-2	PS enhancer-2
PS	presenilin
RA	all-*trans*-retinoic acid
RIP	the regulated intramembrane proteolysis
TM	transmembrane

7. References

Akazawa, C., Y. Sasai, S. Nakanishi and R. Kageyama (1992) Molecular characterization of a rat negative regulator with a basic helix-loop-helix structure predominantly expressed in the developing nervous system. *J Biol Chem.* 267, 21879-85.

Artavanis-Tsakonas, S., K. Matsuno and M. E. Fortini (1995) Notch signaling. *Science.* 268, 225-32.

Artavanis-Tsakonas, S., M. D. Rand and R. J. Lake (1999) Notch signaling: cell fate control and signal integration in development. *Science.* 284, 770-6.

Baek, S. H., K. A. Ohgi, D. W. Rose, E. H. Koo, C. K. Glass and M. G. Rosenfeld (2002) Exchange of N-CoR corepressor and Tip60 coactivator complexes links gene expression by NF-kappaB and beta-amyloid precursor protein. *Cell.* 110, 55-67.

Baker, R. and G. Schubiger (1996) Autonomous and nonautonomous Notch functions for embryonic muscle and epidermis development in Drosophila. *Development.* 122, 617-26.

Bettenhausen, B., M. Hrabe de Angelis, D. Simon, J. L. Guenet and A. Gossler (1995) Transient and restricted expression during mouse embryogenesis of Dll1, a murine gene closely related to Drosophila Delta. *Development.* 121, 2407-18.

Bibel, M., J. Richter, K. Schrenk, K. L. Tucker, V. Staiger, M. Korte, M. Goetz and Y. A. Barde (2004) Differentiation of mouse embryonic stem cells into a defined neuronal lineage. *Nat Neurosci.* 7, 1003-9.

Bland, C. E., P. Kimberly and M. D. Rand (2003) Notch-induced proteolysis and nuclear localization of the Delta ligand. *J Biol Chem.* 278, 13607-10.

Bolos, V., J. Grego-Bessa and J. L. de la Pompa (2007) Notch signaling in development and cancer. *Endocr Rev.* 28, 339-63.

Brou, C., F. Logeat, N. Gupta, C. Bessia, O. LeBail, J. R. Doedens, A. Cumano, P. Roux, R. A. Black and A. Israel (2000) A novel proteolytic cleavage involved in Notch signaling: the role of the disintegrin-metalloprotease TACE. *Mol Cell.* 5, 207-16.

Brown, M. S., J. Ye, R. B. Rawson and J. L. Goldstein (2000) Regulated intramembrane proteolysis: a control mechanism conserved from bacteria to humans. *Cell.* 100, 391-8.

Buoso, E., C. Lanni, G. Schettini, S. Govoni and M. Racchi (2011) beta-Amyloid precursor protein metabolism: focus on the functions and degradation of its intracellular domain. *Pharmacol Res.* 62, 308-17.

Buxbaum, J. D., K. N. Liu, Y. Luo, J. L. Slack, K. L. Stocking, J. J. Peschon, R. S. Johnson, B. J. Castner, D. P. Cerretti and R. A. Black (1998) Evidence that tumor necrosis factor alpha converting enzyme is involved in regulated alpha-secretase cleavage of the Alzheimer amyloid protein precursor. *J Biol Chem.* 273, 27765-7.

Cao, X. and T. C. Sudhof (2001) A transcriptionally [correction of transcriptively] active complex of APP with Fe65 and histone acetyltransferase Tip60. *Science.* 293, 115-20.

Chenn, A. (2005) The simple life (of cortical progenitors). *Neuron.* 45, 817-9.

Cupers, P., I. Orlans, K. Craessaerts, W. Annaert and B. De Strooper (2001) The amyloid precursor protein (APP)-cytoplasmic fragment generated by gamma-secretase is rapidly degraded but distributes partially in a nuclear fraction of neurones in culture. *J Neurochem.* 78, 1168-78.

Dennler, S., S. Itoh, D. Vivien, P. ten Dijke, S. Huet and J. M. Gauthier (1998) Direct binding of Smad3 and Smad4 to critical TGF beta-inducible elements in the promoter of human plasminogen activator inhibitor-type 1 gene. *EMBO J.* 17, 3091-100.

Derynck, R. and Y. E. Zhang (2003) Smad-dependent and Smad-independent pathways in TGF-beta family signalling. *Nature.* 425, 577-84.

Doan, A., G. Thinakaran, D. R. Borchelt, H. H. Slunt, T. Ratovitsky, M. Podlisny, D. J. Selkoe, M. Seeger, S. E. Gandy, D. L. Price and S. S. Sisodia (1996) Protein topology of presenilin 1. *Neuron.* 17, 1023-30.

Dunwoodie, S. L., D. Henrique, S. M. Harrison and R. S. Beddington (1997) Mouse Dll3: a novel divergent Delta gene which may complement the function of other Delta homologues during early pattern formation in the mouse embryo. *Development.* 124, 3065-76.

Edbauer, D., M. Willem, S. Lammich, H. Steiner and C. Haass (2002) Insulin-degrading enzyme rapidly removes the beta-amyloid precursor protein intracellular domain (AICD). *J Biol Chem.* 277, 13389-93.

Ellisen, L. W., J. Bird, D. C. West, A. L. Soreng, T. C. Reynolds, S. D. Smith and J. Sklar (1991) TAN-1, the human homolog of the Drosophila notch gene, is broken by chromosomal translocations in T lymphoblastic neoplasms. *Cell.* 66, 649-61.

Eppert, K., S. W. Scherer, H. Ozcelik, R. Pirone, P. Hoodless, H. Kim, L. C. Tsui, B. Bapat, S. Gallinger, I. L. Andrulis, G. H. Thomsen, J. L. Wrana and L. Attisano (1996) MADR2 maps to 18q21 and encodes a TGFbeta-regulated MAD-related protein that is functionally mutated in colorectal carcinoma. *Cell.* 86, 543-52.

Esch, F. S., P. S. Keim, E. C. Beattie, R. W. Blacher, A. R. Culwell, T. Oltersdorf, D. McClure and P. J. Ward (1990) Cleavage of amyloid beta peptide during constitutive processing of its precursor. *Science.* 248, 1122-4.

Farzan, M., C. E. Schnitzler, N. Vasilieva, D. Leung and H. Choe (2000) BACE2, a beta - secretase homolog, cleaves at the beta site and within the amyloid-beta region of the amyloid-beta precursor protein. *Proc Natl Acad Sci U S A.* 97, 9712-7.

Fitzgerald, K. and I. Greenwald (1995) Interchangeability of Caenorhabditis elegans DSL proteins and intrinsic signalling activity of their extracellular domains in vivo. *Development.* 121, 4275-82.

Fleming, R. J., T. N. Scottgale, R. J. Diederich and S. Artavanis-Tsakonas (1990) The gene Serrate encodes a putative EGF-like transmembrane protein essential for proper ectodermal development in Drosophila melanogaster. *Genes Dev.* 4, 2188-201.

Fortini, M. E. (2009) Notch signaling: the core pathway and its posttranslational regulation. *Dev Cell.* 16, 633-47.

Frise, E., J. A. Knoblich, S. Younger-Shepherd, L. Y. Jan and Y. N. Jan (1996) The Drosophila Numb protein inhibits signaling of the Notch receptor during cell-cell interaction in sensory organ lineage. *Proc Natl Acad Sci U S A.* 93, 11925-32.

Gao, Y. and S. W. Pimplikar (2001) The gamma -secretase-cleaved C-terminal fragment of amyloid precursor protein mediates signaling to the nucleus. *Proc Natl Acad Sci U S A.* 98, 14979-84.

Ghosal, K., D. L. Vogt, M. Liang, Y. Shen, B. T. Lamb and S. W. Pimplikar (2009) Alzheimer's disease-like pathological features in transgenic mice expressing the APP intracellular domain. *Proc Natl Acad Sci U S A.* 106, 18367-72.

Guenette, S. Y. (2002) A role for APP in motility and transcription? *Trends Pharmacol Sci.* 23, 203-5; discussion 205-6.

Guo, M., L. Y. Jan and Y. N. Jan (1996) Control of daughter cell fates during asymmetric division: interaction of Numb and Notch. *Neuron.* 17, 27-41.

Gupta-Rossi, N., E. Six, O. LeBail, F. Logeat, P. Chastagner, A. Olry, A. Israel and C. Brou (2004) Monoubiquitination and endocytosis direct gamma-secretase cleavage of activated Notch receptor. *J Cell Biol.* 166, 73-83.

Haass, C. and D. J. Selkoe (1993) Cellular processing of beta-amyloid precursor protein and the genesis of amyloid beta-peptide. *Cell.* 75, 1039-42.

Hardy, J. (1997) Amyloid, the presenilins and Alzheimer's disease. *Trends Neurosci.* 20, 154-9.

Hardy, J. and D. J. Selkoe (2002) The amyloid hypothesis of Alzheimer's disease: progress and problems on the road to therapeutics. *Science*. 297, 353-6.

Henderson, S. T., D. Gao, E. J. Lambie and J. Kimble (1994) lag-2 may encode a signaling ligand for the GLP-1 and LIN-12 receptors of C. elegans. *Development*. 120, 2913-24.

Henderson, S. T., D. Gao, S. Christensen and J. Kimble (1997) Functional domains of LAG-2, a putative signaling ligand for LIN-12 and GLP-1 receptors in Caenorhabditis elegans. *Mol Biol Cell*. 8, 1751-62.

Hiratochi, M., H. Nagase, Y. Kuramochi, C. S. Koh, T. Ohkawara and K. Nakayama (2007) The Delta intracellular domain mediates TGF-beta/Activin signaling through binding to Smads and has an important bi-directional function in the Notch-Delta signaling pathway. *Nucleic Acids Res*. 35, 912-22.

Ho, A. and T. C. Sudhof (2004) Binding of F-spondin to amyloid-beta precursor protein: a candidate amyloid-beta precursor protein ligand that modulates amyloid-beta precursor protein cleavage. *Proc Natl Acad Sci U S A*. 101, 2548-53.

Hoodless, P. A., T. Haerry, S. Abdollah, M. Stapleton, M. B. O'Connor, L. Attisano and J. L. Wrana (1996) MADR1, a MAD-related protein that functions in BMP2 signaling pathways. *Cell*. 85, 489-500.

Hung, A. Y., E. H. Koo, C. Haass and D. J. Selkoe (1992) Increased expression of beta-amyloid precursor protein during neuronal differentiation is not accompanied by secretory cleavage. *Proc Natl Acad Sci U S A*. 89, 9439-43.

Ikeuchi, T. and S. S. Sisodia (2003) The Notch ligands, Delta1 and Jagged2, are substrates for presenilin-dependent "gamma-secretase" cleavage. *J Biol Chem*. 278, 7751-4.

Imayoshi, I. and R. Kageyama (2011) The role of notch signaling in adult neurogenesis. *Mol Neurobiol*. 44, 7-12.

Iso, T., V. Sartorelli, C. Poizat, S. Iezzi, H. Y. Wu, G. Chung, L. Kedes and Y. Hamamori (2001) HERP, a novel heterodimer partner of HES/E(spl) in Notch signaling. *Mol Cell Biol*. 21, 6080-9.

Itoh, M., C. H. Kim, G. Palardy, T. Oda, Y. J. Jiang, D. Maust, S. Y. Yeo, K. Lorick, G. J. Wright, L. Ariza-McNaughton, A. M. Weissman, J. Lewis, S. C. Chandrasekharappa and A. B. Chitnis (2003) Mind bomb is a ubiquitin ligase that is essential for efficient activation of Notch signaling by Delta. *Dev Cell*. 4, 67-82.

Iwatsubo, T. (2004) The gamma-secretase complex: machinery for intramembrane proteolysis. *Curr Opin Neurobiol*. 14, 379-83.

Jonk, L. J., S. Itoh, C. H. Heldin, P. ten Dijke and W. Kruijer (1998) Identification and functional characterization of a Smad binding element (SBE) in the JunB promoter that acts as a transforming growth factor-beta, activin, and bone morphogenetic protein-inducible enhancer. *J Biol Chem*. 273, 21145-52.

Joutel, A., C. Corpechot, A. Ducros, K. Vahedi, H. Chabriat, P. Mouton, S. Alamowitch, V. Domenga, M. Cecillion, E. Marechal, J. Maciazek, C. Vayssiere, C. Cruaud, E. A. Cabanis, M. M. Ruchoux, J. Weissenbach, J. F. Bach, M. G. Bousser and E. Tournier-Lasserve (1996) Notch3 mutations in CADASIL, a hereditary adult-onset condition causing stroke and dementia. *Nature*. 383, 707-10.

Justice, N. J. and Y. N. Jan (2002) Variations on the Notch pathway in neural development. *Curr Opin Neurobiol*. 12, 64-70.

Kageyama, R., T. Ohtsuka and T. Kobayashi (2007) The Hes gene family: repressors and oscillators that orchestrate embryogenesis. *Development*. 134, 1243-51.

Kageyama, R., T. Ohtsuka, H. Shimojo and I. Imayoshi (2008) Dynamic Notch signaling in neural progenitor cells and a revised view of lateral inhibition. *Nat Neurosci.* 11, 1247-51.

Kang, J., H. G. Lemaire, A. Unterbeck, J. M. Salbaum, C. L. Masters, K. H. Grzeschik, G. Multhaup, K. Beyreuther and B. Muller-Hill (1987) The precursor of Alzheimer's disease amyloid A4 protein resembles a cell-surface receptor. *Nature.* 325, 733-6.

Kimberly, W. T., J. B. Zheng, S. Y. Guenette and D. J. Selkoe (2001) The intracellular domain of the beta-amyloid precursor protein is stabilized by Fe65 and translocates to the nucleus in a notch-like manner. *J Biol Chem.* 276, 40288-92.

Kimberly, W. T., J. B. Zheng, T. Town, R. A. Flavell and D. J. Selkoe (2005) Physiological regulation of the beta-amyloid precursor protein signaling domain by c-Jun N-terminal kinase JNK3 during neuronal differentiation. *J Neurosci.* 25, 5533-43.

Kimble, J. and P. Simpson (1997) The LIN-12/Notch signaling pathway and its regulation. *Annu Rev Cell Dev Biol.* 13, 333-61.

Koo, E. H. and R. Kopan (2004) Potential role of presenilin-regulated signaling pathways in sporadic neurodegeneration. *Nat Med.* 10 Suppl, S26-33.

Kopan, R., E. H. Schroeter, H. Weintraub and J. S. Nye (1996) Signal transduction by activated mNotch: importance of proteolytic processing and its regulation by the extracellular domain. *Proc Natl Acad Sci U S A.* 93, 1683-8.

Kopan, R. and M. X. Ilagan (2004) Gamma-secretase: proteasome of the membrane? *Nat Rev Mol Cell Biol.* 5, 499-504.

Kopan, R. and M. X. Ilagan (2009) The canonical Notch signaling pathway: unfolding the activation mechanism. *Cell.* 137, 216-33.

Kopczynski, C. C., A. K. Alton, K. Fechtel, P. J. Kooh and M. A. Muskavitch (1988) Delta, a Drosophila neurogenic gene, is transcriptionally complex and encodes a protein related to blood coagulation factors and epidermal growth factor of vertebrates. *Genes Dev.* 2, 1723-35.

Kretzschmar, M., F. Liu, A. Hata, J. Doody and J. Massague (1997) The TGF-beta family mediator Smad1 is phosphorylated directly and activated functionally by the BMP receptor kinase. *Genes Dev.* 11, 984-95.

Lammich, S., E. Kojro, R. Postina, S. Gilbert, R. Pfeiffer, M. Jasionowski, C. Haass and F. Fahrenholz (1999) Constitutive and regulated alpha-secretase cleavage of Alzheimer's amyloid precursor protein by a disintegrin metalloprotease. *Proc Natl Acad Sci U S A.* 96, 3922-7.

Laping, N. J., E. Grygielko, A. Mathur, S. Butter, J. Bomberger, C. Tweed, W. Martin, J. Fornwald, R. Lehr, J. Harling, L. Gaster, J. F. Callahan and B. A. Olson (2002) Inhibition of transforming growth factor (TGF)-beta1-induced extracellular matrix with a novel inhibitor of the TGF-beta type I receptor kinase activity: SB-431542. *Mol Pharmacol.* 62, 58-64.

LaVoie, M. J. and D. J. Selkoe (2003) The Notch ligands, Jagged and Delta, are sequentially processed by alpha-secretase and presenilin/gamma-secretase and release signaling fragments. *J Biol Chem.* 278, 34427-37.

Lee, M. K., H. H. Slunt, L. J. Martin, G. Thinakaran, G. Kim, S. E. Gandy, M. Seeger, E. Koo, D. L. Price and S. S. Sisodia (1996) Expression of presenilin 1 and 2 (PS1 and PS2) in human and murine tissues. *J Neurosci.* 16, 7513-25.

Leimeister, C., A. Externbrink, B. Klamt and M. Gessler (1999) Hey genes: a novel subfamily of hairy- and Enhancer of split related genes specifically expressed during mouse embryogenesis. *Mech Dev.* 85, 173-7.

Levitan, D. and I. Greenwald (1995) Facilitation of lin-12-mediated signalling by sel-12, a Caenorhabditis elegans S182 Alzheimer's disease gene. *Nature.* 377, 351-4.

Levy-Lahad, E., W. Wasco, P. Poorkaj, D. M. Romano, J. Oshima, W. H. Pettingell, C. E. Yu, P. D. Jondro, S. D. Schmidt, K. Wang and et al. (1995) Candidate gene for the chromosome 1 familial Alzheimer's disease locus. *Science.* 269, 973-7.

Lewis, J. (1998) Notch signalling and the control of cell fate choices in vertebrates. *Semin Cell Dev Biol.* 9, 583-9.

Leyssen, M., D. Ayaz, S. S. Hebert, S. Reeve, B. De Strooper and B. A. Hassan (2005) Amyloid precursor protein promotes post-developmental neurite arborization in the Drosophila brain. *EMBO J.* 24, 2944-55.

Lindsell, C. E., C. J. Shawber, J. Boulter and G. Weinmaster (1995) Jagged: a mammalian ligand that activates Notch1. *Cell.* 80, 909-17.

Logeat, F., C. Bessia, C. Brou, O. LeBail, S. Jarriault, N. G. Seidah and A. Israel (1998) The Notch1 receptor is cleaved constitutively by a furin-like convertase. *Proc Natl Acad Sci U S A.* 95, 8108-12.

Lorenzo, A., M. Yuan, Z. Zhang, P. A. Paganetti, C. Sturchler-Pierrat, M. Staufenbiel, J. Mautino, F. S. Vigo, B. Sommer and B. A. Yankner (2000) Amyloid beta interacts with the amyloid precursor protein: a potential toxic mechanism in Alzheimer's disease. *Nat Neurosci.* 3, 460-4.

Lu, J., Y. Wu, N. Sousa and O. F. Almeida (2005) SMAD pathway mediation of BDNF and TGF beta 2 regulation of proliferation and differentiation of hippocampal granule neurons. *Development.* 132, 3231-42.

McCarthy, J. V., C. Twomey and P. Wujek (2009) Presenilin-dependent regulated intramembrane proteolysis and gamma-secretase activity. *Cell Mol Life Sci.* 66, 1534-55.

McCright, B., J. Lozier and T. Gridley (2002) A mouse model of Alagille syndrome: Notch2 as a genetic modifier of Jag1 haploinsufficiency. *Development.* 129, 1075-82.

Mello, C. C., B. W. Draper and J. R. Priess (1994) The maternal genes apx-1 and glp-1 and establishment of dorsal-ventral polarity in the early C. elegans embryo. *Cell.* 77, 95-106.

Miyazawa, K., M. Shinozaki, T. Hara, T. Furuya and K. Miyazono (2002) Two major Smad pathways in TGF-beta superfamily signalling. *Genes Cells.* 7, 1191-204.

Nagase, H., C. S. Koh and K. Nakayama (2011) gamma-Secretase-regulated signaling pathways, such as notch signaling, mediate the differentiation of hematopoietic stem cells, development of the immune system, and peripheral immune responses. *Curr Stem Cell Res Ther.* 6, 131-41.

Nakao, A., T. Imamura, S. Souchelnytskyi, M. Kawabata, A. Ishisaki, E. Oeda, K. Tamaki, J. Hanai, C. H. Heldin, K. Miyazono and P. ten Dijke (1997) TGF-beta receptor-mediated signalling through Smad2, Smad3 and Smad4. *EMBO J.* 16, 5353-62.

Nakayama, K., K. Nagase, Y. Tokutake, C. S. Koh, M. Hiratochi, T. Ohkawara and N. Nakayama (2004) Multiple POU-binding motifs, recognized by tissue-specific nuclear factors, are important for Dll1 gene expression in neural stem cells. *Biochem Biophys Res Commun.* 325, 991-6.

Nakayama, K., H. Nagase, M. Hiratochi, C. S. Koh and T. Ohkawara (2008a) Similar mechanisms regulated by gamma-secretase are involved in both directions of the bi-directional Notch-Delta signaling pathway as well as play a potential role in signaling events involving type 1 transmembrane proteins. *Curr Stem Cell Res Ther.* 3, 288-302.

Nakayama, K., T. Ohkawara, M. Hiratochi, C. S. Koh and H. Nagase (2008b) The intracellular domain of amyloid precursor protein induces neuron-specific apoptosis. *Neurosci Lett.* 444, 127-31.

Nakayama, K., H. Nagase, C. S. Koh and T. Ohkawara (2011) gamma-Secretase-Regulated Mechanisms Similar to Notch Signaling May Play a Role in Signaling Events, Including APP Signaling, Which Leads to Alzheimer's Disease. *Cell Mol Neurobiol.* 31, 887-900.

Ni, C. Y., M. P. Murphy, T. E. Golde and G. Carpenter (2001) gamma -Secretase cleavage and nuclear localization of ErbB-4 receptor tyrosine kinase. *Science.* 294, 2179-81.

Oda, T., A. G. Elkahloun, B. L. Pike, K. Okajima, I. D. Krantz, A. Genin, D. A. Piccoli, P. S. Meltzer, N. B. Spinner, F. S. Collins and S. C. Chandrasekharappa (1997) Mutations in the human Jagged1 gene are responsible for Alagille syndrome. *Nat Genet.* 16, 235-42.

Ohkawara, T., H. Nagase, C. S. Koh and K. Nakayama (2011) The amyloid precursor protein intracellular domain alters gene expression and induces neuron-specific apoptosis. *Gene.* 475, 1-9.

Okochi, M., H. Steiner, A. Fukumori, H. Tanii, T. Tomita, T. Tanaka, T. Iwatsubo, T. Kudo, M. Takeda and C. Haass (2002) Presenilins mediate a dual intramembranous gamma-secretase cleavage of Notch-1. *EMBO J.* 21, 5408-16.

Pan, D. and G. M. Rubin (1997) Kuzbanian controls proteolytic processing of Notch and mediates lateral inhibition during Drosophila and vertebrate neurogenesis. *Cell.* 90, 271-80.

Park, J. H., D. A. Gimbel, T. GrandPre, J. K. Lee, J. E. Kim, W. Li, D. H. Lee and S. M. Strittmatter (2006) Alzheimer precursor protein interaction with the Nogo-66 receptor reduces amyloid-beta plaque deposition. *J Neurosci.* 26, 1386-95.

Pierfelice, T., L. Alberi and N. Gaiano (2011) Notch in the vertebrate nervous system: an old dog with new tricks. *Neuron.* 69, 840-55.

Qi, H., M. D. Rand, X. Wu, N. Sestan, W. Wang, P. Rakic, T. Xu and S. Artavanis-Tsakonas (1999) Processing of the notch ligand delta by the metalloprotease Kuzbanian. *Science.* 283, 91-4.

Rebay, I., R. J. Fleming, R. G. Fehon, L. Cherbas, P. Cherbas and S. Artavanis-Tsakonas (1991) Specific EGF repeats of Notch mediate interactions with Delta and Serrate: implications for Notch as a multifunctional receptor. *Cell.* 67, 687-99.

Roehl, H., M. Bosenberg, R. Blelloch and J. Kimble (1996) Roles of the RAM and ANK domains in signaling by the C. elegans GLP-1 receptor. *EMBO J.* 15, 7002-12.

Rogaev, E. I., R. Sherrington, E. A. Rogaeva, G. Levesque, M. Ikeda, Y. Liang, H. Chi, C. Lin, K. Holman, T. Tsuda and et al. (1995) Familial Alzheimer's disease in kindreds with missense mutations in a gene on chromosome 1 related to the Alzheimer's disease type 3 gene. *Nature.* 376, 775-8.

Rohn, J. L., A. S. Lauring, M. L. Linenberger and J. Overbaugh (1996) Transduction of Notch2 in feline leukemia virus-induced thymic lymphoma. *J Virol.* 70, 8071-80.

Ryan, K. A. and S. W. Pimplikar (2005) Activation of GSK-3 and phosphorylation of CRMP2 in transgenic mice expressing APP intracellular domain. *J Cell Biol.* 171, 327-35.

Sarkar, N. H., S. Haga, A. F. Lehner, W. Zhao, S. Imai and K. Moriwaki (1994) Insertional mutation of int protooncogenes in the mammary tumors of a new strain of mice derived from the wild in China: normal- and tumor-tissue-specific expression of int-3 transcripts. *Virology.* 203, 52-62.

Schnabel, J. (2009) Alzheimer's theory makes a splash. *Nature.* 459, 310.

Schroeter, E. H., J. A. Kisslinger and R. Kopan (1998) Notch-1 signalling requires ligand-induced proteolytic release of intracellular domain. *Nature.* 393, 382-6.

Schulz, J. G., W. Annaert, J. Vandekerckhove, P. Zimmermann, B. De Strooper and G. David (2003) Syndecan 3 intramembrane proteolysis is presenilin/gamma-secretase-dependent and modulates cytosolic signaling. *J Biol Chem.* 278, 48651-7.

Selkoe, D. J. (2001) Alzheimer's disease: genes, proteins, and therapy. *Physiol Rev.* 81, 741-66.

Selkoe, D. and R. Kopan (2003) Notch and Presenilin: regulated intramembrane proteolysis links development and degeneration. *Annu Rev Neurosci.* 26, 565-97.

Selkoe, D. J. and M. S. Wolfe (2007) Presenilin: running with scissors in the membrane. *Cell.* 131, 215-21.

Shah, S., S. F. Lee, K. Tabuchi, Y. H. Hao, C. Yu, Q. LaPlant, H. Ball, C. E. Dann, 3rd, T. Sudhof and G. Yu (2005) Nicastrin functions as a gamma-secretase-substrate receptor. *Cell.* 122, 435-47.

Shawber, C., J. Boulter, C. E. Lindsell and G. Weinmaster (1996) Jagged2: a serrate-like gene expressed during rat embryogenesis. *Dev Biol.* 180, 370-6.

Sherrington, R., E. I. Rogaev, Y. Liang, E. A. Rogaeva, G. Levesque, M. Ikeda, H. Chi, C. Lin, G. Li, K. Holman, T. Tsuda, L. Mar, J. F. Foncin, A. C. Bruni, M. P. Montesi, S. Sorbi, I. Rainero, L. Pinessi, L. Nee, I. Chumakov, D. Pollen, A. Brookes, P. Sanseau, R. J. Polinsky, W. Wasco, H. A. Da Silva, J. L. Haines, M. A. Perkicak-Vance, R. E. Tanzi, A. D. Roses, P. E. Fraser, J. M. Rommens and P. H. St George-Hyslop (1995) Cloning of a gene bearing missense mutations in early-onset familial Alzheimer's disease. *Nature.* 375, 754-60.

Shimojo, H., T. Ohtsuka and R. Kageyama (2011) Dynamic expression of notch signaling genes in neural stem/progenitor cells. *Front Neurosci.* 5, 78-84.

Shutter, J. R., S. Scully, W. Fan, W. G. Richards, J. Kitajewski, G. A. Deblandre, C. R. Kintner and K. L. Stark (2000) Dll4, a novel Notch ligand expressed in arterial endothelium. *Genes Dev.* 14, 1313-8.

Sisodia, S. S., E. H. Koo, P. N. Hoffman, G. Perry and D. L. Price (1993) Identification and transport of full-length amyloid precursor proteins in rat peripheral nervous system. *J Neurosci.* 13, 3136-42.

Six, E., D. Ndiaye, Y. Laabi, C. Brou, N. Gupta-Rossi, A. Israel and F. Logeat (2003) The Notch ligand Delta1 is sequentially cleaved by an ADAM protease and gamma-secretase. *Proc Natl Acad Sci U S A.* 100, 7638-43.

Soba, P., S. Eggert, K. Wagner, H. Zentgraf, K. Siehl, S. Kreger, A. Lower, A. Langer, G. Merdes, R. Paro, C. L. Masters, U. Muller, S. Kins and K. Beyreuther (2005) Homo- and heterodimerization of APP family members promotes intercellular adhesion. *EMBO J.* 24, 3624-34.

Spana, E. P. and C. Q. Doe (1996) Numb antagonizes Notch signaling to specify sibling neuron cell fates. *Neuron.* 17, 21-6.

Sparrow, D. B., M. Clements, S. L. Withington, A. N. Scott, J. Novotny, D. Sillence, K. Kusumi, R. S. Beddington and S. L. Dunwoodie (2002) Diverse requirements for Notch signalling in mammals. *Int J Dev Biol.* 46, 365-74.

Struhl, G. and A. Adachi (2000) Requirements for presenilin-dependent cleavage of notch and other transmembrane proteins. *Mol Cell.* 6, 625-36.

Suzuki, A., C. Chang, J. M. Yingling, X. F. Wang and A. Hemmati-Brivanlou (1997) Smad5 induces ventral fates in Xenopus embryo. *Dev Biol.* 184, 402-5.

Tax, F. E., J. J. Yeargers and J. H. Thomas (1994) Sequence of C. elegans lag-2 reveals a cell-signalling domain shared with Delta and Serrate of Drosophila. *Nature.* 368, 150-4.

Terry RD, K. R., Bick KL, Sisodia SS (1999) *Alzheimer's disease.*, Lippincott, Williams & Wilkins, Philadelphia

Thinakaran, G., D. R. Borchelt, M. K. Lee, H. H. Slunt, L. Spitzer, G. Kim, T. Ratovitsky, F. Davenport, C. Nordstedt, M. Seeger, J. Hardy, A. I. Levey, S. E. Gandy, N. A. Jenkins, N. G. Copeland, D. L. Price and S. S. Sisodia (1996) Endoproteolysis of presenilin 1 and accumulation of processed derivatives in vivo. *Neuron.* 17, 181-90.

Vassar, R., B. D. Bennett, S. Babu-Khan, S. Kahn, E. A. Mendiaz, P. Denis, D. B. Teplow, S. Ross, P. Amarante, R. Loeloff, Y. Luo, S. Fisher, J. Fuller, S. Edenson, J. Lile, M. A. Jarosinski, A. L. Biere, E. Curran, T. Burgess, J. C. Louis, F. Collins, J. Treanor, G. Rogers and M. Citron (1999) Beta-secretase cleavage of Alzheimer's amyloid precursor protein by the transmembrane aspartic protease BACE. *Science.* 286, 735-41.

Vazquez, M. C., L. M. Vargas, N. C. Inestrosa and A. R. Alvarez (2009) c-Abl modulates AICD dependent cellular responses: transcriptional induction and apoptosis. *J Cell Physiol.* 220, 136-43.

Wallberg, A. E., K. Pedersen, U. Lendahl and R. G. Roeder (2002) p300 and PCAF act cooperatively to mediate transcriptional activation from chromatin templates by notch intracellular domains in vitro. *Mol Cell Biol.* 22, 7812-9.

Wang, Y. and Y. Ha (2004) The X-ray structure of an antiparallel dimer of the human amyloid precursor protein E2 domain. *Mol Cell.* 15, 343-53.

Wharton, K. A., K. M. Johansen, T. Xu and S. Artavanis-Tsakonas (1985) Nucleotide sequence from the neurogenic locus notch implies a gene product that shares homology with proteins containing EGF-like repeats. *Cell.* 43, 567-81.

Wu, L., J. C. Aster, S. C. Blacklow, R. Lake, S. Artavanis-Tsakonas and J. D. Griffin (2000) MAML1, a human homologue of Drosophila mastermind, is a transcriptional co-activator for NOTCH receptors. *Nat Genet.* 26, 484-9.

Yochem, J. and I. Greenwald (1989) glp-1 and lin-12, genes implicated in distinct cell-cell interactions in C. elegans, encode similar transmembrane proteins. *Cell.* 58, 553-63.

Yoshikai, S., H. Sasaki, K. Doh-ura, H. Furuya and Y. Sakaki (1990) Genomic organization of the human amyloid beta-protein precursor gene. *Gene.* 87, 257-63.

Yu, G., M. Nishimura, S. Arawaka, D. Levitan, L. Zhang, A. Tandon, Y. Q. Song, E. Rogaeva, F. Chen, T. Kawarai, A. Supala, L. Levesque, H. Yu, D. S. Yang, E. Holmes, P. Milman, Y. Liang, D. M. Zhang, D. H. Xu, C. Sato, E. Rogaev, M. Smith, C. Janus, Y. Zhang, R. Aebersold, L. S. Farrer, S. Sorbi, A. Bruni, P. Fraser and P. St George-Hyslop (2000) Nicastrin modulates presenilin-mediated notch/glp-1 signal transduction and betaAPP processing. *Nature.* 407, 48-54.

Zhang, Y., X. Feng, R. We and R. Derynck (1996) Receptor-associated Mad homologues synergize as effectors of the TGF-beta response. *Nature.* 383, 168-72.

Zheng, H. and E. H. Koo (2006) The amyloid precursor protein: beyond amyloid. *Mol Neurodegener.* 1, 5.

Zhong, W., J. N. Feder, M. M. Jiang, L. Y. Jan and Y. N. Jan (1996) Asymmetric localization of a mammalian numb homolog during mouse cortical neurogenesis. *Neuron.* 17, 43-53.

Zhong, W., M. M. Jiang, G. Weinmaster, L. Y. Jan and Y. N. Jan (1997) Differential expression of mammalian Numb, Numblike and Notch1 suggests distinct roles during mouse cortical neurogenesis. *Development.* 124, 1887-97.

10

Role of Growth Factor Receptors in Neural Stem Cells Differentiation and Dopaminergic Neurons Generation

Lucía Calatrava, Rafael Gonzalo-Gobernado, Antonio S. Herranz,
Diana Reimers, Maria J. Asensio, Cristina Miranda and Eulalia Bazán
Department of Neurobiology, Ramón y Cajal Institute for Health Research, Madrid
Spain

1. Introduction

Neural stem cells (NSCs) are defined as clonogenic cells with self-renewal capacity and multilineage potential (Bazán et al., 2004). Cells with these characteristics have been isolated from the embryonic and adult Central Nervous System (CNS) (Gil-Perotin et al., 2009; Merkle & Alvarez-Buylla, 2006; Weiss et al., 1996). Under specific conditions, these cells proliferate in culture as cell clusters, called neurospheres, and differentiate into neurons, glia, and non-neural cell types (Kennea & Mehmet, 2002; Lobo et al., 2003; Reynolds & Weiss, 1992; Vescovi et al., 2002; Arias-Carrión & Yuan, 2009). Moreover, these cultures represent a potential source for cell replacement therapies in neurological diseases such as Parkinson's disease (PD) (Bjugstad et al., 2008; Pluchino et al., 2005; Reimers et al., 2011; Zhu et al, 2009).

Both basic fibroblast growth factor (bFGF) and epidermal growth factor (EGF) promote the proliferation of NSCs (Ciccolini & Svendsen, 1998; Gritti et al., 1996, 1999; Reynolds et al., 1992; Palmer et al., 1999). Moreover, growth factors (GFs) and intracellular mechanisms have been reported to influence or even determine NSCs phenotypic choice "in vivo" and "in vitro" (Daadi & Weiss, 1999; Hagg, 2005, 2009; Ninkovic & Götz, 2007; Redondo et al., 2007; Reimers et al., 2001, 2008). Thus, bFGF in combination with agents that increase cAMP levels and/or protein kinase C (PKC) activators induced the expression of tyrosine hydroxylase (TH), which is the rate-limiting enzyme involved in the synthesis of catecholaminergic neurotransmitters (Lopez-Toledano et al., 2004).

Growth factors exert their action through their interaction with specific receptors. A subset of FGF receptors (FGFRs) have been described in NSCs and their progeny (Reimers et al., 2001, Lobo et al., 2003), but to present nothing is known regarding the role played by these different FGFRs subtypes in the TH-inductive effect of bFGF above described. NSCs also express a 170 kD protein corresponding to the EGF receptor (EGFR) (Lobo et al., 2003). Since bFGF modulates EGF responsiveness in striatal precursors (Ciccolini & Svendsen, 1998), we wonderer whether TH induction in NSCs progeny could be associated with changes in EGFR protein expression and/or cellular localization.

2. Material and methods

2.1 Isolation of neural stem cells from the embryonic rat striatum

Striatal primordia from E15 Sprague-Dawley rat embryos were dissected and mechanically dissociated. Cells were grown in suspension in a defined medium (DF12) composed of Dulbecco's modified Eagle's medium and Ham's F-12 (1:1), 2 mM L-glutamine, 1 mM sodium piruvate (all from Gibco BRL, Life Technologies Inc, Grand Island, NY), 0.6% glucose, 25 µg/ml insulin, 20 nM progesterone, 60 µM putrescine, and 30 nM sodium selenite (all from Sigma Chemical Co, St Louis, MO), 100 µg/ml human transferrin (Boehringer Mannheim GmbH, Germany) and 20 ng/ml human recombinant EGF (PreproTech EC Ltd., London, England). After 48-72 hr in vitro, the cells grew as free-floating neurospheres and were passaged by mechanical dissociation every 2-3 days (Lobo et al., 2003; Reimers et al., 2001).

After a minimum of 4 and a maximum of 5 passages, neurospheres were dissociated and plated at a density of 20,000–30,000 cells/cm2 on 15µg/ml poly l-ornithine (Sigma)-coated round glass cover slips (ø12 mm) or plastic dishes (ø 35 mm). Cultures were maintained in DF12 and 20 ng/ml EGF for 3 days and then switched to DF12 without EGF for longer culture periods (control group). At 7 days postplating (dpp), parallel cultures were treated with 10 ng/ml human recombinant bFGF (Boehringer Mannheim) and 1 mM dibutyryladenosine 3,5-cyclic monophosphate (bFGF + dbcAMP) in the absence (vehicle group), or presence of 20µM PD98058 or 10^{-7}M staurosporin. Cellular phenotypes were determined immunocytochemically 24 hr later using antibodies to β-tubulin isotype III (β-tubulin III) for neurons, glial fibrillary acidic protein (GFAP) for astrocytes, A2B5, which stains bipotential O2A glial progenitors (Raff et al. 1984; Schnitzer & Schachner 1982) as well as subsets of neurons (Schnitzer & Schachner 1982), O4 for immature oligodendrocytes, O1 for mature oligodendrocytes, and TH for catecholaminergic phenotypes.

2.2 Immunocytochemical staining

The polyclonal antibodies used in this study were anti-β-tubulin III (BabCO; Richmond, CA), anti-TH (Chemicon International;Temecula, CA), anti-DOPA-decarboxilase (Sigma, Missouri, USA), anti-dopamine transporter (DAT, Chemicon), anti-vesicular monoamine transporter 2 (VMAT2, Pel-Freez, Arkansas LLC, USA) and anti-GFAP (Dako; Glostrup, Denmark). The antibodies used for the detection of FGF receptors (FGFR1, FGFR2, FGFR3), and EGF receptor (EGFR) were from Santa Cruz Biotechnology Inc., Burlingame, CA, USA. Monoclonal antibodies against β-tubulin III were obtained from Sigma, anti-TH was obtained from Chemicon, and anti-nestin (clone Rat 401) was from the Developmental Studies Hybridoma Bank (University of Iowa, Iowa City, IO). Monoclonal antibodies against A2B5, O4, and O1 were obtained in our laboratory as hybridoma supernatants. The secondary antibodies used were: biotinylated goat anti-mouse IgG (Zymed Laboratories; South San Francisco, CA), streptavidin–biotin–peroxidase complex (DakoCytomation), diaminobenzidine (DAB) + substrate–chromogen system (both from DakoCytomation), Alexa Fluor-568 goat anti-mouse IgG, Alexa Fluor-488 donkey anti-rat IgG, and Alexa Fluor-488 goat anti-rabbit IgG (1:400; all from Molecular Probes; Eugene, OR), Fluorescein-conjugated goat anti-mouse IgG (1:25; Jackson ImmunoResearch Laboratories Inc, West Grove, PA), Cy3-conjugated donkey anti-guinea pig IgG (1:500, Jackson ImmunoResearch Laboratories Inc.), and Rhodamine-conjugated goat anti-rabbit IgG (1:100, Chemicon International Inc.).

For immunocytochemical studies, cells were fixed with 4% paraformaldehyde for 10 min and immunostained for A2B5 (1:10), O4 (1:10), O1 (1:10), FGFR1 (1:100), FGFR2 (1:100), FGFR3 (1:50) and EGFR (1:50) as previously described (Reimers et al., 2001). Permeabilization for GFAP (1:500), β-tubulin III (1:200 for monoclonal and 1:3000 for polyclonal anti-β-tubulin III, and TH (1:500) was achieved by treating cultures with 0.05% Triton X-100 at 4°C for 5min. Immunofluorescent procedures were applied for neural antigens and FGFR3 detection, and immunoperoxidase methods for FGFR1 and FGFR2 visualization. Cover slips were mounted in a medium containing p-phenylenediamine and bis-Benzimide (Hoechst 33342; Sigma).

2.3 Western blot protein analysis

NSCs progeny were treated for 24 hr with TH inducers, in the absence or presence of 20 μM PD98058 or 10^{-7}M staurosporin, and proteins were processed for Western blot analysis to determine the relative levels of growth factor receptors (GFRs) and neural antigens. Cells were lysed with 0.5 M Tris-HCl buffer (pH 7.4) containing 0.24% Triton X-100, 10 mg/ml leupeptin, and 0.5 mM PMSF, all from Sigma. After 1 hr at 4°C, samples were centrifuged at 12,000g for 30 min. Total protein content was quantified using a BCA kit (Pierce; Rockford, IL). Aliquots of 30 μg of protein were separated by electrophoresis on 10% SDS-polyacrylamide minigels and transferred to nitrocellulose filters. Membranes were soaked in blocking solution (0.2 M Tris-HCl, 137 mM NaCl, and 3–5% dry skimmed milk, pH 7.6) and incubatedwith primary antibodies diluted in the same blocking solution: anti-FGFR1 (1:200), anti-FGFR3 (1:200), anti EGFR (1:250), anti-TH (1:10,000), and anti-GFAP (1:1000), anti-β-tubulin III (1:10,000), and anti-CNPasa (1:1000). After extensive washing membranes were incubated with the peroxidase-conjugated secondary antibodies diluted 1:1000 in blocking solution. The filters were developed with enhanced chemiluminescence Western blotting analysis, following the procedure described by the manufacturer (Amersham, Buckinghamshire, England). Membranes were immunolabeled for control charge using mouse anti-β actine (1:5000; Sigma Aldrich). Autoradiograms were quantified by computer-assisted videodensitometry.

2.4 Data analysis and cell counting

For Western blot analysis, results are expressed as mean ± SEM from two to four independent experiments. Where indicated, data represent the mean ± SEM of several cover slips. For each cover slip, stereological sampling of 25 visual fields (magnification of 200x or 400x) was performed by fluorescence microscopy. The number of cells was corrected for cover slip area. Statistical analyses were performed using Student's t-test or one-way ANOVA followed by Newman-Keuls multiple comparison test, and differences were considered significant at $p \leq 0.05$.

3. Results and discussion

3.1 Acquisition of a dopaminergic phenotype in the progeny of neural stem cells

Previously, we demonstrated that bFGF in combination with the PKA activator dbcAMP induced TH immunoreactivity in a subset of neurons and A2B5-positive progenitors derived from striatal EGF-expanded NSCs (striatal EGF-NSCs) (Lopez-Toledano et al., 2004). However, to present nothing is known regarding the ability of bFGF + dbcAMP to promote the expression of other features of dopaminergic mature neurons in these cells. As shown in Fig. 1A, bFGF + dbcAMP treatment increased by 1.5-fold TH protein expression in the progeny derived from striatal EGF-NSCs.

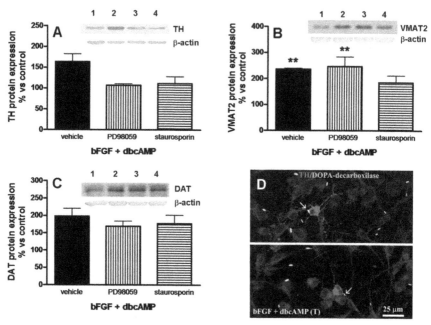

Fig. 1. Induction of a dopaminergic phenotype in the progeny derived from striatal EGF-NSCs. As shown in A-C, bFGF + dbcAMP treatment (black bars) increased the expression of TH (A), VMAT2 (B) and DAT (C). Note how 20 μM PD98059 (vertical line bars) and 10^{-7}M staurosporin (horizontal line bars) prevented TH protein overexpression (A). Line 1, control cultures, line 2, bFGF + dbcAMP treated cultures, line 3, bFGF + dbcAMP in the presence of PD98059, line 4, bFGF + dbcAMP in the presence of staurosporin. Results represent the mean ± SEM of 2 independent experiments. **$p \leq 0.01$ vs control. D shows how in bFGF + dbcAMP treated cultures DOPA-decarboxilase immunoreactivity (D, green) associates with TH-positive cells (D, red, white arrows).

In the presence of 20 μM PD98059 or 10^{-7} M staurosporin, which are inhibitors of the mitogen activated protein kinase/extracellular signal-regulated kinase (MAPK/ERK1/2) and PKC, respectively, the raise in TH protein levels promoted by bFGF + dbcAMP treatment was prevented (Fig. 1A). These results are in agreement with our previous studies showing that the activation of the MAPK/ERK1/2 signaling pathway and PKC activity were required for the generation of TH-positive cells in striatal EGF-NSCs progeny (Lopez-Toledano et al., 2004). Besides TH, bFGF + dbcAMP treated cultures also showed DOPA-decarboxilase immunoreactivity that in some cases was associated with TH-positive cells (Fig. 1D). This enzyme catalyzes the conversion of levodopa (L-DOPA) in dopamine, so we may consider that under TH-inductive conditions striatal EGF-NSCs progeny is able to synthesize this neurotransmitter which deficit is involved in the progression of PD (Aron et al, 2011). As a matter of fact, our preliminary studies indicate that bFGF + dbcAMP treatment significantly increases L-DOPA levels by 1.7-fold ($p \leq 0.01$ vs control). Moreover, in the presence of the DOPA-decarboxilase inhibitor NSD-1015, L-DOPA levels were significantly higher than those observed under control conditions ($p \leq 0.001$), or bFGF + dbcAMP treatment ($p \leq 0.01$). Altogether, these results strongly suggest that under our experimental conditions TH and DOPA-decarboxilase are active enzymes.

We also analyzed the effect of the TH-inductive treatment in the expression of other dopaminergic markers such as VMAT2 and DAT. Thus, bFGF + dbcAMP increased by 2-fold VMAT2 and DAT protein levels (Fig. 1B, C). The expression of both proteins was not regulated by the MAPK/ERK1/2 signaling pathway or PKC activity because neither PD98059, nor staurosporin prevented VMAT2 or DAT upregulation (Fig. 1C, D). In our cultures, bFGF + dbcAMP treatment increased the phosphorylation of the cyclic AMP response element binding protein (CREB) probably through the activation of PKA by dbcAMP (Lopez-Toledano et al., 2004). Because this transcription factor regulates the expression of catecholamine biosynthetic enzymes and transporters (Lewis-Tuffin et al., 2004; Lim et al., 2000; Watson et al., 2001), its activation could be responsible for the increase in VMAT2 and DAT protein levels observed in this study. Besides, bFGF + dbcAMP could stimulate striatal EGF-NSCs to release neurotrophins that are able to increase the expression of TH and monoamine transporters in neural precursors (Maciaczyk et al., 2008; Sun et al., 2004), and in the damaged brain (Emborg et al., 2008).

3.2 Dopaminergic inductors modulate the expression and cellular localization of fibroblast growth factor receptors in the progeny of neural stem cells

Striatal EGF-NSCs and their progeny express a subset of FGFRs, so we were interested in to determine the role played by the different FGFR subtypes in the acquisition of dopaminergic features in these cells. FGFR1 is expressed in nestin-positive neural precursors (Lobo et al, 2003), and was down-regulated during their differentiation in neurons and glial cells (Reimers et al., 2001). Under dopaminergic-inductive conditions, FGFR1 immunoreactivity was higher than in controls (Fig.2A, C). Similarly, FGFR1 protein expression was significantly raised by more than 10-fold in bFGF + dbcAMP treated cultures (Fig. 2B). FGFR1 up-regulation was not affected in the presence of MAPK/ERK1/2 or PKC inhibitors (Fig. 2B, D), indicating that other signaling pathways are involved in FGFR1 over-expression. Growth factors are able to stimulate the phosphatidylinositol 3-kinase (PI3K)/Akt signaling transduction pathway in NSCs to promote their proliferation, survival and differentiation (Lim et al., 2007; Meng et al, 2011; Nguyen et al., 2009; Torroglosa et al., 2007). As mentioned above, FGFR1 is expressed in nestin-positive neural precursors. In our cultures, bFGF + dbcAMP treatment significantly increased nestin protein expression by 2-fold ($p \leq 0.05$ vs control), and neither PD98059 nor staurosporin were able to abolish this effect. Because similar results were observed under bFGF treatment (Reimers et al., 2001), our results strongly suggest that the GF promotes the survival and/or proliferation of resting FGFR1-/nestin-positive neural precursors probably through the stimulation of PI3K/Akt signaling pathway.

Dopaminergic-inductive conditions modulate FGFR3 protein expression and cellular localization. Under control conditions, FGFR3 was localized in the membrane of GFAP-positive astrocytes (Fig. 3A), in the cell bodies of β-tubulin III-positive neurons (Fig. 3B), and in the nuclei of O4-positive preoligodendrocytes (Fig. 3C). Western blot analysis revealed that FGFR3 levels were significantly up-regulated by bFGF + dbcAMP treatment (Fig. 3D). This experimental condition changed the morphology of GFAP-positive cells that showed longer and thinner processes where FGFR3 immunoreactivity was observed (Fig. 3E). Moreover, FGFR3 immunostaining was also detected in their nuclei (Fig. 3E). bFGF + dbcAMP treatment also affected to the morphology of O4-positive cells and increased FGFR3 immunoreactivity in their nuclei (Fig. 3G). Besides, some TH-positive cells showing a neuronal morphology co-expressed FGFR3 in their cell bodies (Fig. 3F). Other authors have shown the presence of two forms of FGFR3 in the nucleus of malignant and non-malignant epithelial cells (Johnston et al., 1995; Zammit et al., 2001). However, to our knowledge this is the first study reporting the nuclear localization of FGFR3 in neural cells. From our results, it is difficult to determine whether the higher levels of FGFR3 nuclear staining observed in GFAP-positive cells are due to the increase in protein expression, or to the translocation of FGFR3 to perinuclear localization.

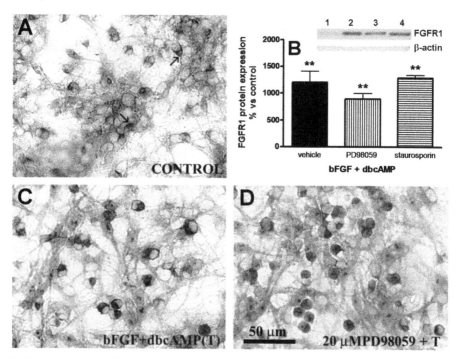

Fig. 2. Tyrosine hydroxylase inductors upregulate FGFR1 protein expression in the progeny derived from striatal EGF-NSCs. A, C an D show FGFR1 immunocytochemical staining in control conditions (A), and in cultures treated with bFGF + dbcAMP (T) in the absence (C) or presence of 20 μM PD98059 (D). Note how in the presence of TH-inductors FGFR1 immunoreactivity is increased (C). bFGF + dbcAMP treatment also upregulates FGFR1 protein expression (B, black bar), and this effect is not prevented by 20 μM PD98059 (B, vertical lines bar) or 10^{-7}M staurosporin (B, horizontal lines bar). Line 1, control cultures, line 2, bFGF + dbcAMP treated cultures, line 3, bFGF + dbcAMP in the presence of PD98059, line 4, bFGF + dbcAMP in the presence of staurosporin. Results represent the mean ± SEM of 2 independent experiments. **$p \leq 0.01$ vs control.

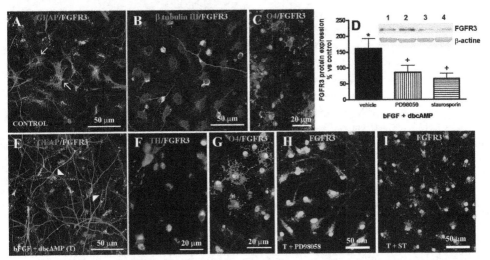

Fig. 3. Tyrosine hydroxylase inductors modulate FGFR3 protein expression and cellular localization in the progeny derived from striatal EGF-NSCs. A-C show how under control conditions FGFR3 immunoreactivity (green) is localized in the membranes of GFAP-positive astrocytes (A, white arrows), cell bodies of β-tubulin III-positive neurons (B, yellow), and nuclei of O4-positive preoligodendrocytes (C). E-I show FGFR3 immunostaining in basic FGF + dbcAMP treated cultures (T). Under TH-inductive conditions, FGFR3 is localized in the nuclei of GFAP-positive astrocytes (E, white arrowheads) and preoligodendrocytes (G), and in the cell bodies of TH-positive neurons (F, yellow). Note, how astrocytes (E, red) and O4-positive cells (G, red) show longer and thinner extensions in bFGF + dbcAMP treated cultures, and how FGFR3 immunoreactivity is decreased in the presence of 20 µM PD98059 (H, green) and 10^{-7}M staurosporin (I, green). TH inductors also upregulate FGFR3 protein expression (D, black bar), and this effect is prevented by 20 µM PD98059 (D, vertical lines bar) or 10^{-7}M staurosporin (D, horizontal lines bar). Line 1, control cultures, line 2, bFGF + dbcAMP treated cultures, line 3, bFGF + dbcAMP in the presence of PD98059, line 4, bFGF + dbcAMP in the presence of staurosporin. Results represent the mean ± SEM of 4 independent experiments. *$p \leq 0.05$ vs control, +$p \leq 0.05$ vs vehicle.

Interestingly, the nuclear translocation of FGFRs in response to bFGF has been reported in reactive astrocytes (Clarke et al., 2001) and Swiss 3T3 fibroblasts (Maher, 1996). Moreover, the antibody used in this study recognizes a 135 kDa form of FGFR3 that showed a mix of nuclear and cytoplasmic localization in epithelial cells that depends on its degree of activation by different members of the FGF family (Zammit et al., 2001).

Similarly to TH protein expression, FGFR3 up-regulation was not observed in the presence of 20 µM PD98059 or 10^{-7}M staurosporin (Fig. 3D). FGFR3 immunoreactivity was also reduced in both experimental conditions (Fig. 3H, I). Moreover, PKC inhibition prevented the morphological changes promoted by bFGF + dbcAMP treatment (Fig. 3I). These results suggest that the modulation of FGFR3 and TH induction are two events closely associated. As a matter of fact, FGFRs nuclear localization has been related with the differentiation of neural progenitor cells (Fang et al., 2005; Stachowiak et al., 2003), and TH gene expression

(Peng et al., 2002). We should comment that not all TH-positive cells were FGFR3 immunoreactive (our unpublished observations), so it seems that they are not direct targets for bFGF. Under our TH-inductive conditions, GFAP protein expression was significantly raised by more than 1.6-fold ($p \le 0.05$ vs control). GFAP over-expression and morphological changes are features of reactive glia which is able to synthesize trophic factors involved in neuronal survival and differentiation (Barreto et al., 2011). Because glial derived factors are also involved in the differentiation of NSCs in TH-immunoreactive dopaminergic neurons (Anwar et al., 2008; Maciaczyk et al., 2008; Sun et al., 2004), from our results we propose that stimulation of FGFR3 localized in glial cells mediate the release of several unknown factors that in combination with PKA activators stimulate TH-induction in the target cells. In fact, glial conditioned medium in combination with PKA activators elicits the expression of TH in the progeny of striatal EGF-NSCs (Reimers et al., 2008).

We have also analyzed the effects of bFGF + dbcAMP treatment in FGFR2 expression. Under the experimental conditions presented in this study, FGFR2 nuclear localization and FGFR2 protein expression were not affected (data not shown), indicating that probably this FGFR is not involved in the acquisition of a dopaminergic phenotype in striatal EGF-NSCs progeny.

3.3 Tyrosine hydroxylase-inducing cues trigger nuclear epidermal growth factor receptor accumulation in the progeny of neural stem cells

EGFR stimulation is essential for the proliferation of striatal EGF-NSCs (Bazán et al., 1998, 2006; Reimers et al., 2001). EGFR protein expression has been detected during the differentiation of these cells in neurons and glia (Lobo et al., 2003); however, to present nothing is known regarding its cellular localization, and the role, if any, played by this receptor in the differentiation of striatal EGF-NSCs to TH-immunopositive cells. As shown in Fig. 4A, EGFR-positive cells were observed in 8 dpp control cultures. At this experimental time, EGFR imuunoreactivity was localized in the cell bodies of β-tubulin III- (Fig. 4B) and O4-positive cells (Fig. 4D). Moreover, EGFR immunostaining was also observed in the membrane of GFAP-positive astrocytes (Fig. 4C). TH-inductive conditions did not affect EGFR protein expression (Fig. 4K), but promoted the translocation of EGFR to the nuclei in many cells (Fig. 4E). Nuclear EGFR immunoreactivity was observed in small spots, suggesting that the EGFR could be localized in the nucleolar compartment. Functional nuclear EGFR have been described in normal and tumoral cells (Jaganathan et al., 2011; Lo & Hung, 2007; Xu et al., 2009), but to our knowledge this is the first study reporting the nuclear localization of EGFR in NSCs and its derived progeny. Interestingly, a recent report discusses the possibility that proliferation and differentiation of NSCs could be controlled by nuclear receptors (Katayama et al., 2005). Moreover, NSCs proliferation seems to be regulated by a nucleolar mechanism that involves the interaction of proteins located in their nucleoli (Tsai & McKay, 2002). Neither EGFR protein expression (Fig. 4K), nor nuclear localization (Fig. 4I) were affected in the presence of PD98059. However, both parameters were significantly reduced in the presence of the PKC inhibitor staurosporin (Fig. 4J, K). As a matter of fact, a recent report demonstrates that PKC activation triggers nuclear EGFR accumulation in a bronchial carcinoma cell line (Wanner et al., 2008). Besides, the nuclear translocalization of EGFR may require its phosphorylation at Ser-229 by Akt (Huang et al., 2011). Further experiments are warranted to determine whether the PI3K/Akt signaling pathway mediates bFGF + dbcAMP-induced EGFR nuclear translocalization in striatal EGF-NSCs.

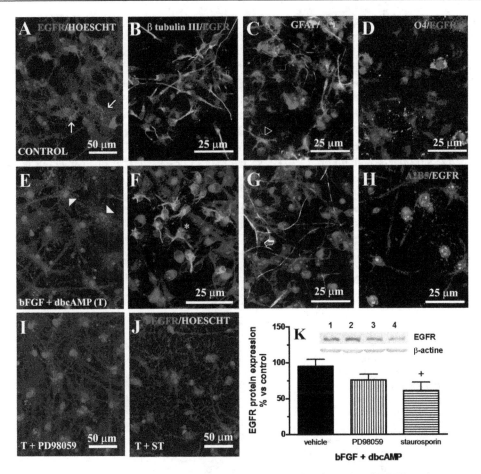

Fig. 4. Tyrosine hydroxylase inductors elicit nuclear translocalization of EGFR in the progeny derived from striatal EGF-NSCs. In control cultures EGFR immunoreactivity is localized the cell bodies (A, red), and in membranes (A, white arrows). Under this condition, EGFR is expressed in the cell bodies of neurons (B, yellow) and O1-positive oligodendrocytes (D), and in the membranes of GFAP-positive astrocytes (C, open triangle). Note how bFGF + dbcAMP (T) translocates EGFR to the nuclear compartment (E, white arrowheads), and how nuclear EGFR is observed in a few β-tubulin III-positive neurons (F, white star), a few astrocytes (G, open arrow), and in many A2B5-positive progenitors (H). Neither EGFR immunoreactivity nor nuclear EGFR localization are affected in the presence of 20 μM PD98059 (I, red), but 10^{-7} M staurosporine significantly decreases both parameters (J, red). bFGF + dbcAMP treatment in the absence (K, black bar) or presence of 20 μM PD98059 (K, vertical lines bar) does not affect EGFR protein expression; however, 10^{-7} M staurosporin significantly reduces EGFR levels (K, horizontal lines bar). Line 1, control cultures, line 2, bFGF + dbcAMP treated cultures, line 3, bFGF + dbcAMP in the presence of PD98059, line 4, bFGF + dbcAMP in the presence of staurosporin. Results represent the mean ± SEM of 2 independent experiments. +p ≤ 0.05 vs vehicle.

Double immunostaining showed that some neurons (Fig. 4F) and a few GFAP-positive astrocytes (Fig.4G) presented nuclear EGFR immunoreactivity. Besides, a population of cells showing EGFR nuclear localization colabeled with A2B5-positive cells (Fig.4H). Emerging evidence suggest that EGFR nuclear translocalization regulates gene expression and mediate other cellular processes such as DNA repair (Chen & Nirodi, 2007; Dittmann et al., 2010; Lo, 2010). Its transcriptional activity depends on its C-terminal transactivation domain, and its physical and functional interaction with other transcription factors that lead the activation of genes (Lo & Hung, 2006). Under our experimental conditions TH is expressed in 4% of the total population of β-tubulin III-positive neurons, and 20% of the TH-positive cells colabel with A2B5 (Lopez-Toledano et al., 2004), so we may hypothesize that nuclear EGFR could regulate TH gene expression in both cell types.

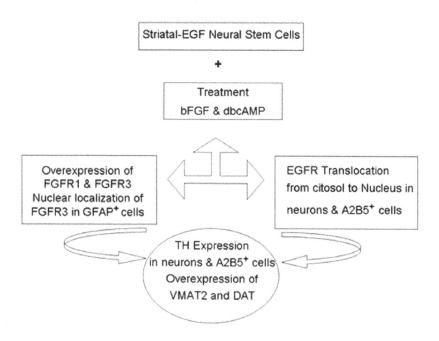

Fig. 5. Schematic diagram illustrating how bFGF + dbcAMP treatment induces the expression of specific features of dopaminergic neurons in the progeny derived from striatal EGF-NSCs through the modulation of GFRs expression and cellular localization.

4. Conclusions

1. In striatal EGF-NSCs, bFGF + dbcAMP treatment up-regulates the expression of the specific dopaminergic markers TH, DAT and VMAT2.
2. FGFR1 and nestin protein levels are significantly raised in bFGF + dbcAMP treated cultures, suggesting the survival and/or proliferation of undifferentiated neural precursors under this experimental condition.

3. bFGF + dbcAMP treatment increases FGFR3 protein expression and FGFR3 immunoreactivity in the glial progeny derived from striatal-EGF-NSCs. Moreover, this experimental condition up-regulates GFAP protein levels, and elicits the translocalization of FGFR3 to the nucleus in reactive GFAP-positive astrocytes.
4. In the presence of MAPK/ERK1/2 or PKC inhibitors, TH protein expression, FGFR3 up-regulation, and glial reactivity are partially prevented, suggesting that in bFGF + dbcAMP treated cultures, the modulation of FGFR3 in glial cells and TH induction are two events closely associated.
5. Under bFGF + dbcAMP treatment, EGFR immunostaining shows a nuclear localization in β-tubulin III-positive neurons and in A2B5-positive precursors derived from striatal EGF-NSCs. Because both cell types are able to express TH, we hypothesize that the nuclear translocalization of EGFR is necessary for the induction of TH in these cells.

As summarize in Fig. 5, our results demonstrate that in striatal EGF-NSCs, bFGF and dbcAMP treatment induces TH protein expression through the stimulation of FGFR3 expressed in glia, and nuclear translocalization of EGFR in the target cells. Under these TH-inductive conditions, striatal EGF-NSCs progeny acquire other specific features of mature dopaminergic neurons, so they can be considered as an excellent tool for stem cell-based replacement therapies in PD.

5. Acknowledgment

The authors wish to acknowledge the editorial for its invitation to contribute with a full chapter for the book under the working title "Neural Stem Cells", ISBN 978-953-307-795-6. This work was supported by the Fondo de Investigaciones Sanitarias (FISS PI060315) and Agencia Laín Entralgo (NDG7/09). RG-G and CM were the recipients of a FiBio HRyC fellowship, and LC was the recipient of an Agencia Laín Entralgo fellowship. We thank Macarena Rodríguez for technical help, and Dr. Maria José Casarejos for the determination of L-DOPA levels by HPLC.

6. References

Anwar MR, Andreasen CM, Lippert SK, Zimmer J, Martinez-Serrano A & Meyer M (2008). Dopaminergic differentiation of human neural stem cells mediated by co-cultured rat striatal brain slices. *J Neurochem.*,Vol. 105, No. 2, (April 2008), pp.(460-70), ISSN 0022-3042.

Arias-Carrión O & Yuan TF (2009). Autologous neural stem cell transplantation: A new treatment option for Parkinson's disease? *Med Hypotheses.*, Vol. 73, No. 5, (November 2009), pp. (757-759), ISSN 0306-9877.

Aron L & Klein R (2011). Repairing the parkinsonian brain with neurotrophic factors. *Trends Neurosci.*, Vol. 34, No. 2, (February 2011), pp. (88-100), ISSN 0166-2236.

Barreto GE, Gonzalez J, Torres Y & Morales L (2011). Astrocytic-neuronal crosstalk: Implications for neuroprotection from brain injury. *Neurosci Res.*, (June 2011) [Epub ahead of print]

Bazán E, López-Toledano MA, Redondo C, Alcázar A, Paíno CL & Herranz AS. (1998). Characterization of rat neural stem cells from embryonic striatum and mesencephalon during in vitro differentiation. In: *Understanding glial cells,*

Castellano B, González B, Nieto-Sampedro M, editors, pp. 133–147. Kluwer Academic Publishers, ISBN 0-7923-8140-8, Dordrecht, The Netherlands.

Bazán E, Alonso FJ, Redondo C, López-Toledano MA, Alfaro JM, Reimers D, Herranz AS, Paíno CL, Serrano AB, Cobacho N, Caso E & Lobo MV (2004). In vitro and in vivo characterization of neural stem cells. *Histol Histopathol,*Vol. 19, No. 4, (October 2004), pp. (1261-75), ISSN 0213-3911.

Bazán E, Herranz AS, Reimers D, Lobo MVT, Redondo C, López-Toledano MA, Gonzalo-Gobernado R, Asensio MJ & Alonso R. (2006). Neural stem cells and taurine. In: *Neural stem cell research*, Greer EV, editor, pp 99–114. Nova Science Publishers, Inc, ISBN 1-59454-846-3, New York.

Bjugstad KB, Teng YD, Redmond DE Jr, Elsworth JD, Roth RH, Cornelius SK, Snyder EY & Sladek JR Jr (2008). Human neural stem cells migrate along the nigrostriatal pathway in a primate model of Parkinson's disease. *Exp Neurol.*, Vol. 211, No. 2, (June 2008), pp. (362-369), ISSN 0014-4886.

Chen DJ & Nirodi CS (2007). The epidermal growth factor receptor: a role in repair of radiation-induced DNA damage. *Clin Cancer Res.*, Vol. 13, No. 22 Pt 1,(November 2007), pp. (6555-6560), ISSN 0008-5472.

Ciccolini F & Svendsen CN (1998). Fibroblast growth factor 2 (FGF-2) promotes acquisition of epidermal growth factor (EGF) responsiveness in mouse striatal precursor cells: Identification of neural precursors responding to both EGF and FGF-2. *J Neurosci.*, Vol. 18, No. 19, (October 1998), pp. (7869–7880), ISSN 0270-6474.

Clarke WE, Berry M, Smith C, Kent A & Logan A (2001).Coordination of fibroblast growth factor receptor 1 (FGFR1) and fibroblast growth factor-2 (FGF-2) trafficking to nuclei of reactive astrocytes around cerebral lesions in adult rats. *Mol Cell Neurosci*, Vol 17, No. 1, (January 2001), pp. (17-30), ISSN 1044-7431.

Daadi MM & Weiss S (1999). Generation of tyrosine hydroxylase-producing neurons from precursors of the embryonic and adult forebrain. *J Neurosci.*, Vol. 19, No. 11,(June 1999), pp. (4484-97), ISSN 0270-6474.

Dittmann K, Mayer C & Rodemann HP (2010). Nuclear EGFR as novel therapeutic target: insights into nuclear translocation and function. *Strahlenther Onkol.*, Vol. 186, No.1, (January 2010), pp.(1-6), ISSN 0179-7158.

Emborg ME, Ebert AD, Moirano J, Peng S, Suzuki M, Capowski E, Joers V, Roitberg BZ, Aebischer P & Svendsen CN (2008). GDNF-secreting human neural progenitor cells increase tyrosine hydroxylase and VMAT2 expression in MPTP-treated cynomolgus monkeys. *Cell Transplant.* Vol. 17, No. 4, pp, (383-95), E-ISSN 1555-3892.

Fang X, Stachowiak EK, Dunham-Ems SM, Klejbor I & Stachowiak MK (2005). Control of CREB-binding protein signaling by nuclear fibroblast growth factor receptor-1: a novel mechanism of gene regulation. *J Biol Chem.*, Vol. 280, No. 31, (August 2005), pp. (28451-28462), ISSN 0021-9258.

Gil-Perotín S, Alvarez-Buylla A & García-Verdugo JM (2009). Identification and characterization of neural progenitor cells in the adult mammalian brain. *Adv Anat Embryol Cell Biol.*, Vol. 203, pp.(1-101), ISSN 0301-5556.

Gritti A, Parati EA, Cova L, , Frölichsthal-Schoeller P, Galli R, Wanke E, Faravelli L, Morassutti DJ, Roisen F, Nickel DD & Vescovi AL (1996). Multipotent stem cells from the adult mouse brain proliferate and self-renewing response to basic

.broblast growth factor. *J Neurosci.*, Vol. 16, No. 3, (February 1996), pp.(1091–1100), ISSN 0270-6474.

Gritti A, Frölichsthal-Schoeller P, Galli R, Paraati EA, Cova L, Pagano SF, Bjornson CR & Vescovi AL (1999). Epidermal and fibroblast growth factors behave as mitogenic regulators for a single multipotent stem cell-like population from the subventricular region of the adult mouse forebrain. *J Neurosci.*, Vol. 19, No. 9,(May 1999), pp. (3287–3297), ISSN 0270-6474.

Hagg T (2005). Molecular regulation of adult CNS neurogenesis: an integrated view. *Trends Neurosci.*, Vol. 28, No. 11, (November 2005), pp.(589-595), ISSN 0166-2236.

Hagg T (2009). From neurotransmitters to neurotrophic factors to neurogenesis. *Neuroscientist.*, Vol. 15, No. 1, (February 2009), pp.(20-27), ISSN 1073-8584.

Huang WC, Chen YJ, Li LY, Wei YL, Hsu SC, Tsai SL, Chiu PC, Huang WP, Wang YN, Chen CH, Chang WC, Chang WC, Chen AJ, Tsai CH & Hung MC (2011). Nuclear translocation of epidermal growth factor receptor by Akt-dependent phosphorylation enhances breast cancer-resistant protein expression in gefitinib-resistant cells. *J Biol Chem*, Vol. 286, No. 23, (June 2011), pp. (20558-68), ISSN 0021-9258.

Jaganathan S, Yue P, Paladino DC, Bogdanovic J, Huo Q & Turkson J (2011). A functional nuclear epidermal growth factor receptor, SRC and Stat3 heteromeric complex in pancreatic cancer cells. *PLoS One.*, Vol. 6, No. 5, (May 2011), e19605, ISSN 1932-6203.

Johnston CL, Cox HC, Gomm JJ & Coombes RC (1995). Fibroblast growth factor receptors (FGFRs) localize in different cellular compartments. A splice variant of FGFR-3 localizes to the nucleus. *J Biol Chem*, Vol. 270, No. 51 (December 1995), pp. (30643-50), ISSN 0021-9258.

Katayama K, Wada K, Nakajima A, Kamisaki Y & Mayumi T (2005).Nuclear receptors as targets for drug development: the role of nuclear receptors during neural stem cell proliferation and differentiation. *J Pharmacol Sci*, Vol. 97, No. 2, (February 2005), pp. (171-6), ISSN 1347-8613.

Kennea NL & Mehmet H (2002). Neural stem cells. *J Pathol.*, Vol. 197 , No. 4, (July 2002), pp. (536-550), ISSN 1096-9896.

Lewis-Tuffin LJ, Quinn PG & Chikaraishi DM (2004). Tyrosine hydroxylase transcription depends primarily on cAMP response element activity, regardless of the type of inducing stimulus. *Mol Cell Neurosci.*,Vol. 25, No. 3, (March 2004), pp. (536-547), ISSN 1044-7431.

Lim J, Yang C, Hong SJ & Kim KS (2000). Regulation of tyrosine hydroxylase gene transcription by the cAMP-signaling pathway: involvement of multiple transcription factors. *Mol Cell Biochem* , Vol. 212, No. 1-2, (September 2000), pp. (51-60), ISSN 0300-8177.

Lim MS, Nam SH, Kim SJ, Kang SY, Lee YS & Kang KS (2007). Signaling pathways of the early differentiation of neural stem cells by neurotrophin-3. *Biochem Biophys Res Commun.*, Vol. 357, No. 4, (June 2007), pp. (903-909), ISSN 0006-291X.

Lo HW & Hung MC (2006). Nuclear EGFR signalling network in cancers: linking EGFR pathway to cell cycle progression, nitric oxide pathway and patient survival. *Br J Cancer*, Vol. 94, No. 2, (January 2011), pp. (184-8), ISSN 0007-0920

Lo HW & Hung MC (2007). Nuclear EGFR signalling network in cancers: linking EGFR pathway to cell cycle progression, nitric oxide pathway and patient survival. *Br J Cancer* ,Vol. 96 Suppl, pp. (16-20), ISSN 0007-0920.

Lo HW (2010). Nuclear mode of the EGFR signaling network: biology, prognostic value, and therapeutic implications. *Discov Med.*,Vol 10, No 50, (July 2010), pp. (44-51), ISSN 1539-6509.

Lobo MV, Alonso FJ, Redondo C, López-Toledano MA, Caso E, Herranz AS, Paíno CL, Reimers D & Bazán E (2003). Cellular characterization of epidermal growth factor-expanded free-floating neurospheres. *J Histochem Cytochem* ,Vol. 51, No. 1, (January 2003), pp. (89-103), ISSN 0022-1554.

López-Toledano MA, Redondo C, Lobo MV, Reimers D, Herranz AS, Paíno CL & Bazán E (2004). Tyrosine hydroxylase induction by basic fibroblast growth factor and cyclic AMP analogs in striatal neural stem cells: role of ERK1/ERK2 mitogen-activated protein kinase and protein kinase C. *J Histochem Cytochem.*, Vol. 52, No. 9, (September 2004), pp. (1177-1189), ISSN 0022-1554.

Maciaczyk J, Singec I, Maciaczyk D & Nikkhah G (2008). Combined use of BDNF, ascorbic acid, low oxygen, and prolonged differentiation time generates tyrosine hydroxylase-expressing neurons after long-term in vitro expansion of human fetal midbrain precursor cells. *Exp Neurol.*, Vol. 213, No. 2, (October 2008), pp. (354-362), ISSN 0014-4886.

Maher PA (1996). Nuclear Translocation of fibroblast growth factor (FGF) receptors in response to FGF-2. J Cell Biol, Vol. 134, No. 2, (July 1996), pp. (529-36), ISSN 0021-9525.

Meng X, Arocena M, Penninger J, Gage FH, Zhao M & Song B (2011). PI3K mediated electrotaxis of embryonic and adult neural progenitor cells in the presence of growth factors. *Exp Neurol.*, Vol. 227, No. 1, (January 2011), pp. (210-217), ISSN 0014-4886.

Merkle FT & Alvarez-Buylla A (2006). Neural stem cells in mammalian development. *Curr Opin Cell Biol.*, Vol 18, No. 6, (December 2006), pp. (704-709), ISSN 0955-0674.

Nguyen N, Lee SB, Lee YS, Lee KH & Ahn JY (2009). Neuroprotection by NGF and BDNF against neurotoxin-exerted apoptotic death in neural stem cells are mediated through Trk receptors, activating PI3-kinase and MAPK pathways. *Neurochem Res.*,Vol. 34, No. 5, (May 2009), pp. (942-951), ISSN 1573-6903.

Ninkovic J & Gotz M (2007). Signaling in adult neurogenesis: from stem cell niche to neuronal networks. *Curr Opin Neurobiol.*, Vol. 17, No. 3, (June 2007), pp. (338-344), ISSN 0959-4388.

Palmer TD, Markakis EA, Willhoite AR, Safar F & Gage FH (1999). Fibroblast growth factor-2 activates a latent neurogenic program in neural stem cells from diverse regions of the adult CNS. *J Neurosci.*, 19, No. 19, (October 1999), pp. (8487–8497), ISSN 0270-6474.

Peng H, Moffett J, Myers J, Fang X, Stachowiak EK, Maher P, Kratz E, Hines J, Fluharty SJ, Mizukoshi E, Bloom DC & Stachowiak MK (2001). Novel nuclear signaling pathway mediates activation of fibroblast growth factor-2 gene by type 1 and type 2 angiotensin II receptors. *Mol Biol Cell.*, Vol. 12, No. 2, (February 2001), pp. (449-462), ISSN 1059-1524.

Pluchino S, Zanotti L, Deleidi M & Martino G (2005). Neural stem cells and their use as therapeutic tool in neurological disorders. *Brain Res Brain Res Rev.*, Vol. 48, No. 2, (April 2005), pp. 211-219, ISSN 0165-0173.

Raff MC, Abney ER, Miller RH (1984) Two glial cell lineages diverge prenatally in rat optic nerve. *Dev Biol* .,Vol. 106, No. 1, (November 1984), pp.(53–60), ISSN 0012-1606.

Redondo C, López-Toledano MA, Lobo MV, Gonzalo-Gobernado R, Reimers D, Herranz AS, Paíno CL & Bazán E (2007). Kainic acid triggers oligodendrocyte precursor cell proliferation and neuronal differentiation from striatal neural stem cells. *J Neurosci Res.*,Vol. 85, No. 6, (May 2007), pp. (1170-1182), ISSN 0360-4012.

Reimers D, López-Toledano MA, Mason I, Cuevas P, Redondo C, Herranz AS, Lobo MV & Bazán E (2001). Developmental expression of fibroblast growth factor (FGF) receptors in neural stem cell progeny. Modulation of neuronal and glial lineages by basic FGF treatment. *Neurol Res.*, Vol. 23, No. 6, (September 2001), pp. (612-621), ISSN 0161-6412.

Reimers D, Gonzalo-Gobernado R, Herranz AS, Osuna C, Asensio MJ, Baena S, Rodríguez M & Bazán E (2008). Driving neural stem cells towards a desired phenotype. *Curr Stem Cell Res Ther.*,Vol. 3, No. 4, (December 2008), pp.(247-253), ISSN 1574-888X.

Reimers D, Osuna C, Gonzalo-Gobernado R, Herranz AS, Díaz-Gil JJ, Jiménez-Escrig A, Asensio MJ, Miranda C, Rodríguez-Serrano M & Bazán E (2010). Liver Growth Factor Promotes the Survival of Grafted Neural Stem Cells in a Rat Model of Parkinson's Disease. *Curr Stem Cell Res Ther.*, (December 2010), [Epub ahead of print], ISSN 1574-888X.

Reynolds BA & Weiss S (1992). Generation of neurons and astrocytes from isolated cells of the adult mammalian central nervous system. *Science.*, Vol. 255, No. 5052, (March 1992), pp. (1707-1710), ISSN 0036-8075.

Reynolds BA, Tetzlaff W & Weiss S (1992). A multipotent EGF responsive striatal embryonicprogenitor cell produces neurons and astrocytes. *J Neurosci.*, Vol. 12, No. 11, (November 1992), pp. (4565–4574), ISSN 0270-6474.

Schnitzer J & Schachner M (1982) Cell type specificity of a neural cell surface antigen recognized by the monoclonal antibody A2B5. *Cell Tissue Res.*, Vol. 224, No. 3, pp. (625–636), ISSN 0302-766X.

Stachowiak EK, Fang X, Myers J, Dunham S & Stachowiak MK (2003). cAMP-induced differentiation of human neuronal progenitor cells is mediated by nuclear fibroblast growth factor receptor-1 (FGFR1). *J Neurochem.*, Vol. 84, No. 6, (March 2003), pp. (1296-1312), ISSN 0022-3042.

Sun ZH, Lai YL, Li P, Zuo HC & Xie ZP (2004). GDNF augments survival and differentiation of TH-positive neurons in neural progenitor cells. *Cell Biol Int.*, Vol. 28, No. 4, pp. (323-325), ISSN 1065-6995.

Torroglosa A, Murillo-Carretero M, Romero-Grimaldi C, Matarredona ER, Campos-Caro A & Estrada C (2007). Nitric oxide decreases subventricular zone stem cell proliferation by inhibition of epidermal growth factor receptor and phosphoinositide-3-kinase/Akt pathway. *Stem Cells* Vol. 25, No. 1, (January 2007), pp. (88-97), ISSN 1066-5099.

Tsai RY & McKay RD (2002). A nucleolar mechanism controlling cell proliferation in stem cells and cancer cells. *Genes Dev*, Vol. 16, No. 23, (December 2002), pp. (2991-3003), ISSN 0890-9369.

Vescovi AL, Rietze R, Magli MC, Bjornson C (2002). Hematopoietic potential of neural stem cells. *Nat Med.*, Vol. 8, No. 6, (June 2002), pp. (535; author reply 536-537), ISSN 1078-8956.

Wanner G, Mayer C, Kehlbach R, Rodemann HP & Dittmann K (2008). Activation of protein kinase Cepsilon stimulates DNA-repair via epidermal growth factor receptor nuclear accumulation. *Radiother Oncol.*, Vol. 86, No. 3, (March 2008), pp. (383-390), ISSN 0167-8140.

Watson F, Kiernan RS, Deavall DG, Varro A & Dimaline R (2001). Transcriptional activation of the rat vesicular monoamine transporter 2 promoter in gastric epithelial cells: regulation by gastrin. *J Biol Chem.,*Vol. 276, No. 10, (March 2001), pp. (7661-7671), ISSN 0021-9258.

Weiss S, Reynolds BA, Vescovi AL, Morshead C, Craig CG & van der Kooy D (1996). Is there a neural stem cell in the mammalian forebrain? *Trends Neurosci.*, Vol. 19, No. 9, (September 1996), pp. (387-393), ISSN 0166-2236.

Xu Y, Shao Y, Zhou J, Voorhees JJ & Fisher GJ (2009). Ultraviolet irradiation-induces epidermal growth factor receptor (EGFR) nuclear translocation in human keratinocytes. *J Cell Biochem.*, Vol. 107, No. 5, (August 2009), pp. (873-880), ISSN 0730-2312.

Zammit C, Barnard R, Gomm J, Coope R, Shousha S, Coombes C & Johnston C (2001). Altered intracellular localization of fibroblast growth factor receptor 3 in human breast cancer. *J Pathol*, Vol. 194, No. 1, (May 2001), pp (27-34), ISSN 1096-9896.

Zhu Q, Ma J, Yu L & Yuan C (2009). Grafted neural stem cells migrate to substantia nigra and improve behavior in Parkinsonian rats. *Neurosci Lett.*, Vol. 462, No. 3, (October 2009), pp. (213-218), ISSN 0304-3940.

11

Active Expression of Retroelements in Neurons Differentiated from Adult Hippocampal Neural Stem Cells

Slawomir Antoszczyk, Kazuyuki Terashima, Masaki Warashina,
Makoto Asashima and Tomoko Kuwabara
Research Center for Stem Cell Engineering,
National Institute of Advanced Industrial Science and Technology (AIST)
Japan

1. Introduction

In the mammalian brain, neurogenesis constitutively occurs in the subventricular zone (SVZ), the olfactory bulb, and the hippocampus throughout adulthood (Kuhn et al., 1996; Lois and Alvarez-Buylla, 1993; Gage, 2000; Pagano et al., 2000; Gritti et al., 2002), and adult hippocampal neurogenesis plays an important role in learning and memory (Deng *et al.*, 2010). In the hippocampus, multipotent neural stem cells (NSCs) reside in the inner layer of the subgranular zone (SGZ) of the dentate gyrus (Gage, 2000; Suh *et al.*, 2007). Undifferentiated NSCs express the high mobility group (HMG)-box transcription factor Sox2 (D'Amour and Gage, 2003; Suh *et al.*, 2007). Sox2 is an SRY-related transcription factor encoding an HMG DNA-binding motif, and is expressed in embryonic stem (ES) cells and neural epithelial cells during development (Avilion et al., 2003; Ferri et al., 2004). Sox2 is essential for the multipotency and self-renewal capacity of NSCs and also functions in pluripotent ES cells (Bylund et al., 2003; Graham et al., 2003; Ferri et al., 2004). Sox2 is known to prevent neurogenesis during development and is thought to be critical for maintaining NSC populations in the neonatal brain (Bylund et al., 2003; Graham et al., 2003; Bani-Yaghoub et al., 2006). In the dentate gyrus of the hippocampus, Sox2 expression is found in the undifferentiated stem cell population with self-renewal capacity, and these Sox2-positive stem cells are exclusive with TUJ1-positive early stage of neurons (Fig. 1).

Fate-tracing studies showed that Sox2-positive cells in the SGZ of the adult hippocampus have the potential to give rise to neurons and astrocytes, revealing their multipotency at both the cell population and single cell levels (Suh et al., 2007). Moreover, a subpopulation of Sox2-positive cells gives rise to cells that retain Sox2, highlighting the importance of Sox2-positive cells as a primary source of adult NSCs (Suh et al., 2007). In response to intracellular or extracellular signals, Sox2-positive NSCs undergo cell division, giving rise to more Sox2-positive NSCs as well as neuronal precursors (Avilion et al., 2003; Ferri et al., 2004). Adult hippocampal neural stem cells express receptors and signaling components for Wnt proteins, which are key regulators of NSCs (Lie et al., 2005).

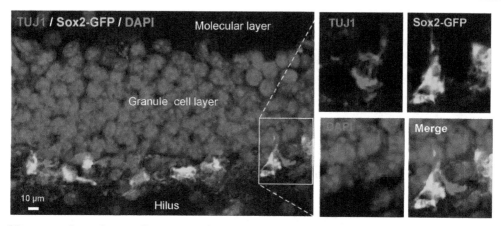

Hippocampal neural stem cells express multipotent marker Sox2. Sox2-positive cells (Sox2-GFP: green; immunohistochemistry analysis using Sox2 promoter-driven EGFP transgenic mice) are exclusive with early stage of neurons expressing β tubulin III (TUJ1: red). DAPI; blue.

Fig. 1. Adult neural stem cells in dentate gyrus of hippocampus

2. Wnt3 promotes the active expression of retroelements in adult hippocampal neurogenesis

Astrocytes are an essential cell population defining the hippocampal niche (Song *et al.*, 2002), and Wnt3 factors secreted from these cells are instructive in promoting adult neurogenesis (Lie *et al.*, 2005). The deletion of *Wnt3a* (*Wnt3a-/-* mice) prevents the formation of the dentate gyrus, which is the site of adult neurogenesis (Lee et al., 2000). Other Wnt proteins (Wnt1, Wnt2, Wnt5a, and Wnt7a/b) are detected and actively function in mature hippocampal neurons (Miyaoka T *et al.*, 1999; Gogolla et al., 2009; Cuitino et al., 2010; Okamoto *et al.*, 2010), suggesting that other Wnt proteins work in an autocrine manner to control neuronal functions, activities in the neuronal network, and synaptic connectivity in mature neurons. In contrast, astrocyte-secreted Wnt3/Wnt3a (Lie et al., 2005) acts in a paracrine manner to induce neurogenesis in NSCs by direct activation of the proneuronal gene neurogenic differentiation 1 (*NeuroD1*), and to generate diversity in newborn neurons through retroelements (i.e., retrotransposons) (Kuwabara et al., 2009).

2.1 Astrocytes-secreting Wnt3 initiates the expression of retroelements in adult neural stem cells

We recently reported that Wnt3/Wnt3a released from underlying astrocytic layers in the dentate gyrus has an important role in triggering neuronal differentiation of hippocampal NSCs. *NeuroD1*, a target gene of Wnt signaling in the coding region of the mammalian genome, is a proneural basic helix-loop-helix (bHLH) transcription factor that is essential for the development of the CNS, particularly for the generation of granule cells in the hippocampus (Miyata et al., 1999; Liu et al., 2000; Deisseroth et al., 2004; Tozuka et al., 2005). The deletion of β-catenin leads to substantial loss of NeuroD1-positive cells, while the stem cell compartment remains intact in vivo, suggesting that Wnt/β-catenin-mediated neuronal differentiation is dependent on NeuroD1 (Kuwabara et al., 2009).

Importantly, paracrine Wnt factors secreted from astrocytes simultaneously target the genomic noncoding region through long interspersed nuclear elements (LINE-1, L1) (Kuwabara et al., 2009). L1 is a large family of mobile elements that constitutes up to 17% of the mammalian genome (Han and Boeke, 2005) and was recently found to be actively retrotransposed in the course of adult neurogenesis in rodents (Muotri et al., 2005) and humans (Coufal et al., 2009). The regulatory sequence recognized by both Sox2 and TCF/LEF/β-catenin is present in the promoter region of NeuroD1 and L1 (Kuwabara *et al.*, 2009). Sox2 can suppress L1 expression in adult NSCs. In contrast, canonical Wnt/β-catenin signaling triggers the active expression of NeuroD1 and L1, indicating the essential role of Sox2 and Wnt in balancing self-renewal of NSCs and neuronal differentiation in the adult hippocampal dentate gyrus (Kuwabara et al., 2009).

The balance of asymmetric lineage control of adult NSCs in maintaining the constant size of the neural stem cell pools and producing newly born neurons relies on the definitive molecular mechanism of Wnt target genes: the Sox/LEF overlapping regulatory sequence on NeuroD1 and L1 functions as a "molecular switch" between Sox2-mediated repression and Wnt signaling-mediated activation of target genes (Fig. 2).

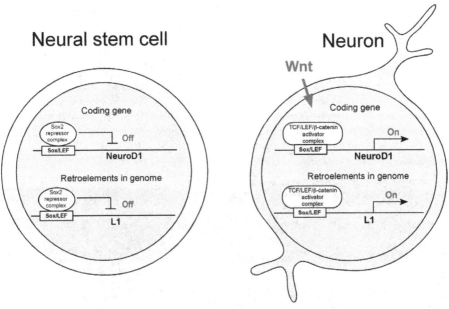

Overlapping Sox/LEF binding site is shown in yellow box. The overlapping DNA regulatory consensus sequence (A/T-A/T-C-A-A-A-G; yellow box) recognized by both Sox2 (A/T-A/T-C-A-A-A/T-G) and TCF/LEF (A/T-A/T-C-A-A-A). When Wnt3/Wnt3a stimulate NSCs, the Wnt-signaling activate NeuroD1 gene and L1 gene.

Fig. 2. Schematic representation of Wnt-mediated regulation in adult hippocampal NSCs.

The Sox/LEF regulatory elements reside within the 5' UTR sequences of human, rat, and mouse L1. Several Sox/LEF-binding sites are also present throughout the entire L1 sequence, including several sites in the second open reading frame (ORF2). The discovery that L1 retroelements embedded in the mammalian genome can function as bidirectional promoters suggests that Sox/LEF regulatory sites may represent a general mechanism for transcriptional regulation. This led us to examine whether other retroelements have a similar ability, thereby expanding the role of retroelements in adult hippocampal neurogenesis.

2.2 Expression of B1 SINE RNA and B2 SINE RNAs in adult hippocampus

The human and rodent genomes harbor numerous non-autonomous retrotransposons, termed short interspersed elements (SINEs). SINEs are highly abundant components of mammalian genomes and are propagated via retrotransposition (Ferrigno et al., 2001). Non-autonomous SINEs recruit L1-encoded proteins for their own mobilization. Alu elements are the major SINEs in the human genome, whereas B1 and B2 elements are the major SINE families in the mouse genome. The B2 SINE family constitutes approximately 0.7% of total mouse genomic DNA (Bennett et al., 1984). These retroelements are widely distributed throughout the genome, although many are heavily truncated and only a few are thought to be active and able to retrotranspose.

We first investigated B2 SINE RNA expression in the adult hippocampus by in situ hybridization. Brains were dissected from freshly euthanized Fisher 344 rats and placed in ice-cold saline. The brains were then placed in plastic blocks in OCT compound (Tissue Tek) and frozen. Sections were cut at 15 μm thickness with a cryostat (LEICA CM1850, Leica). Brain sections on the slide glass were hybridized with labeled riboprobes. Following the in situ hybridization of B2 SINE RNA, immunohistochemical analysis of the L1 protein (1:300; rabbit antibody against LINE-1, SantaCruz) was carried out. We observed that hippocampal granule neurons extensively express L1 RNA, as well as B2 SINE RNA (Fig. 3). Strong signals were also observed in neuronal layers (granule cell layers) but were not found in cells at the innermost layer of the dentate gyrus where astrocytes and undifferentiated neural stem cells reside (Fig. 3).

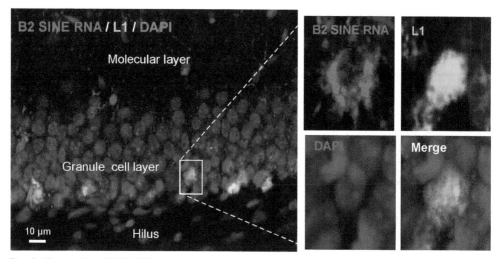

Fig. 3. Expression B2 SINE RNA and L1 in DG of adult hippocampus.

In situ hybridization for B2 SINE RNA (red) and immunohistochemistry of L1 protein (green) was carried out simultaneously on the DG of adult rat hippocampus. Hippocampal granule neurons extensively express both B2 SINE RNA and L1. The SINE RNA and L1 protein double-positive cells in the white square are magnified in the right panels. B2 SINE RNA: red, L1 protein: green, DAPI: blue.

2.3 Wnt-signaling regulatory sites on B1 SINE and B2 SINE DNA sequences

We identified that the 2 major classes of non-coding retroelements, B1 and B2 SINEs (B1 SINE, GenBank accession number X62249; B2 SINE, M31441) also carry Wnt-responsive elements (Fig. 4). SINEs originate from retrotransposition events of small RNAs (Batzer and Deininger, 2002; Hasler & Strub, 2006; Nishihara et al., 2006). Both Alu and B1 elements are derived from the 7SL RNA (Ullu & Tschudi; 1984), whereas B2 and most other SINEs are derived from tRNA genes. The eukaryotic RNA polymerase III (Pol III) system is responsible for synthesizing transfer RNA molecules and other transcripts, which in yeast include the U6 spliceosomal RNA, 7SL RNA, 5S ribosomal RNA, snr52 small nucleolar RNA, and the RNA component of RNaseP (Paule & White, 2000; Geiduschek & Kassavetis, 2001; Huang & Maraia, 2001). Transcription Factor for polymerase III C (TFIIIC) binds to 2 intragenic (lying within the transcribed DNA sequence) control sequences, the A-Box and B-Box (Fig. 4).

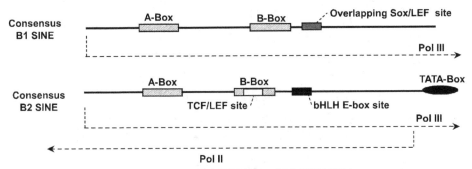

Fig. 4. Transcriptional regulation of B1 SINE RNA and B2 SINE RNA.

RNA polymerase III (also called Pol III) transcribes DNA by recognizing A-box and B-box (grey boxes). Overlapping Sox/LEF sequence (dark grey box) is contained in B1 SINE RNA. TCF/LEF regulatory sequence (white box) is involved in the B-box sequence of consensus B2 SINE RNA. The DNA of B2 SINE RNA contains also the bHLH transcription factor recognizing E-box sequence (black box). B2 SINE also carries an active RNA polymerase II (pol II) regulatory site that is located outside the tRNA region (Ferrigno et al., 2001). TATA box of the pol II promoter is indicated in black oval box.

As Figure 4 indicates, DNA sequences of both B1 SINE RNA and B2 SINE RNA include a Wnt signaling responsive element (Sox/LEF site in B1 SINE and TCF/LEF site in B2 SINE). Interestingly, the DNA sequence of B2 SINE RNA also contains an E-box sequence, which is recognized by a bHLH transcription factor, such as NeuroD1 (Fig. 4). The expression of NeuroD1 is triggered by Wnt-signaling, suggesting that B2 SINE RNA has additional active sites for NeuroD1 regulation in the adult neuronal lineage-differentiation. To explore the expression profile of these retroelement RNAs (B1 SINE RNA and B2 SINE RNA) in a lineage-specific manner in the adult hippocampus, we cultured adult hippocampal NSCs.

Undifferentiated neural stem cells

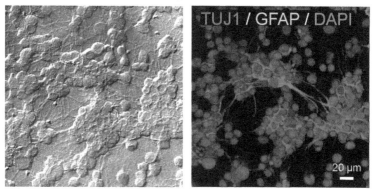

Neurons

Astrocytes

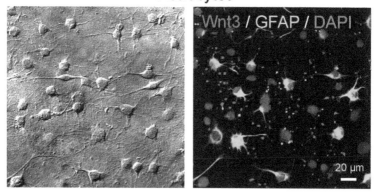

Neural stem cells (top), neurons (middle) and astrocyte cells (bottom) were examined by the immunohistochemistry analysis. TUJ1 (top and middle) and Wnt3 (bottom): red, GFAP: green, DAPI: blue.

Fig. 5. *In vitro* culture system of adult hippocampal neural stem cells

2.4 Expression of B1 SINE RNA and B2 SINE RNA in adult hippocampal neural stem cell culture

Adult hippocampal NSCs were round and retained their shape when expanded as a monolayer (top panels, Fig. 5). These neural progenitor cells have stem cell properties in vitro: (1) they undergo self-renewal in the presence of basic FGF-2; (2) single genetically marked clones can differentiate into neurons, oligodendrocytes, and astrocytes in vitro and when grafted back to the adult hippocampus in vivo; and (3) they express progenitor cell markers such as Sox2 and nestin (Gage et al., 1995; Palmer et al., 1997). Undifferentiated NSCs were negative for the neuronal marker β-tubulin III (TUJ1) and the astrocyte lineage marker glial fibrillary acidic protein (GFAP) (Fig. 5). Under neuronal differentiation conditions, we added 1 μM retinoic acid and 5 μM forskolin to the culture. The expression of β-tubulin III was remarkably up-regulated, as confirmed by the immunohistochemistry analysis. GFAP was found to be absent in the immunohistochemistry analysis, indicating that the adult NSCs in culture were committed to a neuronal lineage specifically (middle panels, Fig. 5). Differentiation into the astrocyte lineage was stimulated by the addition of 50 ng/mL leukemia inhibitory factor (LIF) and 50 ng/mL bone morphogenetic protein 2 (BMP2). Astrocytes prepared in vitro expressed Wnt3 factors, consistent with in vivo data (Lie et al., 2005; Kuwabara et al., 2009; Okamoto et al, 2011).

2.5 Neuronal-specific expression of B1 SINE RNA and B2 SINE RNA in the adult hippocampal neural stem cell culture

By using an *in vitro* culture system of adult hippocampal NSCs (Fig. 5), we investigated the relative expression levels of B1 SINE and B2 SINE RNA. Neurons differentiated from adult neural stem cells expressed high levels of both B1 RNA and B2 RNA, although the expression level of B2 SINE RNA was higher (Fig. 6).

Total RNAs were extracted cells and expression levels of B1 SINE RNA (black bars) and B2 SINE RNA (white bars) ware examined by quantitative real-time PCR (Q-PCR analysis). A) The level was normalized internal control gene GAPDH and platted in the graph. The expression level of B1 SINE RNA in undifferentiated neural stem cells (NSCs) was taken as 100% (asterisk; black bars). B) Time course analysis of B1 SINE RNAs and B2 SINE RNAs.

In the astrocyte lineage, the basal expression of B1 SINE RNA and B2 SINE RNA from undifferentiated cells was largely diminished (Fig. 6A). The neuronal specific expression of B2 SINE RNA by quantitative real-time PCR (QPCR) analysis in vitro was consistent with the results of in situ hybridization (Fig. 3).

Time course of B1 SINE RNA and B2 SINE RNA expression during the early stages of neurogenesis in cultured adult NSCs was assessed by QPCR analysis. Following neuronal differentiation in vitro, B1 SINE RNA and B2 SINE RNA expression peaked at 24 h after neuronal induction (20-fold increase in B1 SINE RNA, 50-fold increase in B2 SINE RNA). These expression levels gradually decreased until they reached a plateau by 48 h after neuronal induction (Fig. 6B). Both NeuroD1 and L1 expression was highest at 24 h after neuronal induction and gradually declined during neuronal differentiation (Kuwabara et al., 2009), similar to the expression profile of B1 SINE RNA and B2 SINE RNA, suggesting that these genes are under similar transcriptional regulation. Combined expression analysis of in situ hybridization and immunohistochemistry of B2 SINE RNA and L1 showed that early stage neuronal progenitors (i.e., neuroblast cells) contained high levels of L1 and B2 SINE RNAs (Fig. 3; inner layer of dentate gyrus, cells indicated by the white square). In the mature neuronal layer of the dentate gyrus (deeper neuronal layer of SGZ), the L1 and B2 SINE RNA signals were still clearly observed, although it was weaker than those in neuroblast cells. The in vivo expression profile obtained from in situ hybridization and the in vitro expression profile obtained from the time course analysis using adult NSC culture are consistent (Fig. 3 and Fig. 6).

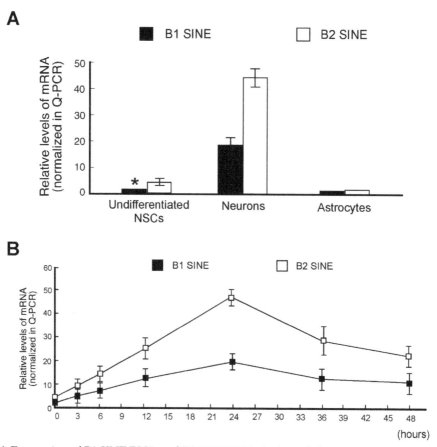

Fig. 6. Expression of B1 SINE RNA and B2 SINE RNA during adult neurogenesis.

2.6 Effect of Wnt3 on the expression of B1 SINE RNA and B2 SINE RNA

Next, we examined the effect of the Wnt3a ligand on the expression of B1 SINE RNA and B2 SINE RNA. Wnt3a ligands were added to the NSC culture at different concentrations (0 ng/mL, 10 ng/mL, 20 ng/mL, and 50 ng/mL of Wnt3a), and the expression levels of B1 SINE RNA and B2 SINE RNA were up-regulated in a dose-dependent manner (Fig. 7).

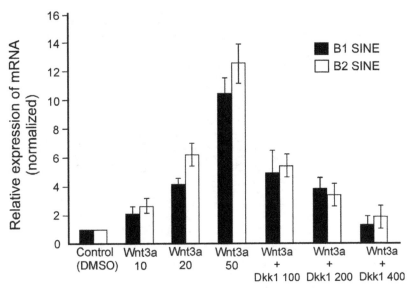

Fig. 7. Wnt signaling increases the expression of B1 SINE RNA and B2 SINE RNA in adult neural stem cell cultures. Ligand of Wnt3a and Dkk1 was added in the adult NSC cultures. Ligand concentration is indicated in the graph (ng/mL). The expression levels of B1 SINE RNA and B2 SINE RNA were normalized with internal control GAPDH. Cells treated with DMSO were taken as control and the relative value of the normalized expression of B1 SINE RNA and B2 SINE RNA was plotted in the graph. B1 SINE RNA: black bars, B2 SINE RNA: white bars.

To evaluate the observed positive effects of Wnt3a on the expression of B1 SINE RNA and B2 SINE RNA, the Wnt antagonist Dickkopf1 (Dkk1) was added into the adult hippocampal NSC culture. As the antagonist concentration was increased (0 ng/mL, 100 ng/mL, 200 ng/mL, and 400 ng/mL of Dkk1 with 50 ng/mL Wnt3a), Wnt3a-mediated activation of B1 SINE RNA and B2 SINE RNA was diminished (Fig. 7). From these data, we confirmed the contribution of Wnt signaling to the transcriptional activation of B1 SINE RNA and B2 SINE RNA in adult hippocampal NSCs.

2.7 Effect of Wnt-signaling on the chromatin regulation of B1 SINE RNA and B2 SINE RNA

To assess protein association on the regulatory region of B1 SINE RNA and B2 SINE RNA, we performed chromatin immunoprecipitation (ChIP). Association levels were quantitatively evaluated using real-time PCR (ChIP-QPCR). From in situ hybridization / immunohistochemistry in vivo data (Fig. 3) and the time course expression profile in vitro (Fig. 6), coordinated expression between SINE RNAs and L1 was observed. Therefore, we performed ChIP-QPCR analysis for SINE RNAs and L1 in parallel.

Addition of Wnt3a into the adult NSC culture promoted the enrichment of trimethyl histone H3 lysine 4 (triMetK4), a modified histone mark associated with gene activation, by more than 15-fold at the B1 SINE RNA locus and by more than 20-fold at the B2 SINE RNA locus, compared to the control cells treated with DMSO (Fig. 8).

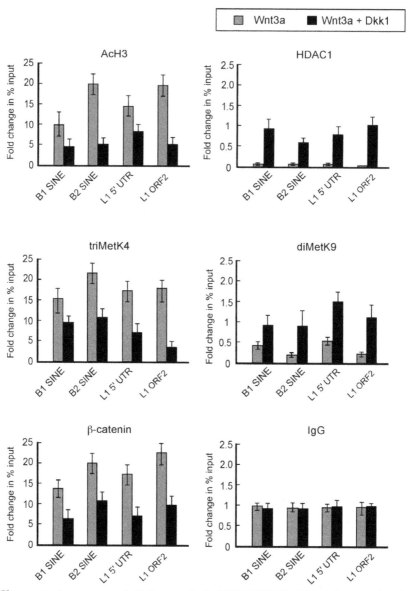

Fig. 8. Chromatin immunoprecipitation analysis (ChIP-QPCR) of retroelements in adult neural stem cells stimulated with Wnt3a and the antagonist Dkk1. PCR primers were designed to surround the Sox/LEF sequence on the L1 promoter. PCR primers for B1 SINE RNAs were designed to surround the Sox/LEF sequence on the B1 SINE DNA (Fig. 4). PCR primers for B2 SINE RNAs were designed to surround the TCF/LEF sequence and bHLH E-box sequence on the B2 SINE DNA (Fig. 4). From these results, we confirmed that similar molecular mechanism controlled SINE RNAs and L1 in the adult hippocampal neurogenesis and Wnt3 has essential role to activate the transcription of these retroelements.

The association of acetylated histone H3 (Ac-H3) and β-catenin increased with the Wnt3a treatment. Dimethylated H3 lysine 9 (diMetK9) and histone deacetylase 1 (HDAC1) were rarely associated, suggesting that the Wnt3a treatment promotes an active chromatin state (Fig. 6A). In contrast, the addition of Dkk1 inhibited the Wnt3a-mediated activation of chromatin at the B1 SINE RNA and B2 SINE RNA loci. We found that β-catenin, Ac-H3, and triMetK4 were associated at the L1 5′ UTR region and L1 ORF2 region, both of which include the Sox/LEF regulatory sequence (Kuwabara et al., 2009), similar to their association on the B1 SINE RNA and B2 SINE RNA loci. In contrast, Dkk1 diminished the Wnt3a-mediated activation process, as seen in the case of the B1 SINE RNA and B2 SINE RNA loci (Fig. 8).

2.8 Promoter activity of B2 SINE RNA in vivo

Although we determined the global expression of B2 SINE RNA in neuronal cells by in situ hybridization (Fig. 3), we further examined the detailed expression of B2 SINE RNA in the adult hippocampus. The transcriptional activity of B2 SINE RNA is controlled by regulatory sequences present on the internal promoter (Fig. 4). We prepared a lentivirus construct that carries the B2 SINE promoter sequence (not including termination sequences) and EGFP reporter cassette (B2 SINE promoter driven EGFP; LV SINE GFP).

SINE GFP lentivirus was stereotactically injected into the dentate gyrus of young adult rats. Three weeks later, mice were injected with BrdU daily for 10 days. Notably, we observed that SINE GFP expression was restricted to neurogenic areas, and that GFP-positive cells colocalized with NeuroD1-positive neuronal progenitors (Fig. 9). We also detected SINE GFP–positive cells that migrated further into the granule cell layer where NeuN-positive mature neurons reside.

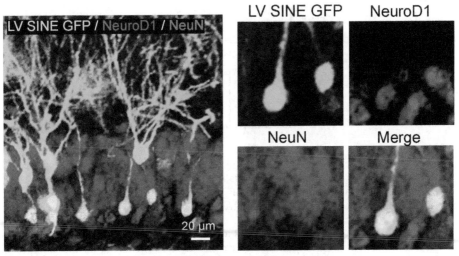

Fig. 9. Activity of B2 SINE as a promoter in adult rat hippocampus.

We examined the activity and specificity of the B2 SINE–based promoter in adult rat hippocampus. EGFP-expressing lentivirus, under the control of the B2 SINE–based promoter, was stereotactically microinjected into the dentate gyrus of adult rats and the population of GFP-positive cells (green) was analyzed by immunohistochemistry using antibodies to NeuroD1 (red) and NeuN (blue).

To identify the composition of cell types in which the B2 SINE-based promoter activity was turned on, we quantified the results of the immunohistochemical analysis. The number of SINE GFP and the lineage marker double-positive cells was counted and graphically plotted (Fig. 10).

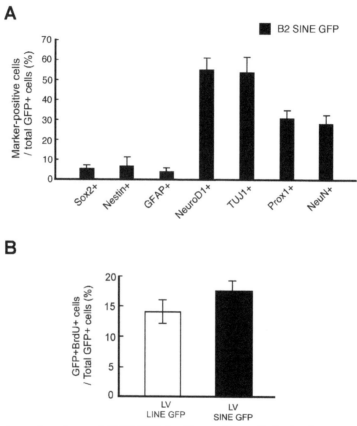

Fig. 10. Numbers of marker and SINE GFP double-positive cells in the dentate gyrus of adult rat. A) Quantitative immunohistochemistry analysis of B2 SINE promoter-active cells in dentate gyrus. B) Quantification of SINE GFP-positive and BrdU-positive cells in dentate gyrus of adult rat (black bar). LINE GFP-positive cells were also examined (white bar).

To examine SINE GFP-positive cells in the stem cell compartment, we stained the cells with Sox2 and nestin, a marker of radial stem-like cells. The proportion of Sox2 and SINE GFP double-positive cells was 6.4% of the total SINE GFP-positive cells. The proportion of nestin and SINE GFP double-positive cells was 7.4% of the total SINE GFP-positive cells. To examine SINE GFP-positive cells in the glial cell compartment, we stained the cells with GFAP. The proportion of GFAP and SINE GFP double-positive cells was 3.7% of total SINE GFP-positive cells.

In contrast, SINE GFP-positive cells in the neuronal cell compartment comprised a majority of the total GFP-positive cells (Fig. 10A). B2 SINE-based promoter activity was up-regulated in cells at the early stage of neuronal lineage, such as NeuroD1- and TUJ1-positive cells. The proportion of NeuroD1 and SINE GFP double-positive cells was 56% of the total SINE GFP-positive cells. The up-regulated activity of the SINE GFP promoter was retained in mature neurons (Prox-1- and NeuN-positive cells), but the proportion was almost half of neuroblast cells (NeuroD1-positive cells). Furthermore, SINE GFP-positive cells were labeled by BrdU, and the proportion of double-positive cells was found to be higher than that with LINE-GFP and BrdU staining (Fig. 10B), suggesting that the B2 SINE RNA-expressing cells actively proliferated in the adult hippocampus.

3. Conclusion

Our data indicate that both B1 SINE RNA and B2 SINE RNA are up-regulated during adult hippocampal neurogenesis, and that Wnt induction is required as the driving force. The specific response of these retroelements to paracrine Wnt factors is coupled with the differentiation progress of adult hippocampal NSCs into the neuronal pathway. Upon Wnt-mediated neuronal induction, the β-catenin activation complex up-regulated NeuroD1 and L1, as well as SINEs in adult hippocampal NSCs in vitro, while the Wnt antagonist Dkk1 down-regulated SINE RNA expression.

In ChIP-QPCR analysis, the association of β-catenin, triMetK4, and Ac-H3 in B1 and B2 SINEs was stimulated in cells treated with the Wnt3a ligand, suggesting that the genomic DNA of B1 and B2 SINEs was positively activated by canonical Wnt signaling. From these data, we propose that the activation of various genomic loci, where L1 and SINE fragments are present, may occur during adult hippocampal neurogenesis. Expression of retroelement RNAs are identified generally in neurogenic region in adult brain, although only hippocampal dentate gyrus is determined as the region that the retrotransposition (" jumping") occurs. Since various transcriptional activators are found in other neurogenic region in adult brain, not solely Wnt-signaling pathway but also other multiple molecules may control the expression of retroelement RNAs. We will actively extend current research to further determine potent regulators and the role of retroelement RNA during adult neurogenesis.

Since retroelement sequences are scattered throughout the genome and contain Wnt-responsive regulatory elements, retroelements retain the ability to act as promoters inducing the activity of nearby chromatin loci during adult neurogenesis. The functional relevance of adult hippocampal neurogenesis has been extensively studied, and the fact that physiological and behavioral events, such as aging, stress, diseases, seizures, learning, and exercise, can modulate neurogenesis is of particular interest. This suggests that the chromatin state at SINE/L1 loci potentially changes depending on paracrine stimuli. These epigenetic mechanisms may act as genomic "sensors" of environmental changes and function as fine modulators of adult hippocampal neurogenesis.

4. Acknowledgment

We thank Hideto Takimoto for providing assistance in the care of animals and in the experiments. SA, MW, KT, MA and TK were supported by various grants from AIST. TK was partly supported by the Grant-in-Aid for Young Scientists (B).

5. References

Avilion, . AA. Et al. (2003) Multipotent cell lineages in early mouse development depend on SOX2 function. *Genes & Development*, Vol. 17, No. 1, (January 1), 126-140, ISSN 0890-9369

Bani-Yaghoub, M. et al. (2006) Role of Sox2 in the development of the mouse neocortex. *Developmental Biology*, Vol. 295, No. 1, (July 1), pp. 52-66, ISSN 0012-1606

Batzer, M. A. & Deininger, P. L. (2002) Alu repeats and human genomic diversity. *Nature Reviews Genetics*, Vol. 3, No. 5, (May), pp. 370-379, ISSN 1471-0056

Bennett, K.L. *et al.* (1984) Most highly repeated dispersed DNA families in the mouse genome. *Molecular and Cellular Biology.* Vol. 4, No. 8, (August) 1561-1571, ISSN 0270-7306

Bylund, M. et al. (2003) Vertebrate neurogenesis is counteracted by Sox1-3 activity. *Nature Neuroscience*, Vol. 6, No. 11, (November), pp. 1162-1168, ISSN 1097-6256

Coufal, N. G. et al. (2009) L1 retrotransposition in human neural progenitor cells. *Nature,* Vol. 460, No. 7259, (August 27), pp. 1127-1131, ISSN 0028-0836

Cuitino, L. N. et al. (2010) Wnt5a is found to modulate recycling of functional GABAA receptors on hippocampal neurons. *The Journal of Neuroscience*, Vol. 30, No. 25, (June 23), pp. 8411-8420, ISSN 0270-6474

Deisseroth, K. et al. (2004) Excitation-neurogenesis coupling in adult neural stem/progenitor cells. *Neuron* Vol. 42, No. 4, (May 27), pp. 535-552, ISSN 0896-6273

Deng, W. et al. (2010) New neurons and new memories: how does adult hippocampal neurogenesis affect learning and memory? *Nature Reviews Neuroscience*, Vol.11, No.5, (May 11), pp. 339-350, ISSN 1471-0048

Ferri, A. L. et al. (2004) Sox2 deficiency causes neurodegeneration and impaired neurogenesis in the adult mouse brain. *Development*, Vol. 131, No. 15, (August), pp. 3805-3819, ISSN 1011-6370

Ferrigno, O. et al. (2001) Transposable B2 SINE elements can provide mobile RNA polymerase II promoters. *Nature Genetics,* Vol. 28, No. 1, (May 28), pp. 77-81, ISSN 1061-4036

Gage, F. H. (2000) Mammalian neural stem cells. *Science* Vol.287, No.5457, (February 25), pp.1433-1438, ISSN 1095-9203.

Gage, F. H. et al. (1995) Survival and differentiation of adult neuronal progenitor cells transplanted to the adult brain. *Proceedings of the National Academy of Sciences*, Vol. 92, No.25, (December 5), pp. 11879-11883, ISSN 1091-6490

Geiduschek, E. P. & Kassavetis, G. A. (2001) The RNA polymerase III transcription apparatus. Journal of Molecular Biology Vol. 310, No. 1, (June 29), pp. 1-26, ISSN 0022-2836

Gogolla, N. et al. (2009) Wnt signaling mediates experience-related regulation of synapse numbers and mossy fiber connectivities in the adult hippocampus. *Neuron* Vol. 62, No. 4, (May 28), pp. 510-525, ISSN 0896-6273

Graham, V. et al. (2003) SOX2 functions to maintain neural progenitor identity. *Neuron*, Vol. 39, No. 5, (August 28) pp. 749-765, ISSN 0896-6273

Gritti, A. et al. (2002) Multipotent neural stem cells reside into the rostral extension and olfactory bulb of adult rodents. *The Journal of Neuroscience,* Vol.22, No.2, (January 15), pp. 437-445, ISSN 0270-6474

Han, J. S. & Boeke, J. D. (2005) LINE-1 retrotransposons: modulators of quantity and quality of mammalian gene expression? *Bioessays,* Vo. 27, No. 8, (August), pp. 775-784, ISSN 1521-1878

Häsler, J. & Strub, K. (2006) Alu elements as regulators of gene expression. *Nucleic Acids Research,* Vol. 34, No. 19, pp. 5491-5497, ISSN 0305-1048

Huang, Y. & Maraia, RJ. (2001) Comparison of the RNA polymerase III transcription machinery in Schizosaccharomyces pombe, Saccharomyces cerevisiae and human. *Nucleic Acids Research,* Vol. 29, No. 13, (July 1), pp. 2675-2690, ISSN 0305-1048

Kuhn, H. G. et al. (1996) Neurogenesis in the dentate gyrus of the adult rat: age-related decrease of neuronal progenitor proliferation. *The Journal of Neuroscience,* Vol.16, No.6, (March 15), pp. 2027-2033, ISSN 0270-6474

Kuwabara, T. et al. (2009) Wnt-mediated activation of NeuroD1 and retro-elements during adult neurogenesis. *Nature Neuroscience,* Vol. 12, No. 9, (September), pp. 1097-1105, ISSN 1097-6256

Lee, S. M. et al. (2000) A local Wnt-3a signal is required for development of the mammalian hippocampus. *Development,* Vol. 127, No. 3, (February), pp. 457-467, ISSN 1011-6370

Lie, D. C. et al. (2005) Wnt signalling regulates adult hippocampal neurogenesis. *Nature,* Vol. 437, No. 7063, (October 27), pp. 1370-1375, ISSN 0028-0836

Liu, M. et al. (2000) Loss of BETA2/NeuroD leads to malformation of the dentate gyrus and epilepsy. *Proceedings of the National Academy of Sciences,* Vol.97, No2, (January 18), pp. 865-870, ISSN 1091-6490

Lois, &Alvarez-Buylla, A. (1993) Proliferating subventricular zone cells in the adult mammalian forebrain can differentiate into neurons and glia. *Proceedings of the National Academy of Sciences,* Vol.90, No.5, (March 1), pp. 2074-2077, ISSN 1091-6490

Miyaoka, T., Seno, H., and Ishino, H. (1999) Increased expression of Wnt-1 in schizophrenic brains. *Schizophrenia Research,* Vol. 38, No. 1, (July 27), pp. 1-6, ISSN 0920-9964

Miyata, T. et al. (1999) NeuroD is required for differentiation of the granule cells in the cerebellum and hippocampus. *Genes & Development,* Vol. 13, No. 13, (Jury 1), 1467-1652, ISSN 0890-9369

Muotri, A. R. et al. (2005) Somatic mosaicism in neuronal precursor cells mediated by L1 retrotransposition. *Nature,* Vol. 435, No. 7044, (June 16), pp. 903-910, ISSN 0028-0836

Nishihara, H. et al. (2006) Functional noncoding sequences derived from SINEs in the mammalian genome. *Genome Research,* Vol. 16, No. 7, (July), pp. 864-874, ISSN 1088-9051

Okamoto, H. et al. (2010) Wnt2 expression and signaling is increased by different classes of antidepressant treatments. *Biological Psychiatry,* Vol. 68, No. 6, (September 15), pp. 521-527, ISSN 0006-3223

Okamoto, M. et al. (2011) Reduction in paracrine Wnt3 factors during aging causes impaired adult neurogenesis. *The FASEB Journal,* Vol. 25, No. 8, (August), pp. xx-xx, ISSN 0892-6638

Pagano S. F. et al. (2000) Isolation and characterization of neural stem cells from the adult human olfactory bulb. *Stem Cells.* Vo.18, No.4, pp. 295-300, ISSN 1066-5099

Palmer, T. D. et al. (1995) FGF-2-responsive neuronal progenitors reside in proliferative and quiescent regions of the adult rodent brain. *Molecular and Cellular Neuroscience,* Vol. 6, No. 5, (October), pp. 474-486, ISSN 1044-7431

Paule, M. R. & White, R. J. (2000) Survey and summary: transcription by RNA polymerases I and III. *Nucleic Acids Research,* Vol. 28, No. 6, (March 15), pp. 1283-1298, ISSN 0305-1048

Song, H. et al. (2002) Astroglia induce neurogenesis from adult neural stem cells. *Nature,* Vol. 417, No. 6884, (May 2), pp. 39-44, ISSN 0028-0836

Suh, H., et al. (2007) In vivo fate analysis reveals the multipotent and self-renewal capacities of Sox2+ neural stem cells in the adult hippocampus. *Cell Stem Cell*, Vol. 1, No. 5, (November), pp.515-528, ISSN 1934-5909

Tozuka, Y. et al. (2005) GABAergic excitation promotes neuronal differentiation in adult hippocampal progenitor cells. *Neuron* Vol. 47, No. 6, (September 15), pp. 803-815, ISSN 0896-6273

Ullu, E. & Tschudi, C. (1984) Alu sequences are processed 7SL RNA genes. *Nature,* Vol. 312, No. 5990, November 8-14), pp. 171-172, ISSN 0028-0836

Permissions

The contributors of this book come from diverse backgrounds, making this book a truly international effort. This book will bring forth new frontiers with its revolutionizing research information and detailed analysis of the nascent developments around the world.

We would like to thank Tao Sun, for lending his expertise to make the book truly unique. He has played a crucial role in the development of this book. Without his invaluable contribution this book wouldn't have been possible. He has made vital efforts to compile up to date information on the varied aspects of this subject to make this book a valuable addition to the collection of many professionals and students.

This book was conceptualized with the vision of imparting up-to-date information and advanced data in this field. To ensure the same, a matchless editorial board was set up. Every individual on the board went through rigorous rounds of assessment to prove their worth. After which they invested a large part of their time researching and compiling the most relevant data for our readers. Conferences and sessions were held from time to time between the editorial board and the contributing authors to present the data in the most comprehensible form. The editorial team has worked tirelessly to provide valuable and valid information to help people across the globe.

Every chapter published in this book has been scrutinized by our experts. Their significance has been extensively debated. The topics covered herein carry significant findings which will fuel the growth of the discipline. They may even be implemented as practical applications or may be referred to as a beginning point for another development. Chapters in this book were first published by InTech; hereby published with permission under the Creative Commons Attribution License or equivalent.

The editorial board has been involved in producing this book since its inception. They have spent rigorous hours researching and exploring the diverse topics which have resulted in the successful publishing of this book. They have passed on their knowledge of decades through this book. To expedite this challenging task, the publisher supported the team at every step. A small team of assistant editors was also appointed to further simplify the editing procedure and attain best results for the readers.

Our editorial team has been hand-picked from every corner of the world. Their multi-ethnicity adds dynamic inputs to the discussions which result in innovative outcomes. These outcomes are then further discussed with the researchers and contributors who give their valuable feedback and opinion regarding the same. The feedback is then collaborated with the researches and they are edited in a comprehensive manner to aid the understanding of the subject.

Apart from the editorial board, the designing team has also invested a significant amount of their time in understanding the subject and creating the most relevant covers. They scrutinized every image to scout for the most suitable representation of the subject and create an appropriate cover for the book.

The publishing team has been involved in this book since its early stages. They were actively engaged in every process, be it collecting the data, connecting with the contributors or procuring relevant information. The team has been an ardent support to the editorial, designing and production team. Their endless efforts to recruit the best for this project, has resulted in the accomplishment of this book. They are a veteran in the field of academics and their pool of knowledge is as vast as their experience in printing. Their expertise and guidance has proved useful at every step. Their uncompromising quality standards have made this book an exceptional effort. Their encouragement from time to time has been an inspiration for everyone.

The publisher and the editorial board hope that this book will prove to be a valuable piece of knowledge for researchers, students, practitioners and scholars across the globe.

List of Contributors

Jorge Oliver-De la Cruz and Angel Ayuso-Sacido
Regenerative Medicine Program, Centro de Investigación Príncipe Felipe, REIG and Ciberned, Spain

Xinhua Zhang and Guohua Jin
Nantong University, China

Jean-Philippe Hugnot
University of Montpellier 2, INSERM U1051, Institute for Neurosciences of Montpellier, France

Oscar Gonzalez-Perez
Laboratory of Neuroscience, Facultad de Psicología, Universidad de Colima, Department of Neuroscience, Centro Universitario de Ciencias de la Salud, Universidad de Guadalajara, Mexico

Aavo-Valdur Mikelsaar
Institute of General and Molecular Pathology, University of Tartu and LabAs Ltd., Tartu, Estonia

Alar Sünter
Institute of General and Molecular Pathology, University of Tartu, Estonia

Peeter Toomik
Department of Food Science and Hygiene, Estonian University of Life Sciences, Tartu, Estonia

Kalmer Karpson
LabAs Ltd., Tartu, Estonia

Erkki Juronen
Institute of General and Molecular Pathology, University of Tartu, Estonia

Kiyokazu Agata
Department of Biophysics, Graduate School of Science, Kyoto University, Japan

Yoshihisa Kitamura
Department of Neurobiology, Kyoto Pharmaceutical University, Japan

Kaneyasu Nishimura
Department of Biophysics, Graduate School of Science, Kyoto University, Japan
Department of Cell Growth and Differentiation, Center for iPS Cell Research and Application (CiRA), Kyoto University, Japan

Kiyoshi Terakado
Saitama University, Japan

Kenichi Horisawa and Hiroshi Yanagawa
Department of Bioscience and Informatics, Keio University, Japan

Kohzo Nakayama and Takeshi Ohkawara
Department of Anatomy, Japan

Hisashi Nagase
Department of Immunology and Infectious Diseases, Shinshu University, School of Medicine, Japan

Chang-Sung Koh
Department of Biomedical Sciences, Shinshu University, School of Health Sciences, Matsumoto, Japan

Lucía Calatrava, Rafael Gonzalo-Gobernado, Antonio S. Herranz, Diana Reimers, Maria J. Asensio, Cristina Miranda and Eulalia Bazán
Department of Neurobiology, Ramón y Cajal Institute for Health Research, Madrid, Spain

Slawomir Antoszczyk, Kazuyuki Terashima, Masaki Warashina, Makoto Asashima and Tomoko Kuwabara
Research Center for Stem Cell Engineering, National Institute of Advanced Industrial Science and Technology (AIST), Japan

Printed in the USA
CPSIA information can be obtained
at www.ICGtesting.com
JSHW011431221024
72173JS00004B/757

9 781632 410184